Family Medicine OSCE: First Aid to Objective Structured Clinical Examination

Shaima Lari
Shammah Al Memari
Dana Al Marzooqi
Editors

Family Medicine OSCE: First Aid to Objective Structured Clinical Examination

Third Edition

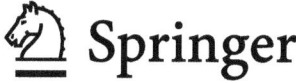 Springer

Editors
Shaima Lari
Family Medicine Consultant
Sheikh Shakhbout Medical City
Abu Dhabi, United Arab Emirates

Shammah Al Memari
Family Medicine Consultant
Abu Dhabi, United Arab Emirates

Dana Al Marzooqi
Family Medicine Consultant
Sheikh Khalifa Medical City
Abu Dhabi, United Arab Emirates

ISBN 978-981-99-5532-9   ISBN 978-981-99-5530-5   (eBook)
https://doi.org/10.1007/978-981-99-5530-5

This Springer imprint is published by the registered company Springer Nature Singapore Pte Ltd.
The registered company address is: 152 Beach Road, #21-01/04 Gateway East, Singapore 189721, Singapore

Paper in this product is recyclable.

Preface

Family medicine is the cornerstone of any healthcare system. As an essential and rewarding field that leads to the provision of comprehensive and continuous care to individuals across their lifespan, being certified at practicing family medicine is challenging as it requires a broad range of knowledge and skills. The Objective Structured Clinical Examination [OSCE] is one of the key components of the medical certification process and an important tool for assessing the competence of medical professionals including medical students and residents.

As a resident preparing for Family Medicine certification examinations, I found that customizing my notes to represent OSCE checklists format attracted my colleague's attention and ignited the idea of this book's authorship. That idea bloomed as one of the most popular tools used by hundreds of Arab Board of Family Medicine OSCE candidates. Soon after the first edition was published by the authors, it was recognized by the national newspaper in an article featuring it as an achievement of 12 Emirati Female Physicians and one-of-a-kind publication across the UAE. With over 2000 copies sold regionally, the editors took the next step to publish it internationally, while covering a wider range of topics, numerous case-based scenarios, and practical tips to succeed in the exam.

We hope that this book will serve as a valuable resource for anyone preparing for Family Medicine OSCE in their journey towards becoming certified family medicine practitioners.

Shaima Lari

Introduction

The "OSCE Preparatory Exam for Family Medicine Residents" is a comprehensive guide designed to aid family medicine residents in preparing for the Arab Board exams. With the collaboration of 12 authors, the book has expanded from its first edition to now include more authors and topics in its third edition.

This book provides a concise and straightforward checklist of essential topics in family medicine, including history-taking, physical examination, and counseling skills, to help residents excel in the OSCE exam. The authors have aimed to create a comprehensive guide that will serve as a useful resource not only for exam preparation but also for general practitioners or family physicians globally.

The book is divided into three parts, each addressing a specific aspect of medical training. Part I covers the techniques of patient history-taking, Part II focuses on physical examination techniques, and the final part concentrates on counseling skills. The third edition features improved content such as an expanded history-taking section with a more comprehensive context and a clinical setting simulation. It also includes a checklist for focused physical examination, differential diagnosis, and main treatment options. The latest edition introduces new emerging health topics, such as telemedicine and obesity, to reflect the latest developments in the field.

The authors emphasize that this book should be used as a guide and preparation tool and is not a substitute for hands-on clinical training and experience. Family medicine residents should be aware that while this book provides comprehensive information to prepare for the OSCE exam, practical experience and hands-on training are equally important.

"We would like to express our heartfelt gratitude to Dr. Maha Al Fahim, the program director of Family Medicine and current Head of Medical Education at Sheikh Khalifa Medical City, for her relentless efforts in encouraging her residents to transform a collection of handouts into this comprehensive medical OSCE book. The book has received widespread recognition and has been used by numerous family medicine residents around the world.

The authors hope that this book will serve as a valuable resource for family medicine residents as they work towards becoming skilled and compassionate healthcare providers. They express their gratitude to the residents for their dedication to their education and hope that this book will help them achieve their goal of excelling in the OSCE exam.

Shammah Al Memari

Acknowledgment

Prof. Wadeia Mohammad Sharief's ongoing support in the publication of the first two editions is essential. It demonstrates a continued commitment to the project and its success.

Contents

Part X   Counseling: Women's Health

Editors and Contributors

About the Editors

Shaima Lari is an Occupational & Environmental Medicine Consultant and chairs the Occupational Safety and Health as well as the Health and Wellbeing Council at Sheikh Shakhbout Medical City in Abu Dhabi, UAE. She is an adjunct faculty in the College of Medicine and Health Sciences at Khalifa University in Abu Dhabi, UAE and a member of the Arab Board of Family Medicine, the Canadian Board of Occupational Medicine and the American band the American Board of Independent Medical Examiners. Dr Lari received her Bachelor of Medicine and General Surgery from Dubai Medical College in Dubai, UAE. She completed her residency training in Family Medicine at Sheikh Khalifa Medical City in Abu Dhabi, UAE followed by fellowship training in Occupational & Environmental Medicine at the University of Toronto in Canada. Further in her journey as a pioneer and leader in the field she has completed her Masters in Business Administration from the United Arab Emirates University, UAE, Masters of Science in Community Health – Occupational and Environmental Health from University of Toronto, Canada and an alumnus of SEHA Leadership Academy. Dr Lari is passionate about teaching and sharing knowledge and experience. She was awarded the Best Resident as a Teacher back in 2014. Currently she Chairs the Scientific Committee of Occupational and Environmental Medicine at the National Institute of Health Specialities in the UAE.

Shammah Al Memari a Family Medicine Consultant in Abu Dhabi Emirate, is a graduate of UAE University with an Arab Board Certification in Family Medicine. Noteworthy achievements include the Harvard Global Clinical Research Scholarship and an MBA from Abu Dhabi School of Government.

Throughout her career, Shammah has played key roles in public health initiatives, policy development, and impactful research during the COVID-19 pandemic. She is recognized for developing the bariatric surgeries standards in 2018 and IFHAS, screening program initiative of Abu Dhabi Emirate.

Shammah is commended for her contributions to the first and second editions of OSCE: First Aid and currently serves as an editor and correspondent author for the upcoming third edition.

Dana Al Marzooqi (MBBCH, EMHCA, MRCGP-Int, CMQ, Arab Board of Family Medicine, Post-graduate Clinical Diploma in psychotherapy and cognitive behavioral therapy, Postgraduate Certificate in medical education, affiliate of American Medical Informatics Association) carries out the tasks of the "Referral Division's Manager" at the Family Care Authority in addition to practicing as a Family Medicine Consultant at SEHA. The wide scope of her current roles allows her to effectively contribute to the "Integrated Case Management" model. Among other things, earlier experiences that Dr Dana has had includes being a member of the Faculty of Family Medicine Residency Program at Sheikh Khalifa Medical City and the Ambulatory Health Services (AHS)'s Clinical Guidelines Committee for 5 years. Additionally, she served as Abu Dhabi's Regional Lead for Premarital Service and Clinical Key Performance Indicators. Moreover, she served as a member of SEHA's Physician Advisory Council that was leading the Electronic Medical Record's enhancements. Furthermore, she has received a couple of peer reviews, published internationally, and delivered numerous oral and posters presentations at international meetings. Dr. Dana is an alumnus of the UAE Government Leaders and SEHA Leadership Academy.

Contributors

Shaima Lari, MBBCh, MBA, MSc, CCBOM, CIME Sheikh Shakhbout Medical City, Abu Dhabi, United Arab Emirates

Dhuha Al Ameri, MBBS Ambulatory Healthcare Services, Abu Dhabi, United Arab Emirates

Kawthar Al Ameri, MBBS, CPHQ Ambulatory Healthcare Services, Abu Dhabi, United Arab Emirates

Faculty of Family Medicine Residency Program, Sheikh Khalifa Medical City, Abu Dhabi, United Arab Emirates

Noora Al Blooshi, MBBS Ambulatory Healthcare Services, Abu Dhabi, United Arab Emirates

Sakina Al Bloushi, MBBS Ambulatory Healthcare Services, Abu Dhabi, United Arab Emirates

Khuloud Al Hammadi, MBBS, MFOM, MPH, CIME Sheikh Khalifa Medical City, Abu Dhabi, United Arab Emirates

Eman Al Hayayi, MBBS Etihad Airways Medical Center, Abu Dhabi, United Arab Emirates

Reem Al Mansoori, MBBCh Emirates Medical Association of Family Medicine, Abu Dhabi, United Arab Emirates

Buthaina Al Maskari, MBBS Ambulatory Healthcare Services, Abu Dhabi, United Arab Emirates

Shammah Al Memari, MBBS Abu Dhabi, United Arab Emirates

Eiman Al Murar, MBBCh Ambulatory Healthcare Services, Abu Dhabi, United Arab Emirates

Abeer Al Naqbi, MBBS Ambulatory Healthcare Services, Abu Dhabi, United Arab Emirates

Halima Al Shehhi, MBBS Ambulatory Healthcare Services, Abu Dhabi, United Arab Emirates

Dana Al Marzooqi, MBBCh, EMHCA, CMQ, MRCGP(INT) Sheikh Khalifa Medical City, Abu Dhabi, United Arab Emirates

Sumiya Taheri, MBBS Ambulatory Healthcare Services, Abu Dhabi, United Arab Emirates

Part I

History-Taking and Management: Adult Health

History Taking and Management of a Patient Presenting with Acne

Khuloud Al Hammadi, Buthaina Al Maskari, and Shammah Al Memari

Learning Objectives
- How to master history taking for patients presenting with acne?
- How to perform a focused exam for patients presenting with acne?
- How to approach and provide management tips for patients with acne?

Focus areas include polycystic ovarian syndrome (PCOS), acne secondary to a medication use (side effect), screen for depression, counseling about medications and their side effects.

1. Introduce yourself.
2. Establish good rapport.
3. Identify the complaint: duration, sites involved, onset, reason for seeking treatment now (preparation for social event), relieving or aggravating factors (exam or stress), previous attempts of treatment in details (type, duration of use, and outcome), associated symptoms or events such as:
   (a) Hirsutism, weight gain, irregular periods, and infertility (consider PCOS).
   (b) Pregnancy or menstrual cycle.

K. Al Hammadi
Sheikh Khalifa Medical City, Abu Dhabi, United Arab Emirates

B. Al Maskari
Ambulatory Healthcare Services, Abu Dhabi, United Arab Emirates

S. Al Memari (✉)
Abu Dhabi, United Arab Emirates

© The Author(s), under exclusive license to Springer Nature Singapore Pte Ltd. 2024
S. Lari et al. (eds.), *Family Medicine OSCE: First Aid to Objective Structured Clinical Examination*, https://doi.org/10.1007/978-981-99-5530-5_1

3

    (c) Use of oral contraceptive pills, androgens, corticosteroids (topical or oral or injectable).

4. Explore patient's ideas, concerns and expectations (ICE):
   (a) Ideas: "what do you know about acne?"
   (b) Concerns: losing friends, not getting married, scars, and discolored skin.
   (c) Expectations: referral to dermatologist, or effects of acne?
5. Explore continuous problems: irregular periods, diabetes mellitus, asthma, or depression.
6. Past medical, surgical, family, and social histories.
7. Examination: inspection of the face, shoulders, back, upper arms and chest looking for acne and evidence of scarring, describe the lesions (comedonal, macular, papular, pustular, and/or nodulocystic), and categorize according to severity (mild, moderate, or severe).
8. Order investigations as indicated: luteinizing hormone, follicle stimulating hormone, testosterone, HbA1c and pelvic ultrasound.
9. Management:
   (a) Ensure shared understanding: summarize and provide with health education.
   (b) Give information on acne: "acne is caused by an expansion of the sebaceous glands (the oil-producing glands in the skin), which become infected with bacteria when they become clogged. It is a widespread problem (particularly among adolescents) where up to 80% of people have had acne at some point in their lives. Its triggers include hormonal changes (such as puberty, menstruation, pregnancy, birth control pills, or stress), usage of oil-based or alcohol-based cosmetics, certain medicines (steroids, testosterone, estrogen, and phenytoin), high humidity, and perspiration. There is no evidence that chocolate, nuts, or oily foods promote acne; nevertheless, a diet high in refined sugar may be associated with acne. It is not connected to personal hygiene, in other words, black or white heads are not dirt, hence scrubbing will not help, it in fact increases oil production from skin when it is lost promptly. It is a chronic condition that requires patience and time to treat."
10. Management (refer to Table 1.1) and health education: advise to use along with sunscreen as they increase photosensitivity.
11. Provide the patient with reading educational materials if any.
12. Discuss health maintenance and screening for age.
13. Arrange for follow up.
14. Communication skills: organized approach, mixed questioning styles (open- and close-ended questions), active listening, clear language, and reflection on patient's ICE.

Table 1.1 Acne treatment options*

Medication	Method of administration	Dose and application	Details	Side effects
Benzoyl peroxide	Topical	To be applied at night	Advise the patient to sleep when it is absorbed completely as it can cause bleaching of the hair, clothes, and bed linens	Peeling, erythema, and dryness
Retinoids	Topical	To be applied at night	Not suitable for pregnant ladies	Peeling, erythema, and dryness
Antibiotics	Oral	Tetracycline (250 or 500 mg BID), or doxycycline (50 or 100 mg BID or 100 mg OD) for a duration of 3 months	– Avoid concomitant administration with iron or dairy products (as they decrease its absorption) – Not suitable for pregnant ladies or children less than 12 years of age	Teeth discoloration, photosensitivity, gastrointestinal upset, and high liver function test (LFT). Additional side effects that are specific for minocycline include dizziness and lupus
Isotretinoin	Oral	0.5–1 mg/kg/day in two divided doses for 15–20 weeks, aiming at a cumulative dose of 120–150 mg/kg	– Discuss in detail: the nature of the medication, the precautions needed, and the importance of dual contraception use for female patients – Need for monthly blood monitoring	Body aches, mucocutaneous dryness, teratogenicity, high LFTs, thrombocytopenia, and hyperlipidemia

*The table includes treatments strongly recommended for acne management. Topical options such as clascoterone, salicylic acid, and azelaic acid, along with oral alternatives like minocycline, sarecycline, combined oral contraceptive (COC) pills, and spironolactone are conditionally recommended based on the guidance provided by the American Academy of Dermatology

History Taking and Management of a Patient Presenting with Pruritus

2

Abeer Al Naqbi and Shammah Al Memari

Learning Objectives
- How to master history taking for patients presenting with pruritus?
- How to perform a focused exam for patients presenting with pruritus?
- How to approach and provide management tips for patients with pruritus?

Focus areas include dermatologic, hepatic (cholestasis), endocrine (hyperthyroidism and diabetes mellitus), malignant (lymphomas and leukemias), infectious, neurologic or psychiatric, rheumatic diseases (Sjogren, scleroderma and dermatomyositis), as well as allergies, or medications.

1. Introduce yourself.
2. Establish good rapport.
3. Identify the complaint (what do you mean by pruritus?, which part of the body is affected?): onset, duration, timing (day or night), site, character, relieving or aggravating factors (known allergies, any new exposure to soap, perfumes, or food), radiation, severity (interfering with sleep and daily activity), associated symptoms (skin changes: describe the rash if any, symptoms of hyperthyroidism, hyperparathyroidism, gout, pregnancy, iron deficiency anemia, or psychological stress).

A. Al Naqbi
Ambulatory Healthcare Services, Abu Dhabi, United Arab Emirates

S. Al Memari (✉)
Abu Dhabi, United Arab Emirates

© The Author(s), under exclusive license to Springer Nature Singapore Pte Ltd. 2024
S. Lari et al. (eds.), *Family Medicine OSCE: First Aid to Objective Structured Clinical Examination*, https://doi.org/10.1007/978-981-99-5530-5_2

4. Rule out red flags:
   (a) Weight loss, fatigue, and night sweats (human immunodeficiency virus (HIV) infection, or malignancy (multiple myeloma, polycythemia, Hodgkins lymphoma)).
   (b) Weakness, numbness, abdominal pain, and jaundice (cholestasis (primary biliary cirrhosis, pregnancy, oral contraception pills, and liver failure)).
   (c) Urinary frequency, excessive thirst, and weight loss (diabetes).
5. Enquire about the patient's or parent's ideas, concerns and expectations (ICE), and the effect of the complaint on the quality of life (interference with sleep, marital life, or work).
6. Explore ongoing problems: diabetes mellitus, chronic liver, or renal or rheumatic disease.
7. Question regular use of medications: aspirin, vitamin B, opiates, amphetamine, quinidine, retinoids, or antibiotics such as doxycycline.
8. Social history: occupation (contact dermatitis and malignancy), smoking, alcohol intake (liver disease).
9. Family or contact history of a similar problem (scabies).
10. Examination: vital signs, general look (weight loss, jaundice, alcoholic odor), skin (any dryness, rash, lesions), enlarged lymph nodes, central nervous system, thyromegaly, cardiovascular system, chest, and abdomen (looking for stigmata of liver disease, or splenomegaly).
11. Order initial investigations:
    (a) Complete blood count to exclude iron deficiency anemia, polycythemia rubra vera, malignancies, and myeloproliferative disease.
    (b) Creatinine, glucose, and blood urea nitrogen levels.
    (c) Erythrocyte sedimentation rate (ESR).
    (d) Liver function test to exclude chronic liver disease.
    (e) Thyroid function test to exclude thyroid disease (Grave's).
12. Consider further investigations:
    (a) Human Immunodeficiency Virus screen and Hepatitis serology.
    (b) Chest X-ray to exclude malignancy (looking for adenopathy).
    (c) Stool analysis to exclude parasitic infestations.
    (d) Fecal immunochemical test to exclude gastrointestinal malignancy.
    (e) Immunoglobulin E level (may help exclude being allergic pruritus if negative)
    (f) Potassium hydroxide if suspecting fungal infection.
    (g) Skin biopsy if unclear diagnosis.
13. Management and education: share diagnosis, treatment options, and prognosis according to the cause:
    (a) Eliminate underlying cause if possible.
    (b) Advise the patient to modify his or her lifestyle by washing with a gentle cleaner and avoiding excessive washing. In dry weather, recommend avoiding excessive heat and using a humidifier. Advise for use of emollients, as dry skin is the most common cause of pruritus.
    (c) Consider antihistamine to control pruritus (if severe).

(d) Consider a course of topical steroids, such as 1% Hydrocortisone, for 3–5 days for localized pruritus when history is suggestive of atopic dermatitis (eczema), contact dermatitis, or inflammatory disease.

(e) If scabies was the cause, recommend Permethrin 5% cream for the patient and all contacts. Instruct the patient to apply the medication to all regions of the body below the neck. "Apply it to all areas between your neck and your toes, including the skin around your nails, the crease between your buttocks, and the skin between your toes." The patient should never apply the medication to the nose, lips, eyelids, or mouth or eye area. Advise the patient to leave it on for 8–14 h before washing it off the following morning. In 1 week, reapply it. Give the patient instructions to administer treatment to his or her family members who sleep in the same room. Additionally, advise to wash all clothing, linens, and towels with hot water the day prior to treatment.

(f) Consider Cognitive Behavioral Therapy (CBT) to cope with persistent symptoms.

14. Provide the patient with reading educational materials if any.
15. Discuss health maintenance and screening for age.
16. Arrange for follow up.
17. Arrange for referral if patient has any red flags or when the diagnosis remains unclear.
18. Communication skills: organized approach, mixed questioning styles (open- and close-ended questions), active listening, clear language, and reflection on patients' ICE.

History Taking and Management of a Patient Presenting with Headache

3

Shaima Lari, Kawthar Al Ameri, and Shammah Al Memari

> **Learning Objectives**
> - How to master history taking for patients presenting with headache?
> - How to perform a focused exam for patients presenting with headaches?
> - How to approach and provide management tips for patients with headache?

> **Focus areas** include Differentiating between primary and secondary causes, identifying red flags or emergencies related to headache, and looking for hidden agenda (depression, anxiety).

1. Introduce yourself and establish good rapport.
2. Identify the complaint: duration, site, onset, character, relieving and aggravating factors timing, radiation, associated symptoms (as flashing lights or vision disturbance), or red flags (use mnemonic **SNNOOP10**: **S**ystemic symptoms (fever, eye squint, projectile vomiting, purpuric rash, or unexplained weight loss), **N**eoplasm history, **N**eurologic deficit (including altered or loss of consciousness), **O**nset being abrupt, **O**lder age (onset after age 50 years), **P**attern

S. Lari
Sheikh Shakhbout Medical City, Abu Dhabi, United Arab Emirates

K. Al Ameri
Ambulatory Healthcare Services, Abu Dhabi, United Arab Emirates

Faculty of Family Medicine Residency Program, Sheikh Khalifa Medical City, Abu Dhabi, United Arab Emirates

S. Al Memari (✉)
Abu Dhabi, United Arab Emirates

© The Author(s), under exclusive license to Springer Nature Singapore Pte Ltd. 2024
S. Lari et al. (eds.), *Family Medicine OSCE: First Aid to Objective Structured Clinical Examination*, https://doi.org/10.1007/978-981-99-5530-5_3

or severity change (including headache waking a patient from sleep), **P**ositional headache, **P**recipitated by sneezing, coughing, or exercise, **P**apilledema, **P**rogressive headache and atypical presentations, **P**erinatal (pregnancy or puerperium), **P**ainful eye with autonomic features, **P**ost-traumatic onset, **P**athology of the immune system such as HIV, **P**ainkiller (analgesic) overuse). Work out your differentials accordingly:

(a) Migraine headache: moderate to severe headache with the features summarized in the mnemonic: **POUND** (**P**ulsating, episodic with duration of each episode between 4 and 72 h**O**urs, **U**nilateral, **N**ausea with or without vomiting, **Disabling** (photophobia, phonophobia, preceding aura (bad or burning smell, seeing spots or zigzag lines)).

(b) Sinusitis: fever, nasal congestion or discharge, facial fullness, or pain.

(c) Meningitis: fever, neck pain or stiffness, photophobia, rash, and recent travel.

(d) Acute angle closure glaucoma: very painful red eye, haloes around the lights, blurred vision, nausea, and vomiting, with history of similar episodes that were aborted in few minutes.

(e) Temporal arteritis: Unilateral temporal headache, dental or facial pain, claudication of jaw and tongue when talking or chewing, or scalp pain.

(f) Transient Ischemic Attack: transient visual loss (amaurosis fugax).

(g) Cervicogenic headache: neck pain or spasm, shoulder pain, numbness in upper extremity.

(h) Trigeminal Neuralgia: recurrent paroxysms of sharp or electric pain that is unilateral, usually affecting the maxillary and mandibular branches of the trigeminal nerve.

(i) Acoustic Neuroma: unilateral hearing loss, tinnitus, and facial palsy.

(j) Subarachnoid Hemorrhage: severe usually worst headache ever, with neck stiffness, vomiting and history of hypertension.

(k) Cluster headache: recurrent severe (ranges from once every other day to up to eight times daily), strictly unilateral, peri-orbital headache (15–180 min), with ipsilateral autonomic features (lacrimation, nasal congestion, rhinorrhea), ipsilateral miosis, ptosis, restlessness, agitation, manifesting in seasonal pattern (clusters of weeks to months with remission for months to periods).

(l) Increased intracranial pressure: occipital headache, increasing with coughing, vomiting or sneezing, associated with dizziness, seizure, and vomiting.

(m) Depression: PHQ-2 reflecting low mood or loss of interest in the past 2 weeks.

3. Explore patient's ideas, concerns, and expectations (ICE) as well as the effect of the problem on the quality of life.

4. Explore ongoing problems: exclude diabetes, hypertension, erectile dysfunction, and coronary artery disease.

5. Question regular use of medications: analgesia, oral contraception, glyceryl-trinitrate, and sildenafil.

6. Social history: stressful events, marital conflicts, domestic violence, job instability, smoking, and alcohol use.
7. Family history of chronic headache or brain tumor.
8. Examination:
   (a) Vital signs: blood pressure and pulse.
   (b) Check temporal and neck arteries. Listen for bruits over carotid arteries.
   (c) Examine the spine, head, and neck muscles.
   (d) Fundoscopy and otoscopy.
   (e) Neurologic exam including gait assessment, Romberg test, and meningeal signs.
9. Consider imaging if patient has high risk features:
   (a) Age more than 50 years.
   (b) Concerning changes in the usual chronic headache pattern of the patient.
   (c) Features typical of secondary headaches.
   (d) New or concerning findings on history or examination.
   (e) High-risk comorbid conditions.
10. Arrange referral as needed:
   (a) Urgently if patient has features of temporal arteritis, meningitis, intracranial mass, or angle closure glaucoma.
   (b) Patient has atypical features.
   (c) Patients not responding to first- and second-line treatments.
11. Management and education: share differential diagnosis and prognosis.
   (a) Encourage the patient to maintain a headache diary that elaborates the headaches' onset (time of the day), duration (length of episode), character, intensity, aura, precipitating factors, associated and relieving symptoms.
   (b) Provide medications if needed as elaborated in Table 3.1.
   (c) Treat underlying pathology and consider antidepressants if needed.
12. Give reading educational materials if any and arrange for follow up.
13. Discuss health maintenance and age-appropriate screening.
14. Communication skills: organized approach, mixed questioning styles (open- and close-ended questions), active listening, clear language, and reflection on patient's ICE.

Table 3.1 Treatment options for different types of headaches

Type of headache	Options		Medication and dose
Tension headache	Abortive drugs		Acetaminophen: 1000 mg every 6–8 h
			Ibuprofen: 400–800 mg every 4–6 hr maximum dose 2400 mg/day.
			Amitriptyline: 10–75 mg at bedtime
Migraine headache	Abortive drugs		Ibuprofen: 200–400 mg every 4–6 h. 400–800 mg every 4–6 hr maximum dose 2400 mg/day.
			Sumatriptan: 25–100 mg orally or 10–20 mg intra-nasally
	Prophylactic drugs: – Reduce 50% of the attacks – Indications: Two or more attacks every month, each lasting for more than 3 days Ineffectiveness, contraindications, or harmful effects of acute therapies. Additionally, the use of abortive medication for episodes occurring more than twice each week. Migraine diseases that are uncommon, such as hemiplegic migraine, migraine with protracted aura, and migrainous infarction	First line treatment	Amitriptyline: 10–150 mg/day at bedtime
			Atenolol: 50–200 mg daily
			Nadolol: 80–160 mg daily
		Second line treatment	Topiramate: 25–200 mg daily
			Candesartan: 16 mg daily
		Third line treatment	Pizotifen
		Advanced treatment (in specialty clinic)	Subcutaneous biologic (calcitonin gene-related peptide (CGRP) receptor antagonists: erenumab, fremanezumab, and galcanezumab)
			Botulinum Toxin is injected topically in the forehead, temples, and occiput
			Occipital nerve block
Cluster headache	Abortive drugs		Oxygen 100%, 7–12 L per minute for 15 min
			Sumatriptan: 6 mg subcutaneously
			Verapamil: 240–960 mg daily

History Taking and Management of an Adult Patient Presenting with Fever

4

Dana Al Marzooqi
and Shammah Al Memari

Learning Objectives
- How to master history taking for patients presenting with fever?
- How to perform a focused exam for patients presenting with fever?
- How to approach and provide management tips for patients with fever?

Focus areas include differential diagnosis includes **infections** (abscess, tuberculosis, granulomata, parasites, bacteria, rheumatic fever, fungi, and viruses), **multisystem diseases** (connective tissue disease, systemic lupus erythematosus, polyarteritis nodosa, sarcoidosis, cranial arteritis, polymyalgia rheumatic, rheumatoid arthritis, still's disease, inflammatory bowel disease), **tumors** (lymphoma, solid tumors), and drug induced fever.

For Child with fever refer to Chap 35.

1. Introduce yourself and establish good rapport.
2. Identify the complaint: duration (acute or chronic), onset (sudden or gradual, post-surgery or trauma, travel, contact with animal, insect bite, contact with patient with upper respiratory tract infection, exposure to heat or transfusion), character (low or high grade), relieving and aggravating factor (response to antipyretics), timing (continuous, intermittent or diurnal variation), progression

---

D. Al Marzooqi
Sheikh Khalifa Medical City, Abu Dhabi, United Arab Emirates

S. Al Memari (✉)
Abu Dhabi, United Arab Emirates

© The Author(s), under exclusive license to Springer Nature Singapore Pte Ltd. 2024
S. Lari et al. (eds.), *Family Medicine OSCE: First Aid to Objective Structured Clinical Examination*, https://doi.org/10.1007/978-981-99-5530-5_4

(deteriorating or improving), associated symptoms (headache, rigors, rash, coryza, diarrhea, vomiting, arthralgia, myalgia and dizziness, ear pain, dysuria, urgency, hesitancy, abdominal or pelvic pain, vaginal discharge, calf pain or pleuritic chest pain, tachypnea, bone pain), red flags (neck stiffness, photophobia, phonophobia, petechial rash, weight loss, headache, confusion, hemoptysis, night sweats, history of recent travel).

3. Explore the patient's or parent's ideas, concerns and expectations (ICE) and the effect of the complaint on the quality of life.
4. Explore ongoing problems: past medical, surgical, and menstrual histories.
5. Any regular use of medications: immunosuppressive medications.
6. Question the appropriateness of the dose of the antipyretics that have been used if any.
7. Social (including history of travel) and family history: availability of family support, access to health care, family history of any cancer, contact with tuberculosis or any other infection, and recent travel to countries endemic in malaria or meningitis-endemic areas.
8. Examination (looking for the focus):
   (a) Vital signs (tachycardia and hypotension suggestive of sepsis).
   (b) Inspect the hands and feet for signs of infective endocarditis.
   (c) Inspect the joints for signs of rheumatological diseases.
   (d) Rule out meningeal signs: inspect for rash and palpate for lymphadenopathy.
   (e) Look for any signs of upper or lower respiratory tract infection, otitis media, or sinusitis.
   (f) Look for any signs of temporal arteritis.
   (g) Abdominal exam: look for hepatomegaly or splenomegaly (suggestive of infection) and signs of appendicitis or pyelonephritis.
   (h) Look for any signs of deep vein thrombosis.
9. Order investigations as indicated: consider complete blood count and differential, blood, urine, sputum culture, urine analysis, CRP (C-Reactive Protein), stool for Ova and Parasite, lumbar puncture, chest X-ray, tuberculin test.
10. Arrange referral to emergency department if needed.
11. Management and education: share differential diagnosis and prognosis.
    (a) Educate the patient on conservative management, including the use of antipyretics, increased fluid intake, and other medications as prescribed based on the diagnosis.
    (b) Inform the patient with warning signs and the condition's prognosis.
    (c) Systemic diseases: consider further work up.
12. Give reading educational materials if any.
13. Discuss health maintenance, age-appropriate screening and arrange for follow-up.
14. Communication skills: organized approach, mixed questioning styles (open- and close-ended questions), active listening, clear language, and reflection on patient's ICE.

History Taking and Management of a Patient Presenting with Red Eye

5

Shaima Lari, Kawthar Al Ameri, and Shammah Al Memari

> **Learning Objectives**
> - How to master history taking for patients presenting with red eye?
> - How to perform a focused exam for patients presenting with red eye?
> - How to approach and provide management tips for patients with red eyes?

> **Focus areas** on cases to be treated in primary care setting: chalazion, stye, subconjunctival hemorrhage, episcleritis, blepharitis, dry eye syndrome, corneal abrasion, as well as viral, bacterial, or allergic conjunctivitis.

1. Introduce yourself.
2. Establish good rapport.
3. Identify the complaint: duration, associated symptoms (pain, itching, discharge and its characteristics, or vision disturbance), relieving and aggravating factors. Work out your differentials accordingly:
   (a) Viral conjunctivitis: presents with history of contact with patient with symptoms of upper respiratory tract infection or conjunctivitis, absent or

S. Lari
Sheikh Shakhbout Medical City, Abu Dhabi, United Arab Emirates

K. Al Ameri
Ambulatory Healthcare Services, Abu Dhabi, United Arab Emirates

Faculty of Family Medicine Residency Program, Sheikh Khalifa Medical City, Abu Dhabi, United Arab Emirates

S. Al Memari (✉)
Abu Dhabi, United Arab Emirates

© The Author(s), under exclusive license to Springer Nature Singapore Pte Ltd. 2024
S. Lari et al. (eds.), *Family Medicine OSCE: First Aid to Objective Structured Clinical Examination*, https://doi.org/10.1007/978-981-99-5530-5_5

minimal discharge, tearing, no visual disturbance, gritty sensation, rash of dermatomal distribution.

(b) Bacterial conjunctivitis: moderate pain, mucopurulent discharge, glued eyes, tearing, no visual disturbance, urethral discharge in males, rash in newborns.

(c) Allergic conjunctivitis: chronic itching, tearing, gritty sensation, chronic sneezing, or coughing, associated history of dry skin or eczema.

(d) Subconjunctival hemorrhage: possible history of a triggering movement (crying, progressive sneezing, or harsh coughing), sudden onset of redness, usually early in the morning, without any other complaint or visual disturbance.

(e) Acute angle closure glaucoma: headache, very painful red eye, haloes around the lights, blurred vision, nausea, and vomiting.

(f) Scleritis and uveitis: ocular pain, disturbed vision, progressive diffuse redness and photophobia, history of arthritis or rheumatologic condition.

(g) Corneal ulcer: history of trauma to the eye, foreign body sensation, possible history of contact-lenses uses, tearing, visual disturbance, photophobia.

(h) Vitreous hemorrhage or retinal detachment: painless visual loss with floaters.

4. Explore the patient's ideas, concerns and expectations (ICE).
5. Identify the effect of complaint on the quality of life.
6. Explore any ongoing problems: exclude diabetes, hypertension, multiple sclerosis, migraine, rheumatologic condition, and bleeding disorders (gum bleeding, epistaxis, or bruising).
7. Obtain a brief social and family history.
8. Examinations: For eye physical examination refer to Chap 71.

(a) Inspection of lids, Conjunctiva (diffuse injection: conjunctivitis), Sclera (hemorrhagic redness: subconjunctival hemorrhage), Cornea (fluorescein stain can be used to rule out corneal abrasions, or keratitis (grayish branching opacity of herpes simplex virus). Check for any discharge (Purulent discharge: bacterial conjunctivitis or bacterial keratitis).

(b) Visual acuity: instead of Snellen chart use reading vision (small versus large print); or vision only (hand motions or fingers' count); or light perception.

(c) Extraocular eye movement.

(d) Tonometer.

(e) Check for color vision.

(f) Visual field.

(g) Pupil size and reactiveness to light. Remember that pinpoint can be seen in corneal abrasion, infectious keratitis, or iritis, while fixed Pupil in mid-dilation can be seen acute angle closure glaucoma.

9. Arrange for referral accordingly: cases of angle closure glaucoma, hypopyon, hyphema, vitreous hemorrhage, and retinal detachment must be seen the same day in the emergency room or ophthalmology clinic, whereas urgent cases (such as iritis, keratitis, or scleritis) can be seen in one week.

10. Management and education:
    (a) Give the patient the differential diagnosis. Advise the patient to follow a conservative course of treatment for self-limiting conditions (such as sub-conjunctival hemorrhage). Emphasize to the patient about lifestyle modification: highlight the importance of regular hand washing for viral conjunctivitis and advise about allergen avoidance for allergic conjunctivitis.
    (b) Prescribe topical treatments as needed: artificial tears for mild irritation and conjunctivitis management, antihistamine, or decongestant drops for allergic conjunctivitis (1–2 drops, to be applied 4 times daily, as needed, for no more than 3 weeks), and topical antibiotic for bacterial conjunctivitis (Erythromycin 5 mg/g ophthalmic ointment).
    (c) Educate patient about red flags (severe pain, periocular edema, blurred vision, headache, photophobia, excessive discharge, floaters, and colored halos) and advise to attend to emergency or come back if any.
11. Give reading educational materials if any.
12. Discuss health maintenance and age-appropriate screening.
13. Order required investigations.
14. Arrange for follow up in 2 days.
15. Communication skills: organized approach, mixed questioning styles (open- and close-ended questions), active listening, clear language, and reflection on patients' ICE.

History Taking and Management of Adult Patient Presenting with Cough

6

Buthaina Al Maskari and Shammah Al Memari

> **Learning Objectives**
> - How to master history taking for patients presenting with cough?
> - How to perform a focused exam for patients presenting with cough?
> - How to approach and provide management tips for patients presenting with cough?

For infant with cough refer to Chap. 41.

> **Focus areas** include the duration of cough and the serious life-threatening conditions that need to be ruled out (pulmonary tuberculosis, pulmonary embolism, congestive heart failure, and malignancy).

1. Introduce yourself, establish good rapport, and take basic demographic information.
2. Identify the complaint: onset (sudden or gradual), duration (acute, subacute, or chronic), diurnal variation (more nocturnally), progression (same, worsening, improving), nature (intermittent or continuous), type (productive or non-productive), relieving and aggravating factors (worse by lying down (posterior nasal drip, esophageal reflux, bronchiectasis, bronchitis, and heart failure), worse by exercise or exposure to allergens (asthma). Refer to (Table 6.1) for

B. Al Maskari
Ambulatory Healthcare Services, Abu Dhabi, United Arab Emirates

S. Al Memari (✉)
Abu Dhabi, United Arab Emirates

© The Author(s), under exclusive license to Springer Nature Singapore Pte Ltd. 2024
S. Lari et al. (eds.), *Family Medicine OSCE: First Aid to Objective Structured Clinical Examination*, https://doi.org/10.1007/978-981-99-5530-5_6

21

Table 6.1 Differential diagnosis of cough based on duration

Acute cough (less than 3 weeks)	Subacute cough (from 3 to 8 weeks)	Chronic cough (more than 8 weeks)
• Upper respiratory infection • Lower respiratory tract infection • Exacerbation of preexisting conditions including asthma, bronchiectasis, chronic obstructive pulmonary disease (COPD), or upper airway cough syndrome • Life-threatening conditions including pulmonary embolism or congestive heart failure	• Post-infectious cough, posterior nasal drip, or upper airway irritation • Mucus accumulation: a manifestation of bronchial hyperresponsiveness that may be associated with asthma • Ongoing allergen or irritant exposure • Lingering effects of an infection with or without pneumonia • Acute exacerbation of chronic bronchitis • Pertussis or whooping cough	• Asthma • Gastroesophageal reflux disease • Upper airway cough syndrome • Angiotensin-converting enzyme inhibitor use (in adults)

differential diagnosis of cough. Associated symptoms that would help point towards the causation as follows:

(a) Sputum, its color, consistency, amount, and frequency if any. Clear sputum is usually found in allergy cases, purulent occurs more in infections, and bloody sputum can be found in tuberculosis, bronchiectasis, heart failure, or cancers.

(b) Hemoptysis, its volume, frequency, nature (fresh, altered blood, or mixed with sputum. The latter being suggestive of chest infection, tumor, tuberculosis, infarction) if any.

(c) Orthopnea, dyspnea, paroxysmal nocturnal dyspnea, and leg swelling are suggestive of heart failure.

(d) Fever: suggestive of infection.

(e) Weight loss: suggestive of cancer or tuberculosis.

(f) Insomnia and daytime somnolence: suggestive of obstructive sleep apnea.

(g) Allergic history and wheezing: suggestive of bronchial asthma or allergic rhinitis.

(h) Throat tickling sensation: suggestive of posterior nasal drip or gastroesophageal reflux.

3. Explore patients ideas, concerns and expectations (ICE) and the effect of the problem on daily activities.

4. Explore ongoing problems: asthma, allergy, heart failure, chronic bronchitis, hypertension, heartburn.

5. Question use of regular medications: Angiotensin-converting-enzyme (ACE) inhibitors, angiotensin receptor blockers, calcium channel blockers (worsen gastroesophageal reflux disease), nonsteroidal anti-inflammatory drugs and

beta blockers (may induce asthma exacerbation), nitrofurantoin (causes lung fibrosis).

6. Social and family history: smoking history, occupational exposure, and recent travel.

7. Examination: vital signs, cardiovascular system, chest, ear, nose, throat, and peak follow meter if needed.

8. Order required investigations as indicated: Peak expiratory flow rate, chest X-Ray, and Monteux test.

9. Arrange referral: as required for cardiology, oncology, respirology, or infectious disease.

10. Explain possible diagnoses, along with treatment and education:

    (a) In upper airway cough syndrome (including non-allergic causes and allergic rhinitis), advise the patient to avoid allergens and to take oral or intra nasal antihistamines and intra nasal glucocorticoids.

    (b) In congestive heart failure, the patient will require immediate care and cardiology referral.

    (c) Patients with asthma must avoid allergens and triggers, use disease controllers, and adhere to the asthma action plan. If the reason is gastroesophageal reflux disease, recommend lifestyle and dietary modifications such as weight loss, avoidance of food triggers, and the use of antacids, histamine receptors-2 blockers, or proton pump inhibitors.

    (d) Send a nasopharyngeal swab for culture in cases of pertussis. Patients with confirmed whooping cough should be given macrolide antibiotics based on the length of their symptoms and should be isolated for 5 days beginning on the first day of treatment. They are urged to avoid contact with others until at least 5 days of antibiotic treatment have passed.

    (e) Cessation of smoking is nearly always successful in eliminating cough in smokers.

    (f) Antibiotics or corticosteroids should be considered for chronic obstructive pulmonary disease (COPD) exacerbations.

    (g) If the cough is caused by an ACE inhibitor, reassure the patient that it will typically subside after 2 weeks of discontinuing treatment.

11. Give reading educational materials if any.

12. Discuss health maintenance and screening for age and arrange for follow up.

13. Communication skills: organized approach, mixed questioning styles (open- and close-ended questions), active listening, clear language, and reflection on patient's ICE.

History Taking and Management of a Patient Presenting with Sore Throat

7

Abeer Al Naqbi, Buthaina Al Maskari, and Shammah Al Memari

Learning Objectives
- How to master history taking for patients presenting with sore throat?
- How to perform a focused exam for patients presenting with sore throat?
- How to approach and provide management tips for patients presenting with sore throat?

Hints Usually, simulated patients with minor illness appear in the exam to test certain skills. This may include patient demanding referral for tonsillectomy, patient demanding antibiotic inappropriately, smoker for counseling or patient with hidden agenda such as marital problem, parent using the child as presenting complaint, or malingering patient requesting sick leave.

1. Introduce yourself and establish good rapport.
2. Identify the complaint: onset, duration, character, relieving or aggravating factors, associated symptoms (fever, malaise, rash, runny nose, cough, shortness of breath).
3. Rule out red flags:
   (a) Ashen color and drooling child (epiglottitis).
   (b) Signs of meningism (meningitis).
   (c) Unstable vital signs (streptococcal sepsis).

A. Al Naqbi · B. Al Maskari
Ambulatory Healthcare Services, Abu Dhabi, United Arab Emirates

S. Al Memari (✉)
Abu Dhabi, United Arab Emirates

© The Author(s), under exclusive license to Springer Nature Singapore Pte Ltd. 2024
S. Lari et al. (eds.), *Family Medicine OSCE: First Aid to Objective Structured Clinical Examination*, https://doi.org/10.1007/978-981-99-5530-5_7

25

> **Box 7.1 Indications for Tonsillectomy**
>
> (a) Tonsillitis: chronic or recurrent (4–7 episodes in 1 year or more than five episodes per year over 2 consecutive years or more than three episodes per year over 3 consecutive years)
> (b) Obstruction: compromise to airway, voice, or swallowing
> (c) Tonsillar malignancy or suspicion of it
> (d) Uncontrollable hemorrhage from tonsillar blood vessels
> (e) Peritonsillar abscess: more than one episode or one episode with history recurrent tonsillitis
> (f) Chronic pharyngeal carriage of "Group A Beta-Hemolytic Streptococci"
> (g) Refractory halitosis
> (h) PFAPA syndrome (periodic fevers with aphthous stomatitis pharyngitis and adenitis syndrome) that is unresponsive to conservative treatment

    (d) Murmur and heart failure (rheumatic fever).

    (e) Unilateral swelling with marked tenderness and trismus (peritonsillar abscess).

4. Explore patient's and parent's ideas, concerns and expectations (ICE), and effect of the complaint on quality of life.
5. Explore ongoing problems: immunocompromise, diabetes, asthma, or malnutrition.
6. Note vaccination history and any known allergy.
7. Question regular use of medications.
8. Social and family history: smoking, poor social conditions, family history of rheumatic fever.
9. Examination: vital signs, neck (lymph nodes), skin (rash), ENT (ear nose and throat), abdomen (splenomegaly), enlarged lymph nodes, rash, and splenomegaly indicate infectious mononucleosis.
10. Order required investigations as indicated: rapid streptococcal test, throat swab (for culture and sensitivity), complete blood count, infectious mononucleosis test if highly suspected.
11. Decide whether the patient fits the "Modified Centor Criteria." It includes absence of cough, high-grade fever (more than 38 °C), 3 or more tender anterior cervical lymph nodes, tonsillar exudates or swelling, age (3–14 years = +1 point, more than 45 years = −1 point). Classify according to cumulative score: if less than 2, no need for antibiotic or further testing, if 2–3 perform rapid strep test or throat culture, if 4 consider empiric antibiotic.
12. Decide whether the patient has an indication for consideration of tonsillectomy. Refer to Box 7.1.

13. Management and education: share diagnosis; discuss nature of the problem and prognosis.
    (a) For bacterial pharyngitis: use proper dose of appropriate antibiotic, at the right frequency, for the right duration.
    (b) For viral upper respiratory tract infection, describe to the patient or parents that: upper respiratory tract infections can be viral or bacterial. While bacterial infection is treated with antibiotics, viral infection requires symptomatic treatment only. We use a set of clinical indicators to establish whether this infection is viral or bacterial. These items are (mention the Centor criteria). You or your child do not meet the criteria and so do not require an antibiotic. Encourage the use of symptomatic treatments, such as paracetamol for fever, nasal saline spray for nasal congestion, and honey for cough (advice against anti-tussive as cough is a protective mechanism that assists the body to get rid of the microbes). Always remind the patient or parent about the safety net, you may say: Viral infections can lower a patient's immunity, and as a result, he or she may have a secondary bacterial illness. Please return for review if you or your child develop a non-response fever or cannot tolerate oral feeds.
14. Give reading educational materials if any.
15. Discuss health maintenance and screening for age.
16. Arrange for follow up, referral if indicated (to ENT for epiglottitis or tonsillectomy).
17. Communication skills: organized approach, mixed questioning styles (open- and close-ended questions), active listening, clear language, and reflection on patient's ICE.

History Taking and Management of a Patient Presenting with Epistaxis

8

Shaima Lari, Buthaina Al Maskari, and Shammah Al Memari

Learning Objectives
- How to master history taking for patients presenting with epistaxis?
- How to perform a focused exam for patients presenting with epistaxis?
- How to approach and provide management tips for patients presenting with epistaxis?

Focus areas include history of trauma (digital, blunt, foreign bodies), barometric changes, nasal dryness, allergic or viral rhinitis, or exposure to chemicals (cocaine, xylometazoline, nasal steroids). Possibility of malignancy (especially if unilateral in an adolescent male), systemic disease (as in coagulopathies, hypertension, hepatic disease, leukemia, thrombocytopenia), or physiologic congestion in pregnancy (may result in epistaxis which is self-limited).

1. Introduce yourself.
2. Establish good rapport.
3. Identify the complaint: duration, site, onset (illicit onset of any preceding trauma, exposure to extreme weather changes or altitude changes), character

S. Lari
Sheikh Shakhbout Medical City, Abu Dhabi, United Arab Emirates

B. Al Maskari
Ambulatory Healthcare Services, Abu Dhabi, United Arab Emirates

S. Al Memari (✉)
Abu Dhabi, United Arab Emirates

© The Author(s), under exclusive license to Springer Nature Singapore Pte Ltd. 2024
S. Lari et al. (eds.), *Family Medicine OSCE: First Aid to Objective Structured Clinical Examination*, https://doi.org/10.1007/978-981-99-5530-5_8

29

(fresh or old blood), relieving and aggravating factors, timing, frequency, and severity.

4. Explore patient's ideas, concerns and expectations (ICE): trauma, hidden agenda, or asking for sick leave!

5. Explore ongoing problems: allergic rhinitis, nasal dryness, hypertension, bleeding disorder, hepatic disease, leukemia, or pregnancy.

6. Question regular use of medications: Xylometazoline (Otrivin), nasal steroids, aspirin, warfarin.

7. Social and family history: briefly exclude bleeding disorders among males, abuse or domestic violence, smoking, cocaine sniffing, alcohol.

8. Examination:
    (a) Vitals (assessing hemodynamic instability due to excessive blood loss).
    (b) Determine site of bleeding: use topical anesthetic and vasoconstrictor to facilitate exam and use nasal speculum and good lighting.
    (c) Look for other signs of coagulopathy (e.g., ecchymosis, petechiae, telangiectatic lesions).

9. Order investigations as indicated: complete blood count, prothrombin time and Partial thromboplastin time, liver function test.

10. Management (as elaborated in Table 8.1) and health education:
    (a) Share the differential diagnosis and prognosis.
    (b) Explain to the patient strategies that prevent recurrence: lubricating the nostril with olive oil, regular steam inhalation, avoiding excessive blowing, straining, or heavy lifting.
    (c) Explain to the patient strategies of applying first-aid in case of recurrence: start with focusing on maintenance of airway, breathing, and circulation (ABCs). Lean forward and pinch the cartilaginous portion of the nose for 20 min. You can apply cold pack on the upper nose. Remember to breathe through mouth all through.
    (d) Safety-net: remind the patient to come back immediately, for consideration of cauterization, if all above methods fail to control the epistaxis.

Table 8.1 Management of epistaxis

Mild anterior bleeding	Mild posterior bleeding	Significant bleeding
• Conservative measures: position the head forward while squeezing the nasal bridge • Xylometazoline spray (two puffs) • If bleeding persists and the source is identified then cauterize using chemical (silver nitrate) or electrical means • If unsuccessful, then consider anterior nasal packing • If all measures fail, then explore the possibility of posterior bleeding	• Posterior nasal packing by balloon catheter, Foley catheter, or cotton packing • Urgent referral to ENT	• Consider starting intravenous fluids and cross match two units packed RBC

11. Discuss health maintenance and screening for age.
12. Provide the patient with reading educational materials.
13. Arrange for follow up.
14. Arrange urgent referral to Ear-Nose-Throat (ENT) specialist if the patient is vitally unstable, has posterior bleeding or uncontrolled bleed despite packing.
15. Communication skills: organized approach, mixed questioning styles (open- and close-ended questions), active listening, clear language, and reflection on patient's ICE.

History Taking and Management of a Patient Presenting with Dizziness

9

Reem Al Mansoori, Sumiya Taheri, and Shammah Al Memari

Learning Objectives
- How to master history taking for patients presenting with dizziness?
- How to perform a focused exam for patients presenting with dizziness?
- How to approach and provide management tips for patients with dizziness?

Focus areas include medication's side effects, hypoglycemia, orthostatic hypotension, cervicogenic dizziness, or psychiatric origin.

1. Introduce yourself and establish good rapport.
2. Identify the complaint (refer to Table 9.1 for classification of vertigo and Table 9.2 for the prominent of its differential diagnoses):
   (a) Clarify what exactly the patient means by dizziness: true vertigo (spinning of self or environment), light headedness (vague floating sensation), pre-syncope (sense of impending fainting), or disequilibrium (unbalanced).
   (b) Determine: timing (onset, duration, evolution), frequency, previous episodes, relieving or aggravating factors, and triggers (actions, motions, and situations. Examples: arising from bed, change in head position, auricle manipulation, coughing, or sneezing).

R. Al Mansoori
Emirates Medical Association of Family Medicine, Abu Dhabi, United Arab Emirates

S. Taheri
Ambulatory Healthcare Services, Abu Dhabi, United Arab Emirates

S. Al Memari (✉)
Abu Dhabi, United Arab Emirates

© The Author(s), under exclusive license to Springer Nature Singapore Pte Ltd. 2024
S. Lari et al. (eds.), *Family Medicine OSCE: First Aid to Objective Structured Clinical Examination*, https://doi.org/10.1007/978-981-99-5530-5_9

33

Table 9.1 Classification of vertigo

Central vertigo	Peripheral vertigo
• Vertebrobasilar transient ischemic attack • Stroke • Multiple sclerosis • Vestibular migraine • Concussion	• Benign paroxysmal positional vertigo (BPPV) • Meniere's disease • Vestibular neuritis or labyrinthitis • Acoustic neuroma • Otosclerosis

Table 9.2 Symptoms and probable diagnoses of vertigo

Symptoms	Probable diagnosis
Vertigo with fluctuating deafness, tinnitus, ear fullness, nausea, and vomiting	Meniere's disease
Spontaneous episodic vertigo with conductive hearing loss	Otosclerosis
Sudden spontaneous vertigo, unsteadiness, nausea, vomiting, and oscillopsia (items in the visual field appears to oscillate)	Vestibular neuritis
Positional vertigo that lasts for a few seconds, with nausea and vomiting, especially when it wakes the patient from sleep when turning over in bed	BPPV
Spontaneous episodes of vertigo associated with migraine headaches	Vestibular migraine
Lightheadedness with hyperventilation	Psychosomatic dizziness

  (c) Associated symptoms: headache, visual disturbance, hearing loss, tinnitus, otalgia, otorrhea, facial weakness or numbness, difficulty walking, common cold, depression, anxiety, or hyperventilation.
  (d) Relevant history: history of recent travel, upper respiratory tract infection, exposure to toxins or medications that can cause dizziness (antihistamines, antihypertensive, anticonvulsants, narcotics, sedatives, muscle relaxants, antibiotics, aminoglycosides, quinine, and antidepressant), as well as previous ear surgery, trauma to head, or neck.
  (e) Red Flags (refer to Table 9.3).
3. Explore patient's ideas, concerns and expectations (ICE) and the effect of the problem on the quality of life.
4. Explore ongoing problems: including diabetes, hypertension, pregnancy, anemia, heart disease, neurologic disorder, history of stroke or head trauma.
5. Question use of any regular medications.
6. Social and family history: smoking, alcohol, lack of support, home environment, emotional or financial problems.
7. Examination:
  (a) Vital signs: including blood pressure in sitting or supine position and standing to assess for orthostatic hypotension (a drop in systolic blood pressure of 20 mmHg or diastolic blood pressure of up to 10 mmHg or a rise of heart rate of up to 30 beats per minute).

Table 9.3 Vertigo's red flags

Red flags	Probable diagnosis
Vertigo with diplopia, dysarthria, weakness, numbness, confusion, loss of consciousness, swallowing problem, or seizures	Central cause for the vertigo
Presyncope with nausea, vomiting, headache, sweating, or tremors	Hypoglycemia
Presyncope with palpitation or chest pain	Valvular disease or acute coronary syndrome
Chest, back, abdominal or pelvic pain	Intrathoracic or intraabdominal emergency
Vertigo with unilateral tinnitus, hearing loss, progressive facial numbness, weakness	Acoustic neuroma

    (b) Observe patient gait and test for Romberg sign (assess for ataxia, dorsal column dysfunction, and peripheral neuropathy).

    (c) Head-Impulse, Nystagmus and Test of Skew (HINTS): to distinguish central causes (stroke) from peripheral causes (vestibular neuritis).

    (d) Full ear, nose, throat examination: autoscopy, Rinne and Weber tests.

    (e) Cardiovascular exam: pulse, carotids for bruits, heart sounds, or murmurs.

    (f) Central nervous system exam: cranial nerves, gait, cerebellar signs, motor, and sensory.

    (g) Dix-Hallpike maneuver: (refer to Chap. 72 for further details).

8. Order required investigations as indicated:

    (a) Patient with chronic illness: glucose, complete blood count, electrolytes.

    (b) Patient with cardiac symptoms: electrocardiogram, Holter monitor, carotid doppler.

    (c) Patient with hearing loss: audiometry.

    (d) Patient with neurological signs: brain MRI.

9. Management and education:

    (a) Refer case to the emergency department if red flags are present.

    (b) Otherwise, reassure: "I understand that these symptoms are frightening. However, I would like to reassure you as most causes of vertigo are not serious health threats." Give general advice on what to do while feeling dizzy or vertiginous: ask the patient to lie still in a darkened room and avoid head movement. Advise the patient to avoid provocative movement and ensure patient safety (address driving and dealing with heavy machinery).

    (c) Discuss the differential diagnosis with the patient, explain the most probable diagnosis and treatment in simple words (refer to Table 9.4).

10. Give reading educational materials (How to perform Apply's exercise).

11. Arrange for follow up and referral if indicated (neurologist if central cause, cardiologist if cardiac cause, ENT if medical treatment fails).

12. Discuss health maintenance and age-appropriate screening.

13. Communication skills: organized approach, mixed questioning styles (open- and close-ended questions), active listening, clear language, and reflection on patients ICE.

Table 9.4 Vertigo's management and patient education

Diagnosis	Explaining it to the patient in simple language	Treatment
Meniere's disease	A disorder of the inner ear that affect the hearing and balance. symptoms may presents as an episodes of dizziness, hearing loss, and a sensation of fullness or tinnitus in the ear.	– Lifestyle modification (limiting dietary salt intake to less than 2000 mg per day, reducing caffeine intake, and limiting alcohol to one drink per day) – Medications (thiazide diuretics, trans-tympanic injections of glucocorticoids and gentamicin, or vestibular suppressant medications) – Surgery as last option
Vestibular neuritis	A condition sometimes caused by a virus which can affect the inner ear or the nerve in the inner ear. People with this condition have vertigo that comes on quickly and can last several days. They also often feel very sick and off balance	– Vestibular rehabilitation – Medications: antihistamines (Meclizine 12.5–50 mg every 4–6 h), antiemetics (metoclopramide 5–10 mg every 6 h), Benzodiazepines (Diazepam 2–10 mg every 4–6 h). Remember to discuss medication side effects (dry mouth, sedation, blurred vision, amnesia, akathisia)
BPPV	Deep inside the ear, there is a small network of tubes that are filled with fluid. Floating inside that fluid are special calcium deposits. Together, these tubes and deposits make up the "vestibular system." This system tells the brain what position the body is in. It also helps keep you balanced. In BPPV, extra calcium deposits form in the inner ear. This can lead to short episodes of vertigo that happen when you move your head in certain ways	– Canalith repositioning maneuvers: Epley's maneuver (70% success at first attempt and 100% on successive attempts) or Brandt-Daroff exercises – There is no role of vestibular suppressants (might increase risk of fall)

History Taking and Management of a Patient Presenting with Hearing Loss

10

Kawthar Al Ameri, Sumiya Taheri,
and Shammah Al Memari

Learning Objectives
- How to master history taking for patients presenting with hearing loss?
- How to perform a focused exam for patients presenting with hearing loss?
- How to approach and provide management tips for patients presenting with hearing loss?

Focus areas include

Differential diagnosis of conductive hearing loss: cerumen impaction, otitis media, otosclerosis, cholesteatoma, tympanic membrane perforation, Eustachian tube dysfunction, foreign body in the ear canal, benign mass (osteoma, polyp), barotrauma, congenital malformation (external auditory canal atresia, ossicular malformation).

Differential diagnosis of sensorineural hearing loss: presbycusis, congenital infections (syphilis, cytomegalovirus, herpes, rubella, mumps), genetic reasons (syndromic, non-syndromic), noise trauma, ototoxic medications, autoimmune disease, temporal bone fracture, Meniere's disease, meningitis, acoustic neuroma, iatrogenic (middle ear surgery).

K. Al Ameri
Ambulatory Healthcare Services, Abu Dhabi, United Arab Emirates

S. Taheri
Ambulatory Healthcare Services, Abu Dhabi, United Arab Emirates

S. Al Memari (✉)
Abu Dhabi, United Arab Emirates

© The Author(s), under exclusive license to Springer Nature Singapore Pte Ltd. 2024
S. Lari et al. (eds.), *Family Medicine OSCE: First Aid to Objective Structured Clinical Examination*, https://doi.org/10.1007/978-981-99-5530-5_10

1. Introduce yourself.
2. Establish a good rapport.
3. Identify the complaint:
    (a) Onset: Gradual onset suggests age related hearing loss, otosclerosis, or acoustic neuroma. While a rapid onset suggests perforated tympanic membrane, trauma, or idiopathic sudden sensorineural hearing loss.
    (b) Laterality (unilateral or bilateral).
    (c) Frequency and progression (worsening, improving, or unchanged).
    (d) Aggravating and relieving factors.
    (e) Associated symptoms: Otologic symptoms like otalgia, itching, fullness of the ear, pulling of the ears, ear discharge, tinnitus, and vertigo. Neurologic symptoms like headache, weakness or asymmetry of the face, and abnormal sense of taste. Other symptoms like fever, upper respiratory tract infection features, or vomiting (children "Otitis Media"). Mention red flags (See Table 10.1).
4. Explore patient's ideas, concerns, expectations, and impact of hearing difficulty on the patient's life: consider depression, keep in mind hearing loss stigma, cost, and inconvenience.
5. Explore ongoing problems: diabetes, chronic infections, renal failure, or atherosclerosis.
6. Medications intake: antibiotics (like aminoglycosides, macrolides, or quinolones), analgesics (like aspirin or non-steroidal anti-inflammatory drugs), diuretics (like furosemide), beta blockers (like metoprolol or bisoprolol), ACE inhibitors (like ramipril), and hydroxychloroquine.
7. Allergies history.
8. Family history of hearing loss or brain tumor.
9. Social history: marital status, smoking, alcohol, employment (military, planes).
10. Physical examination:
    (a) Ear: look at the auricle and the external auditory canal for obstruction by cerumen or foreign body.
    (b) Head: look for signs of trauma or masses.
    (c) Neck: look for lymphadenopathy or masses.
    (d) Neurologic examination: testing cranial nerves and cognitive function. (Refer to Chap. 69).

Table 10.1 Red flags for hearing loss	• Sudden onset of hearing loss in case of head trauma
	• History of preceding exposure to noise (occupational noise exposure, gunshot, or explosion)
	• Visual impairment that may be suggestive of intra-cranial tumor
	• Delay in speech, language, or motor development in children

(e) Otoscopy: Is the tympanic membrane (TM) perforated, retracted, bulging, or erythematous? Any signs of drainage, cholesteatoma, or foreign body?

(f) Whispered voice test.

(g) Weber and Rinne test to narrow down the differential diagnosis by categorizing the hearing loss into conductive or sensorineural hearing loss. (Refer to Chap. 72).

(h) Audiometry and tympanometry: refer to Table 10.2 for details.

(i) Language testing in children with persistent infection or developmental delay.

11. Investigations if patient has unexplained sensorineural deficit:

(a) Blood sugar especially in diabetic patients (consider cochlear ischemia).

(b) Complete blood count.

(c) Thyroid stimulating hormone (TSH).

(d) Syphilis.

(e) Serological testing for Sjogren disease.

(f) CT scan of temporal bone if patient has unexplained conductive hearing loss.

(g) MRI with gadolinium if patient has unilateral or asymmetric sensorineural hearing loss.

12. Arrange referral to:

(a) Otolaryngologist: if patient has sudden sensorineural hearing loss or when in need for hearing aids.

(b) Rehabilitation: for "communication therapy" programs.

13. Management and education: share the deferential diagnosis with the patient and explain accordingly:

(a) Child with hearing loss: explain that "hearing problems are common in children. The most common cause of hearing problems is a 'glue ear', which is a build-up of sticky fluid in the middle ear following middle-ear infections. The external ear canal can get blocked with things such as wax and foreign objects put in there by the child."

(b) Cerumen impaction: Options of management are watchful waiting, manual removal, or cerumenolytic agents and advise patient against use of cotton swabs and ear candles.

(c) Otitis media: treat with antibiotic: Amoxicillin (child dose: 80–90 mg/kg/day) if resistant Macrolide, Clindamycin, or Cephalosporins.

Table 10.2 Interpretation of tympanometry graphs

Graph type	Most probable cause
Type A	Normal
Type B: little or no mobility	Fluid behind the TM
Type C: negative pressure in middle ear	A retracted TM
Type AS: very stiff middle ear	Myringosclerosis or otosclerosis
Type AD: highly compliant TM	Ossicular-chain discontinuity

(d) Presbycusis: Educate the patient and the family regarding methods to improve communication including minimizing background noise, ensuring face-to-face conversation, and asking for summary or rephrase of wording when not heard. You can advise on hearing aids or Cochlear implant in case of severe hearing-loss based on outcome of the ear examination (Refer to Chap. 72).

14. Give reading educational materials if any.
15. Discuss health maintenance and screening for age.
16. Arrange for follow up, safety netting, and reflecting on patient's ideas, concerns, and expectations (ICE).
17. Communication skills: organized approach, mixed questioning styles (open- and close-ended questions), active listening, clear language, and reflection on patient's ICE.

History Taking and Management of a Patient Presenting with Fatigue

11

Kawthar Al Ameri, Buthaina Al Maskari, and Shammah Al Memari

Learning Objectives
- How to master history taking for patients presenting with fatigue?
- How to perform a focused exam for patients presenting with fatigue?
- How to approach and provide management tips for patients with fatigue?

Focus areas include physiologic fatigue, chronic fatigue syndrome, risky behaviors, depression, sleeping disorders, chronic diseases, life-threatening conditions (cancer), hypothyroidism, and rheumatologic diseases (as in fibromyalgia, and polymyalgia rheumatic).

---

1. Introduce yourself.
2. Establish good rapport.
3. Identify the complaint:
   (a) Clarify the symptom "what do you mean by fatigue?": lack of energy, mental exhaustion, or poor muscle endurance.

K. Al Ameri
Ambulatory Healthcare Services, Abu Dhabi, United Arab Emirates

Faculty of Family Medicine Residency Program, Sheikh Khalifa Medical City, Abu Dhabi, United Arab Emirates

B. Al Maskari
Ambulatory Healthcare Services, Abu Dhabi, United Arab Emirates

S. Al Memari (✉)
Abu Dhabi, United Arab Emirates

© The Author(s), under exclusive license to Springer Nature Singapore Pte Ltd. 2024
S. Lari et al. (eds.), *Family Medicine OSCE: First Aid to Objective Structured Clinical Examination*, https://doi.org/10.1007/978-981-99-5530-5_11

41

    (b) Onset and course: (acute: less than 1 month, subacute: 6 months, chronic: more than 6 months).

    (c) Frequency and duration: (chronic fatigue syndrome: lasting hours or days).

    (d) Aggravating and relieving factors.

    (e) Evaluate sleep quality and quantity: hours, falling asleep (reading, watching, or talking), sleeping environment, and habit.

    (f) Associated symptoms: weight gain or loss, steatorrhea, cold or heat intolerance, heavy periods, nausea, vomiting, shortness of breath, snoring, fever, night sweating, joint pain, headaches, sore throat, cough, rectal bleeding, polyuria, polydipsia.

    (g) Patient health questionnaire-9 (PHQ-9) assessing depression.

    (h) CAGE questions (Cut down, Annoyed, Guilty, Eye-opener) assessing alcohol dependence.

4. Explore patient's ideas concerns and expectation (ICE) and impacts on work performance, family, or social relationships.

5. Explore ongoing problems: past medical (chronic diseases including renal and liver diseases, infections like infectious mononucleosis, HIV, tuberculosis, viral hepatitis) and social histories.

6. Medications: antiarrhythmic, antihypertension, antiepileptic, antihistamine, antidepressants agents, steroids, immunosuppressants, and allergies history.

7. Family history: chronic diseases, cancers, hypothyroidism, rheumatologic conditions.

8. Social history: marital status, smoking, alcohol, and substance abuse, unprotected sexual intercourse, employment.

9. Examination: as indicated by symptoms.

10. Management: treat any contributing medical conditions as indicated. If idiopathic fatigue or chronic fatigue syndrome:

    (a) Trial of antidepressant therapy (SSRI or SNRI)

    (b) Cognitive behavioral therapy (CBT)

    (c) Exercise therapy

History Taking and Management of a Patient Presenting with Hypothyroidism

Khuloud Al Hammadi, Kawthar Al Ameri, and Shammah Al Memari

Learning Objectives
- How to master history taking for patients presenting with hypothyroidism?
- How to perform a focused exam for patients presenting with hypothyroidism?
- How to approach and provide management tips for patients with hypothyroidism?

Focus areas include symptoms, signs and management of hypothyroidism, family history of other autoimmune disorders.

1. Introduce yourself.
2. Establish good rapport.
3. Identify patient complaint, duration, site and radiation, onset, character, relieving or aggravating factors, and associated symptoms:
   (a) **Slowing of metabolic processes:** fatigue, weakness, cold intolerance, dyspnea on exertion, weight gain, decrease concentration, intellectual disability (infantile onset), constipation, and growth failure.

K. Al Hammadi
Sheikh Khalifa Medical City, Abu Dhabi, United Arab Emirates

K. Al Ameri
Ambulatory Healthcare Services, Abu Dhabi, United Arab Emirates

S. Al Memari (✉)
Abu Dhabi, United Arab Emirates

© The Author(s), under exclusive license to Springer Nature Singapore Pte Ltd. 2024
S. Lari et al. (eds.), *Family Medicine OSCE: First Aid to Objective Structured Clinical Examination*, https://doi.org/10.1007/978-981-99-5530-5_12

    (b) **Accumulation of matrix substances:** dry skin, hoarseness, carpal tunnel syndrome, or edema.

    (c) **Others:** decreased hearing, myalgia, paresthesia, depression, menorrhagia, infertility, joint pain, or pubertal delay.

4. Medications: Lithium, immune modulators (like interferon-alpha), iodine containing antiarrhythmic (like Amiodarone).

5. Explore patient's ideas, concerns and expectations (ICE).

6. Explore ongoing problems: diabetes, celiac disease, anemia, vitiligo, rheumatoid arthritis, hypercholesterolemia, depression, Down syndrome, any other autoimmune diseases, cardiac disease.

7. Past medical and surgical history: inquire about thyroidectomy, radiation to the neck, use of radioactive iodine, Graves' disease, de Quervain thyroiditis, or painless (postpartum) thyroiditis.

8. Social and Family history: thyroid dysfunction in the family or any autoimmune disease.

9. Examination:

    (a) Vital signs: pulse rate, blood pressure, respiratory rate.

    (b) Neck examination: inspection (for goiter, dilated veins, or scar from thyroidectomy), palpation (for nodules and lymph nodes), percussion (over the clavicles at the fossa) and auscultation (for bruits).

    (c) Look for signs of reduced metabolism: slow movement, slow speech, coarse voice, delayed relaxation of tendon reflexes, or bradycardia.

    (d) Look for signs of accumulation of matrix substances: coarse skin, puffy facies, dull facial expression, loss of eyebrows, periorbital puffiness, tongue enlargement, Tinel's signs (resulting from carpel tunnel thickening: Flexure retinaculum is thickened by myxedema, and it may entrap the median nerve in the carpal tunnel).

    (e) Look for other possible signs: diastolic hypertension, crackles on auscultation due to pleural and pericardial effusions, ascites, or galactorrhea.

10. Investigations as indicated:

    (a) Thyroid function tests: thyroid stimulating hormone (TSH), triiodothyronine (T3), and thyroxine (T4).

    (b) Thyroid antibodies including thyroid peroxidase antibodies (anti-TPO).

    (c) Lipid panel.

    (d) Complete blood count.

    (e) Ultrasound of the thyroid.

11. Arrange referral to endocrinologist if needed: as in patients with central hypothyroidism (low TSH and low free T4) or hypothyroidism that is unresponsive to treatment.

12. Management and education:
    (a) Replacement therapy with levothyroxine for life. Starting low and going slow, especially for patients who are more than 60 years and those who have ischemic heart disease (IHD).
    (b) Explain to the patient intake instructions: inform the patient to take it either early in the morning on an empty stomach, delaying the breakfast until 30–60 min after taking it, *or* at other times of the day, at least 2 h after the last meal. Advise the patient to void taking it at the same time of taking other medication that would interfere with its absorption; such as proton pump inhibitor, calcium carbonate, or ferrous sulfate.
    (c) Educate the patient about therapy expectation: inform the patient that symptoms may begin to resolve only after 2–3 weeks. Explain that peak TSH concentrations are not achieved for at least 6 weeks. Hence, Full effect may be delayed in terms of feelings improvement up to 8 weeks.
    (d) Educate the patient about common side effects of the medication such as: palpitations, sweating, disturbed sleep, and loose motions.
    (e) Explain to female patients the need to visit back once pregnant as they usually need monitoring of TSH in each trimester with a probable dose increase by 25–50 µg.
    (f) Educate the patient about the possible complications of hypothyroidism (if untreated) such as increased risk of coronary artery disease, secondary hyperlipidemia, depression, and memory decline.
13. Give reading educational materials if any.
14. Discuss health maintenance and screening for age.
15. Assist patient in regards of follow up:
    (a) Provide an appointment to repeat the TSH, 6–8 weeks from the beginning of the treatment.
    (b) TSH and free T4 are to be monitored annually for stable hypothyroid patients.
16. Communication skills: organized approach, mixed questioning styles (open- and close-ended questions), active listening, clear language, and reflection on patient's ICE

History Taking and Management of a Patient Presenting with Tremor

Eiman Al Murar, Sumiya Taheri,
and Shammah Al Memari

Learning Objectives
- How to master history taking for patients presenting with tremor?
- How to perform a focused exam for patients presenting with tremor?
- How to approach and provide management tips for patients with tremor?

Focus areas on essential tremor, alcohol or medication-induced, enhanced physiologic tremor, cerebellar disease, (Multiple Sclerosis, stroke or tumor), hyperthyroidism, Parkinsonism in resting tremor, psychogenic tremor (anxiety), metabolic tremors (as in hepatic encephalopathy, Wilson's disease, and hypoglycemia).

1. Introduce yourself.
2. Establish good rapport.
3. Identify the complaint: "What do you mean by tremor?"
   (a) Onset: sudden (suggests toxic cause or withdrawal) or gradual.
   (b) Age of onset: less than 40 years of age (consider Wilson's disease), whereas more than 60 years of age (consider essential tremor).
   (c) Body parts affected: site (head, neck, or hand) and symmetry (symmetrical or asymmetrical).

E. Al Murar · S. Taheri
Ambulatory Healthcare Services, Abu Dhabi, United Arab Emirates

S. Al Memari (✉)
Abu Dhabi, United Arab Emirates

© The Author(s), under exclusive license to Springer Nature Singapore Pte Ltd. 2024
S. Lari et al. (eds.), *Family Medicine OSCE: First Aid to Objective Structured Clinical Examination*, https://doi.org/10.1007/978-981-99-5530-5_13

Table 13.1 Key symptoms in the differential diagnosis of tremors

Symptoms associated with tremor	Probable diagnosis
Sweating, palpitations, weight loss	Hyperthyroidism
Excessive worries, poor concentration, fatigue, disturbed sleep, irritability	Generalized anxiety disorder
Coarse resting tremors, pill-rolling movements, rigidity, and gait disturbance	Parkinson
Wing-beating, resting tremor with hepatic, neurological, psychiatric, and ocular symptoms	Wilson's disease
Coarse, slow tremor that appears both in rest and with movements	Rubral tremor or Holmes tremor (a subtype of cerebellar tremor)
Tremors that decrease by distraction	Psychogenic causes
Tremor that decreases with alcohol intake	Essential or familial tremor
Immediate limbs jerk after standing	Orthostatic tremor

    (d) Character: resting or kinetic tremor, visible or simply a sensation of tremor.
    (e) Duration and Progression.
    (f) Relieving or aggravating factors
    (g) Associated symptoms: refer to Table 13.1 for details.
4. Explore patients or parent's ideas, concerns and expectations (ICE), and effect of the complaint on quality of life.
5. Explore ongoing problems: cerebellar disease, Parkinson, diabetes, hyperthyroidism, or anxiety. History of chronic diseases such as diabetes and hypertension.
6. Past medical or surgical history: head trauma, multiple sclerosis, or brain tumor.
7. Medication history: cold medication such as Pseudoephedrine, antipsychotics (Lithium), antidepressant, Thyroxine, Albuterol, Corticosteroids or Metoclopramide.
8. Social history: smoking, alcohol use, or illicit drug use.
9. Family history: similar problem in the family (suggests familial tremor).
10. Examination:
    (a) Observe resting tremor (try to provoke it by sustained arm extension if not initially visible). Identify its frequency, amplitude, pattern, and body distribution. Look for cranial tremors in jaw, face, chin, tongue, palate, and voice.
    (b) Assess for kinetic tremor: by asking the patient to perform finger to nose to finger maneuver, pour water from cup to cup, or drink from a cup.
    (c) Look for other neurological signs: assess gait and observe for ataxia (suggests cerebellar diseases), dystonic postures (suggests dystonic tremor), rigidity, and bradykinesia (parkinsonism), or eye movements' abnormalities (brainstem or cerebellar disease).
    (d) Look for relevant systemic signs: exophthalmos (Graves' disease), hepatosplenomegaly and Kayser-Fleischer rings in the cornea (Wilsons disease).

Table 13.2 Management of tremor based on diagnosis

Tremor type	Management
Essential tremor	• First line management: propranolol 10–320 mg per day orally or primidone 25–750 mg per day
	• Second line management: topiramate 25–300 mg per day orally or gabapentin 100–1800 mg per day orally
	• Botulinum toxin injections can be effective for head tremor
Drug-induced tremor	• Stop the offending medication and explain that resolution may take days to weeks
Enhanced-physiological tremor	• Treat associated endocrine disorders
	• Management of stress, anxiety, and fatigue
	• May benefit from a trial of beta blockers
Rest tremor	Consider using Parkinson's medications levodopa/carbidopa

11. Order required investigations:
    (a) Enhanced physiological tremor: rule out hypoglycemia and pheochromocytoma.
    (b) Consider thyroid and liver function if suspecting liver or thyroid disease.
    (c) Consider serum ceruloplasmin and 24-h urine copper if symptoms suggest Wilson disease (especially if patient is less than 40 years old)
    (d) Consider toxin screen for suspected substance use.
    (e) Consider polymyography in case of orthostatic tremor.
    (f) Consider brain imaging MRI or CT when suspecting a lesion.
12. Management and education:
    (a) Explain differential and probable diagnosis, as well as prognosis.
    (b) Treat underlying cause if any identified, otherwise support by symptomatic treatment (refer to Table 13.2 for further details).
13. Give reading educational materials if any.
14. Discuss health maintenance and age-appropriate screening.
15. Arrange referral to neurology or endocrine as indicated.
16. Arrange for follow up.
17. Communication skills: organized approach, mixed questioning styles (open- and close-ended questions), active listening, clear language, reflection on patient's ICE.

History Taking and Management of a Patient Presenting with Chest Pain

14

Kawthar Al Ameri and Shammah Al Memari

Learning Objectives
- How to master history taking for patients presenting with chest pain?
- How to perform a focused exam for patients presenting with chest pain?
- How to approach and provide management tips for patients with chest pain?

Focus areas include life-threatening conditions like acute coronary syndrome (ACS), pulmonary embolism, aortic dissection, esophageal rupture, tension pneumothorax, cardiac arrhythmias, cardiac tamponade. Remember to immediately transfer the patient from triage to the emergency room ensuring urgent evaluation if vitally unstable.

1. Introduce yourself.
2. Establish good rapport.
3. Identify the complaint: site, onset (gradual, or sudden), history of similar pain, duration, frequency, character (constant or intermittent), progression, severity (use scale of 10), radiation, associated symptoms, exacerbating, or relieving factors (exercise, rest), and red flags. Work out your differentials as follows:

K. Al Ameri
Ambulatory Healthcare Services, Abu Dhabi, UAE

Faculty of Family Medicine Residency Program, Sheikh Khalifa Medical City, Abu Dhabi, United Arab Emirates

S. Al Memari (✉)
Abu Dhabi, United Arab Emirates

(a) Increased pain with respirations, movement, or lying supine, radiation to the shoulder, relieved with leaning forward or sitting, with pulsus paradoxus (suggests pericarditis).

(b) Palpitations, sweating, nausea, vomiting, dizziness, radiation to the jaw or shoulder, pain that increases with exertion and decreases with rest, sharp squeezing pain or heaviness (suggests cardiac ischemia).

(c) Shortness of breath and hemoptysis, with history of calf pain, recent travel, pregnancy, post- partum, or use of oral contraception (suggests pulmonary embolism (PE)). Refer to (Table 14.1) for Well's Criteria of PE.

(d) Cough, fever, and sputum (suggests pneumonia or tuberculoses).

(e) Acute chest and back pain that is severe, sharp, and has a tearing quality (suggests aortic dissection).

(f) Heart burn, retrosternal pain, dysphagia, dyspepsia, with or without history of NSAIDs use (suggests gastroesophageal reflux, perforating peptic ulcer disease, or esophageal spasm).

(g) Skin rash with pain (Fire band) (suggests Herpes Zoster or neuralgia).

(h) Localized sharp pain, increased with movement or deep inspiration, history of trauma or fall, heavy exertion (suggests musculoskeletal pain).

(i) Pain and swelling at costo-chondral junctions (suggest costochondritis).

(j) Panic symptoms, signs of malingering or somatoform disorder (suggests psychiatric disorder).

4. Explore patient's ideas, concerns and expectations (ICE), and effect of the pain on quality of life, job, and exercise tolerance.

5. Explore ongoing problems and past history:

(a) Atherosclerotic disease: previous myocardial infarction (MI), CABG (Coronary artery bypass graft surgery), or angioplasty.

(b) History of DVT or PE, recent surgery, current pregnancy, history of malignancy, immobility.

(c) Chronic diseases: diabetes, hypertension, hyperlipidemia, or smoking.

Table 14.1 Modified Wells criteria for pulmonary embolism

Sign and symptoms	Points
History of PE or Deep Venous Thrombosis (DVT)	1.5
Heart rate of more than 100 beats per minute	1.5
Recent immobilization or surgery	1.5
Clinical picture of DVT	3
Other diagnosis unlikely than PE	3
Hemoptysis	1
Cancer	1
Calculate *total score* and classify accordingly:	
– 1 or less (low probability of PE)	
– 2–6 (moderate probability of PE)	
– More than 6 (high probability of PE)	

6. Social history: stressful events, marital conflicts, job instability, smoking, sedentary lifestyle, alcohol.
7. Family history: cardiac event and at what age.
8. Investigations as indicated:
   (a) Electrocardiogram.
   (b) Troponins.
   (c) Lipid profile.
   (d) HbA1c.
   (e) Coagulation panel and D-dimmer.
9. Management and education: share differential and probable diagnosis, as well as prognosis:
   (a) Arrange Referral to emergency department if picture is suggestive of a life-threatening cause. Utilize advanced cardiac life support (ACLS) protocol as needed. For patients with acute MI do that after starting supportive therapy (MONA): Morphine, Oxygen, Nitro sublingual (avoid if patient has low blood pressure, inferior MI, or has taken phosphodiesterase in the last 24 h) and Aspirin (162–325 mg). Keep observing the blood pressure all through. After the acute stabilization, consider: ACE inhibitors, lipid lowering agent (statins), and aspirin.
   (b) If an infectious disease, educate the patient about infection control measure to prevent spread of infection and manage accordingly.
   (c) Emphasize lifestyle modification: healthy diet, exercise, smoking cessation, and weight loss.
   (d) Give reading educational materials if any.
10. Discuss health maintenance and screening for age.
11. Arrange for follow up.
12. Communication skills: organized approach, mixed questioning styles (open- and close-ended questions), active listening, clear language, and reflection on patients' ICE.

History Taking and Management of a Patient Presenting with Palpitation

15

Eiman Al Murar, Sumiya Taheri, and Shammah Al Memari

Learning Objectives
- How to master history taking for a patient presenting with palpitations?
- How to perform a focused exam for patients presenting with palpitations?
- How to approach and provide management tips for patients presenting with palpitations?

Focus areas include *Cardiac causes:* cardiac arrhythmias (sinus tachycardia, supraventricular and ventricular tachycardia (SVT), ventricular ectopic, WPW syndrome, atrial fibrillation, or flutter, long QT syndrome, or structural heart diseases (valvular heart disease, myocardial disease, congenital heart disease, hypertrophic obstructive cardiomyopathy, or cardiac tumors). *Noncardiac causes:* anemia, fever, hypoglycemia, dehydration, thyrotoxicosis, orthostatic hypotension, pheochromocytoma, postmenopausal syndrome, anxiety, somatization disorders, or drug induced.

E. Al Murar · S. Taheri
Ambulatory Healthcare Services, Abu Dhabi, United Arab Emirates

S. Al Memari (✉)
Abu Dhabi, United Arab Emirates

© The Author(s), under exclusive license to Springer Nature Singapore Pte Ltd. 2024
S. Lari et al. (eds.), *Family Medicine OSCE: First Aid to Objective Structured Clinical Examination*, https://doi.org/10.1007/978-981-99-5530-5_15

Table 15.1 Palpitations red flags and suggested etiologies

Associated symptoms	Suggestive etiologies
Chest pain and shortness of breath	Pulmonary embolism or pericarditis
Sweating, tremor, fatigue, weight loss, anxiety, and heat intolerance	Hyperthyroidism
Sweating, headache, and hypertension	Pheochromocytoma
Sweating and syncope	Arrhythmia or pericarditis
Chest pain, sweating, dizziness	Myocardial infarction or Ischemic heart disease
Excessive worries, poor concentration, fatigue, disturbed sleep, irritability, and feeling anxious	Generalized anxiety disorder
Low mood, loss of interest, and other somatic symptoms	Depression
Pallor and history of blood loss	Anemia
Palpitations with sudden posture change	Orthostatic hypotension
Palpitations triggered by physical activity	Atrial fibrillation, SVT, ventricular tachycardia, or mitral valve prolapse

1. Introduce yourself and establish good rapport.
2. Explore patient's ideas, concerns and expectations (ICE).
3. Identify the complaint: "What do you mean by palpitations?":
   (a) Onset: abrupt or gradual.
   (b) Character: rate rhythm and intensity: can be elicited by having patient tap out rhythm with fingers or vocalize perceived rhythm (specifically looking for any fast beat, chest flattering, or skipped beats).
   (c) Course: frequency, duration, and cessation ("how does it end?" (abrupt or gradual), (spontaneous, with vagal maneuvers, or with drugs)).
   (d) Relieving and aggravating factors (exertion, position, or emotional stress).
   (e) Associated symptoms and red flags of chest pain. Refer to (Table 15.1).
4. Drugs and stimulant use: tea, coffee (amount if any?), sympathomimetics, anticholinergics, alcohol, cocaine, recent withdrawal of beta blockers.
5. Past medical and surgical history: cardiac disease, diabetes, hypertension, asthma, depression, anxiety, insomnia, anemia, or thyroid disease.
6. Social history: stressful events, effect of the problem on patient's life, smoking, alcohol, or recreational drug use (cocaine, amphetamines, and marijuana).
7. Family history of heart disease, sudden death, anxiety disorder, or thyrotoxicosis.
8. Examination:
   (a) Vital signs: heart rate, respiratory rate, elevated temperature, blood pressure, and oxygen saturation.
   (b) Perform complete cardiovascular examination (refer to Chap. 74 for details).
   (c) General exam for any signs of anemia, thyroid disease, or endocrine disorders.

9. Order required investigations:
   (a) Electrocardiogram for all patients. Look for any pathognomonic changes: short PR interval and delta waves (suggests Wolff-Parkinson-White syndrome), marked left ventricular hypertrophy with deep septal Q waves in lead I, aVL, and V4 through V6 (suggests the presence of hypertrophic obstructive cardiomyopathy), prolongation of the QT interval and abnormal T-wave morphology (suggests the prolonged QT syndrome).
   (b) Blood tests if suspecting systemic causes: p complete blood count, urea, electrolytes, and thyroid stimulating hormone.
   (c) Holter monitor in patients with repeated symptoms where no cause is identifiable (to rule out episodic arrythmias).
10. Management and education:
   (a) Infrequent palpitations or missed beats with no associated symptoms: reassure and advice patient to avoid precipitating factors (adrenergic agents: alcohol and caffeine, drugs that have been determined to be the cause). Consider psychiatric counseling if patient has recent stressful life events.
   (b) Frequent palpitations with chest pain or dyspnea: perform detailed assessment, follow arrhythmia management algorithms if one is found, and refer the patient accordingly (cardiology or emergency department).
   (c) Safety net: clarify to the patient the need to attend to the nearest emergency department in case of developing any red flags: syncope, chest pain, or dizziness.
   (d) Management of cardiovascular risks: hypertension, diabetes, or hyperlipidemia.
   (e) Give reading educational materials if any.
11. Discuss health maintenance and screening for age.
12. Arrange for follow up.
13. Communication skills: organized approach, mixed questioning styles (open- and close-ended questions), active listening, clear language, and reflection on patient's ICE.

History Taking and Management of a Patient Presenting with Back Pain

16

Kawthar Al Ameri, Sumiya Taheri, and Shammah Al Memari

Learning Objectives
- How to master history taking for patients presenting with back pain?
- How to perform a focused exam for patients presenting with back pain?
- How to approach and provide management tips for patients with back pain?

Focus areas include differentiate between acute (less than 4 weeks), subacute (4–12 weeks), and chronic back pain (more than 12 weeks). Differentiate between muscle strain and mechanical (usually muscle spasm due to wrong posture, prolonged sitting or standing, and or degenerative disc disease, spondylolysis, spondylolis- thesis, spinal stenosis, vertebral compression fracture), misalignment (scoliosis, lordosis and kyphosis), malignant (local and metastatic), infections (osteomyelitis, epidural abscess), inflammatory (ankylosing spondylitis, psoriatic spondylitis), or referred pain (pelvic organ disease (endometriosis, PID), renal disease (nephrolithiasis), gastrointestinal disease (pancreatitis, peptic ulcer disease, acute cholecystitis)).

K. Al Ameri
Ambulatory Healthcare Services, Abu Dhabi, United Arab Emirates

Faculty of Family Medicine Residency Program, Sheikh Khalifa Medical City, Abu Dhabi, United Arab Emirates

S. Taheri
Ambulatory Healthcare Services, Abu Dhabi, United Arab Emirates

S. Al Memari (✉)
Abu Dhabi, United Arab Emirates

© The Author(s), under exclusive license to Springer Nature Singapore Pte Ltd. 2024
S. Lari et al. (eds.), *Family Medicine OSCE: First Aid to Objective Structured Clinical Examination*, https://doi.org/10.1007/978-981-99-5530-5_16

59

1. Introduce yourself and establish good rapport.
2. Identify the complaint: location, severity (1–10 scale), onset (gradual or sudden), duration, character (burning, sharp, constant, or intermittent), radiation, progression, exacerbating and relieving factors, associated symptoms, red flags (age more than 50 years, history of trauma (fall from a height or motor vehicle crash), heavy lifting in osteoporotic patients, major or progressive motor or sensory deficit, new-onset bowel or bladder incontinence or urinary retention, loss of anal sphincter tone, saddle anesthesia, history of cancer metastatic to bone, suspected spinal infection, fever, pain at rest or night, immunosuppression, unexplained weight loss, dermatomal rash, abdominal pain, or pulsatile mass), and risk factors (age above 30, physical inactivity, obesity, osteoporosis, arthritis, pregnancy, smoking, psychological factors (stress, or depression), occupational factors (heavy lifting, twisting, turning, poor posture, or whole-body vibration)). Classify accordingly (refer to Table 16.1 for details).
3. Explore patient's ideas, concerns and expectations (ICE), and effect of the complaint on the quality of life (restrictions and absenteeism from work).
4. Explore ongoing problems: past medical, surgical, and social histories.
5. Question use of any regular medication: opioids, prolonged corticosteroid use, long term use of proton pump inhibitors.
6. Social and family history: stressful events, marital conflicts, job instability, smoking, alcohol intake, sedentary lifestyle, and occupational history.

Table 16.1 Classification of back pain according to its character

Character and associated symptoms		Diagnosis
Fever, chills, severe back pain, recent history of spine surgery, or penetrating back injury		Osteomyelitis of spine
Point tenderness at spinal process, pain worsens with flexion, while pulling up from a supine to sitting position or from a sitting to standing position		Compression fracture
Leg pain is greater than back pain	Worsens when *sitting*, radiating (pain from Lumbar 1 to 3 nerve roots radiates to hip or anterior thigh, while pain from Lumbar 4 to Sacral 1 nerve roots radiates to below the knee)	Herniated disc
	Worsens with *extension* (standing and walking down hill) and improves with flexion (pushing a cart, walking uphill) or rest	Spinal stenosis
Diffuse back pain with or without buttock pain, worsens with movement and improves with rest		Lumbar strain
Back pain radiates posteriorly to knees, worsens with bending, lifting, or twisting		Spondylolisthesis
Gradual onset, morning stiffness, pain improves with exercise, pain does not improve when lying supine		Ankylosing spondylitis

7. Examination:
   (a) Vitals: assess for fever.
   (b) Back examination: inspect for deformities (scoliosis), assess for tenderness (infection, fracture, or neoplasm), range of motion, and provocative tests (refer to "Chap. 77: Back Examination" for further details).
   (c) Examine the legs for neurovascular symptoms and assess anal tone.
8. Investigations as indicated:
   (a) Complete blood count, C-reactive protein (CRP), and erythrocyte sedimentation rate (ESR) if suspecting infection, inflammation, or malignancy.
   (b) Urine analysis and culture if suspecting pyelonephritis or renal colic.
   (c) Back X-ray if patient has been having back pain for more than 1 month, is more than 50 years of age, or in cases where cancer or compression fracture is suspected.
   (d) Back MRI if patient has neurological deficit, or in cases where cauda equina syndrome, or spine infection is suspected.
9. Arrange referral to:
   (a) Spine neurosurgeon: if pain is severe or limits functionality.
   (b) Pain clinic.
   (c) Physiotherapy.
10. Management: (refer to Table 16.2).
11. Health education:
    (a) Backache is usually caused by minor strains in the muscles or ligaments, but more serious lower back pain is usually a result of an injury to one of the many joints at the base of your spine. The joints include the facet joints and discs, which when disturbed can push against painful tissue or nerve roots just behind them. The injury usually happens while bending your spine forwards (flexing it), especially while lifting something heavy.
    (b) Never bend forward with your legs straight to perform any task.
    (c) Avoid lifting anything heavier than 10 kg. Instead, squat close to the load and keep your back straight.
    (d) Do not stoop over the load to get a grip and pick it up. Lift using your knees and legs (not your back) as leverage. Keep your back straight, not bent forwards or backwards.
    (e) Once you have experienced back trouble, it tends to recur, and so be careful to protect your back: adjust your activity to your back discomfort, take care with posture, making beds and so on, perform a set of exercises to strengthen the muscles of your spine and abdomen, avoid sitting for long periods, especially in the car (your knees should be higher than your hips and your back need to remain straight. Maintain the hollow in your back).
12. Give reading educational materials including exercise leaflet if any.
13. Discuss health maintenance and screening for age.
14. Arrange for follow-up, safety net, and reflect on patient's ICE with the goal of relieving pain, improving function, and reducing absenteeism.

Table 16.2 Management of back pain

Measures	Details	
Non-pharmacological measures	Advise the patient to remain active: "this will improve your pain and functional status"	
	Exercise (stretching and graded activity) targeting the following: – Improving motor control. – Core strengthening (experiencing abdominal and trunk extensors). – Flexion and extension movements. – Directional preference (as in McKenzie exercises). – General physical fitness: aerobic exercise and Pilates. – Exercise programs with a mind-body component (as in yoga and Tai Chi). – Functional restoration programs.	
	Heat therapy	
	Massage, acupuncture, and spinal manipulation (has low quality evidence)	
Pharmacological measures	First line therapy	Non-steroidal anti-inflammatory drugs (NSAIDs) like ibuprofen, 400–800 mg, as needed every 8 h (encourage patients to use the lowest effective dose).
		Paracetamol, if NSAIDs are contraindicated (evidence suggests that it is superior to placebo but inferior to NSAIDS in lowering the back pain).
	Second line therapy	Skeletal muscle relaxant (Tizanidine 4–8 mg every 8 h as needed). Inform the patient about the sedative side effect, data lacking about efficacy, and that it might only improve pain for short term.
	Third line therapy	Emphasize that for patients with chronic back pain the goal is to manage their pain, increase their functionality, and maximize their coping skills. This is mainly achieved by non-pharmacological measure. If the above-mentioned pharmacological measures fail to provide adequate relief, the patient can be started on one of the below (weak recommendation, hence always weight risks and benefits): – Duloxetine (SNRI) – Amitriptyline (tricyclics antidepressant), or gabapentin or pregabalin (anticonvulsants) for neuropathic pain – Tramadol – Epidural steroid injection

History Taking and Management of a Patient Presenting with Dyspepsia

17

Eiman Al Murar, Buthaina Al Maskari, and Shammah Al Memari

Learning Objectives
- How to master history taking for patients presenting with dyspepsia?
- How to perform a focused exam for patients presenting with dyspepsia?
- How to approach and provide management tips for patients with dyspepsia?

Focus areas on gastroesophageal reflux disease, peptic ulcer (with or without underlying *Helicobacter pylori* infection, non-steroidal anti-inflammatory drugs (NSAIDS) or steroids use, or stress), functional dyspepsia, or referred pain (cardiac or cholelithiasis).

---

1. Introduce yourself.
2. Establish good rapport.
3. Identify the complaint: onset (new or recurrent), duration, site, character, timing, radiation, progression, and previous management if any.
   (a) Aggravating factors: stressful life events, position (supine or bending), being hungry, or after eating (generally or specifically after heavy or fatty meals).
   (b) Relieving factors: rest, analgesia, antacid, or eating.
   (c) Associated symptoms: heart burn, nausea, vomiting, bloating, irregular bowel habits, or signs of acid regurgitation (throat discomfort, dental erosions, change in voice, chronic cough, shortness of breath, and chest pain).

E. Al Murar · B. Al Maskari
Ambulatory Healthcare Services, Abu Dhabi, United Arab Emirates

S. Al Memari (✉)
Abu Dhabi, United Arab Emirates

© The Author(s), under exclusive license to Springer Nature Singapore Pte Ltd. 2024
S. Lari et al. (eds.), *Family Medicine OSCE: First Aid to Objective Structured Clinical Examination*, https://doi.org/10.1007/978-981-99-5530-5_17

(d) Red flags: more than 50 years of age, non-responsiveness to treatment, gastrointestinal bleeding, melena, unexplained iron deficiency anemia, weight loss, anorexia, dysphagia, odynophagia, hematemesis, palpable mass, or nocturnal pain that wakes the patient from sleep.

4. Explore patient's ideas, concerns and expectations (ICE), and effect of the complaint on quality of life.
5. Explore ongoing problems: diabetes, arthritis, pernicious anemia, depression.
6. Question regular use of medications: NSAIDS, steroids, aspirin, theophylline, calcium channel blockers, anti-cholinergic, or bisphosphonate.
7. Social history: stressful live events, smoking, and alcohol use.
8. Family history: of gastrointestinal problem or gastric cancer.
9. Examination: (refer to "Chap. 76: Abdominal Examination" for further details).
10. Order required investigations (if recurrent):
    (a) *Helicobacter pylori* stool antigen or urea breath test.
    (b) Complete blood count.
    (c) Endoscopy (to rule out peptic ulcer).
    (d) Abdominal ultrasound (to rule out cholelithiasis).
11. Management and education: refer to Table 17.1 for further details.
12. Safety net: "If you develop black stool, bleeding, chest pain or fast heart beats you need to seek medical attention."
13. Give reading educational materials if any.
14. Arrange referral to gastroenterology clinic if patient has red flags: for Esophago-gastro-duodenoscopy (EGD).
15. Discuss health maintenance and screening for age.
16. Arrange for follow up in 2–4 weeks.
17. Communication skills: organized approach, mixed questioning styles, clear language, and reflection on patient's ICE

Table 17.1 Management of dyspepsia

Measures	Details
Non-pharmacological measures	Lifestyle modifications: sleeping with elevated bedhead, smoking and alcohol cessation, avoiding tight fitting clothes, maintaining regular exercise and healthy diet, and applying stress management strategies
	Dietary adjustments include maintaining healthy diet, avoiding spicy, fatty, and heavy meals, and dividing food intake to small frequent meals. Additionally, limit coffee intake to moderation and avoid eating late at night (ideally no food 3 h before bedtime)
	Avoiding aggravating drugs: steroid, ibuprofen
Pharmacological measures	Proton pump inhibitors (PPI): example Omeprazole (20 mg once daily, for 4–8 weeks). Emphasize the need to take it on an empty stomach and delay feeds for 30–60 min after the pill. Formulate a clear plan: "if you improve, the PPI will be continued as needed only (to avoid long term side effects: like iron, vitamin B12 or calcium deficiency)"
	Consider antacids if patient has heart burn
Additional measures	Explain: "If you did not improve with the above strategies, you will need more investigations to rule out *Helicobacter pylori* infection with or without endoscopy"

History Taking and Management of a Patient Presenting with Abdominal Pain

18

Reem Al Mansoori, Kawthar Al Ameri, and Shammah Al Memari

Learning Objectives
- How to master history taking for patients presenting with abdominal pain?
- How to perform a focused exam for a patient presenting with abdominal pain?
- How to approach and provide management tips for a patient with abdominal pain?

Focus areas on referred pain from myocardial infarction, diabetic ketoacidosis, acute cholecystitis, acute pancreatitis, acute appendicitis, irritable bowel syndrome (IBS), perforated viscous, bowel obstruction, ruptured abdominal aortic aneurysm, renal stone, ectopic pregnancy, pelvic inflammatory disease, malignancy, and somatization disorder.

R. Al Mansoori
Emirates Medical Association of Family Medicine, Abu Dhabi, United Arab Emirates

K. Al Ameri
Ambulatory Healthcare Services, Abu Dhabi, United Arab Emirates

Faculty of Family Medicine Residency Program, Sheikh Khalifa Medical City, Abu Dhabi, United Arab Emirates

S. Al Memari (✉)
Abu Dhabi, United Arab Emirates

1. Introduce yourself.
2. Establish good rapport.
3. Identify the complaint: site, onset, character, radiation, duration, timing, progression, relieving and aggravating factors, associated symptoms, and **red flags**. Work out the differential diagnosis accordingly:
   (a) Vomiting, **hyperglycemia**, polyuria, and polydipsia (suggests diabetic ketoacidosis).
   (b) Epigastric pain and **hematemesis** (suggest acute gastrointestinal bleeding).
   (c) Pain increasing increases with eating spicy food (gastric ulcer).
   (d) Pain relieved by eating but recur several hours after a meal (suggests duodenal ulcer).
   (e) Pain increases with fatty meals (cholecystitis).
   (f) Gradual, steady pain that is relieved by sitting up or leaning forward (suggests pancreatitis).
   (g) Pain starts within 1 h of eating (suggests mesenteric Ischemia).
   (h) Abdominal distention, nausea, vomiting, **absent bowel motion**, and history of abdominal surgery (suggests bowel obstruction).
   (i) Sudden onset of sharp pain that increase with movement, forcing the **patient to lie motionless** (suggests peritonitis).
   (j) Alternating diarrhea and constipation, **mucous or blood in stool, sense of incomplete evacuation or need for digitation, perianal lesions**, joint pain, and red eye (suggests inflammatory bowel disease).
   (k) Pain worsens by stress and relieved by defecating (irritable bowel syndrome).
   (l) Dysuria, urgency, frequency, and hematuria (suggests urinary tract infection).
   (m) Pain radiating to the groin (renal colic).
   (n) Dysuria, fever, pain radiating to flanks (suggests pyelonephritis).
   (o) Chronic use of steroids or **orthostatic hypotension** as an early sign of shock (suggests adrenal insufficiency).
   (p) **Amenorrhea, vaginal bleeding**, and dizziness (suggests ectopic pregnancy).
   (q) Cough, shortness of breath, orthopnea, and exertional dyspnea (suggests cardiac or pulmonary etiology).
   (r) **Pain that awakens the patient at night**, fever, nausea, vomiting, **weight loss, change in bowel habits**, anemia, and blood in stool (suggests malignancy).
4. Explore patient's ideas, concerns and expectations (ICE) as well as the effect of the problem on the quality of life.
5. Explore ongoing problems: exclude diabetes and asthma.
6. Question use of any regular medications:
   (a) Drugs inducing gastritis: NSAIDs, anticholinergics, or steroids.
   (b) Drugs that might mask pain: steroids or analgesic.
   (c) Drugs that can increase risk of *Clostridium difficile* infection: recent antibiotics.

7. Social history: smoking, alcohol (liver disease/pancreatitis), stress, marital conflicts, domestic violence, or job instability.
8. Family history: gastrointestinal cancer, inflammatory bowel disease, celiac disease, or rheumatologic disorders.
9. Examination: (refer to "Chap. 76: Abdominal Examination" for further details).
10. Order required investigations as indicated:
    (a) Complete blood count (especially when suspecting acute appendicitis or inflammatory bowel disease. Look for leukocytosis and anemia).
    (b) Pregnancy test to exclude ectopic pregnancy.
    (c) Urinalysis to exclude urinary tract infections.
    (d) Computed tomography scan to exclude masses suggestive of malignancy.
    (e) Ultrasound to exclude ectopic pregnancy or bowel obstruction.
    (f) Tissue transglutaminase level to exclude celiac disease.
    (g) Upper or lower gastrointestinal endoscopy to exclude gastric ulcers or inflammatory bowel disease.
    (h) Fecal occult blood or fecal immunochemical test (FIT) to exclude lower gastrointestinal bleed.
11. Management and education:
    (a) Discuss the nature of problem and the cause.
    (b) Advise for analgesia (enough dose and right frequency).
    (c) Provide written management plan for patients with acute relapse on top of chronic diseases.
    (d) Give reading educational materials if any.
12. Arrange referral if indicated.
13. Discuss health maintenance and age-appropriate screening.
14. Arrange for follow up.
15. Communication skills: organized approach, mixed questioning styles (open- and close-ended questions), active listening, clear language, and reflection on patient's ICE.

History Taking and Management of Adults Presenting with Jaundice

19

Shaima Lari, Noora Al Blooshi, and Shammah Al Memari

Learning Objectives
- How to master history taking for patients presenting with jaundice?
- How to perform a focused exam for patients presenting with jaundice?
- How to approach and provide management tips for patients with jaundice?

For Neonatal jaundice read Chap. 38

Focus areas on acute versus chronic onset, travel to endemic areas, drug users, alcohol consumption, sexually transmitted infections, or history of transfusion.

1. Introduce yourself and establish a good rapport.
2. Identify the complaint (icterus): duration, onset, relieving and aggravating factors, timing, character (same, improving, or worsening), significant recent history (travel to Indian subcontinent or East Asia, participating in sexual tourism or other high risk sexual behaviors, history of new tattoo or intravenous drug abuse), and prior episodes. For differential diagnosis of jaundice refer to (Table 19.1). For classification according to complaint and presentation:

S. Lari
Sheikh Shakhbout Medical City, Abu Dhabi, United Arab Emirates

N. Al Blooshi
Ambulatory Healthcare Services, Abu Dhabi, United Arab Emirates

S. Al Memari (✉)
Abu Dhabi, United Arab Emirates

Table 19.1 Differential diagnosis of jaundice based on underlying causes

Prehepatic	Hemolysis and Gilberts syndrome
Hepatic	Infections, toxins, neoplasia, autoimmune, and genetics
Post-hepatic	Choledocholithiasis, ascending cholangitis, parasitic infection, pancreatic cancer, and cholangiocarcinoma

(a) Fever, nausea, vomiting, abdominal pain, diarrhea, recent travel, street food, and loss of appetite (suggests acute hepatitis).

(b) Onset associated with upper respiratory tract infections, stress, or fasting (suggests Gilbert's disease).

(c) Dyspepsia, mood swings, weight loss, pruritus, urine, and stool color changes (suggests chronic hepatitis).

(d) Alcohol abuse (suggests liver cirrhosis).

(e) Autoimmune disease, renal disease, or history of multiple miscarriages (suggests systemic lupus erythematosus (SLE) or primary biliary cirrhosis).

3. Explore patient's ideas, concerns, and expectations (ICE).

4. Explore ongoing problems: Glucose-6-phosphate dehydrogenase deficiency, sickle cell disease, transfusions, chronic hepatitis B or C viral infection, liver cirrhosis, and history of total parenteral nutrition use.

5. Inquire about Hepatitis B and A vaccination status.

6. Question use of regular medications: any hepatotoxic drugs?

7. Social history: intravenous drug or alcohol abuse, homosexuality, multiple sexual partners, health care professional, and smoking.

8. Family history: hemolytic anemia, mother, or spouse diagnosed with hepatitis infection.

9. Examination:

   (a) General: pallor, icterus, thalassemic facies, cachexia, tattoos, injection sites, muscle wasting (temporal wasting).

   (b) Hand: clubbing, flaps, palmar erythema, Dupuytren's contractures, wasting of thenar muscles.

   (c) Chest: gynecomastia.

   (d) Heart: congestive heart failure secondary to liver dysfunction.

   (e) Abdomen: spider nevi, hepatosplenomegaly, Murphy's sign, caput medusa, ascites, ecchymosis or petechia, Courvoisier's law (jaundice with painless enlarged gallbladder), and rectal examination. Charcot's triad (fever, RUQ tenderness, jaundice).

10. Order required investigations:

   (a) Initial bloods: complete blood count, liver function test, lactate dehydrogenase, G6PD, hepatitis, and human immunodeficiency virus screen.

   (b) Imaging: abdominal ultrasound, computed tomography, or MRI.

   (c) Further testing, as indicated: anti-nuclear antibodies (ANA), anti-smooth muscle, anti-mitochondrial, serum IgG, serum ceruloplasmin, and serum alpha 1 antitrypsin.

11. Arrange referral: as needed for hemolysis, hepatic failure.

12. Management and education: share differential and probable diagnosis, as well as the prognosis:
    (a) Alcohol liver disease: referral for smoking and alcohol cessation, avoid toxic medications like Propylthiouracil (PTU) and colchicine, provide nutritional support especially Thiamin, and start steroids in severe cases.
    (b) Viral hepatitis: consider immunoglobulin, anti-viral medications, and vaccinations.
    (c) Choledocholithiasis: medical or surgical treatment.
    (d) Acute cholangitis: antibiotics and intravenous fluids.
    (e) Acute cholecystitis: nil per mouth (NPO), intravenous fluids, analgesia, antibiotics, and surgical removal within 72 h of acute presentation.
13. Give reading educational materials if any.
14. Discuss health maintenance and screening for age.
15. Arrange for follow up.
16. Communication skills: organized approach, mixed questioning styles (open- and close-ended questions), active listening, clear language, and reflection on patient's ICE.

History Taking and Management of a Patient Presenting with Rectal Bleeding

20

Kawthar Al Ameri and Shammah Al Memari

Learning Objectives
- How to master history taking for patients presenting with rectal bleeding?
- How to perform a focused exam for patients presenting with rectal bleeding?
- How to approach and provide management tips for patients with rectal bleeding?

Focus areas on external or internal hemorrhoids, perianal abscess, anal fissures, anal condylomata, colorectal cancer, inflammatory bowel disease, or diverticulitis.

---

1. Introduce yourself and establish good rapport.
2. Identify the complaint:
   (a) Onset, duration, frequency (and relation with bowel movement), aggravating and relieving factors, and associated symptoms (abdominal pain or cramps, change in bowel habit, dizziness, anal discharge and itching, weight loss, urge to defecate, or prolonged straining, digital evacuation).

K. Al Ameri
Ambulatory Healthcare Services, Abu Dhabi, United Arab Emirates

Faculty of Family Medicine Residency Program, Sheikh Khalifa Medical City, Abu Dhabi, United Arab Emirates

S. Al Memari (✉)
Abu Dhabi, United Arab Emirates

© The Author(s), under exclusive license to Springer Nature Singapore Pte Ltd. 2024
S. Lari et al. (eds.), *Family Medicine OSCE: First Aid to Objective Structured Clinical Examination*, https://doi.org/10.1007/978-981-99-5530-5_20

(b) Red flags: fever, unintended weight loss, sweating, change in bowel habit, fatigue, or age more than 50 years.
3. Explore patient's ideas, concerns, and expectations (ICE).
4. Explore ongoing problems, past medical and surgical histories: diverticulosis or diverticular bleeding, current pregnancy, diabetes mellitus, hypertension, or recent surgical procedures as colonoscopy.
5. Medications (nonsteroidal anti-inflammatory drugs) and allergies.
6. Family history: Colon cancer.
7. Social history: marital state, smoking, alcohol abuse, and employment.
8. Examination: including per rectum exam for anal fissures, ulcers, cauliflower-like lesions, or leakage of stool refer to "Chap. 76: Abdominal Examination" for further details.
9. Investigations:
   (a) Blood: complete blood count, hematocrit levels, erythrocyte sedimentation rate, blood typing, and cross matching.
   (b) Abdominal computed tomography scan.
10. Management and education: share differentials and probable diagnosis, as well as the prognosis. Refer to (Table 20.1).
11. Arrange referral:
    (a) Gastroenterologist for flexible sigmoidoscopy or colonoscopy.
    (b) Emergency department if hemodynamically unstable. Meanwhile resuscitate (with oxygen and fluid).
12. Give reading educational materials if any.
13. Discuss health maintenance and age-appropriate screening.
14. Arrange for follow up and safety net by asking the patient to come back if bleeding persists.
15. Communication skills: ensure organized approach, mixed questioning style (open- and closed-ended questions), active listening, clear language, and reflection on patients' ICE.

Table 20.1 Management of rectal bleeding according to etiology

Etiology	Management
Constipation	– Educate the patient about nutritional adjustments: high-fiber diet and increased water intake – Emphasize need for regular exercise (especially walking) – Prescribe laxatives (for example: lactulose or polyethylene glycol)
Hemorrhoid	– Explain to the patient: "Common, knobby varicose veins of the rectal or anal area, which can prolapse outside the anus and hang as small grape-like lumps. Usually caused by constipation, due to excessive straining" – Pharmacological support: combined topical nifedipine and lidocaine cream are more effective than plain xylocaine cream – Surgical management according to severity grade: rubber band ligation, excisional or stapled hemorrhoidopexy, or excisional or stapled hemorrhoidectomy – Cryotherapy, sclerotherapy, and anal dilatation are less effective
Anal fissure	– Explain to the patient: "A crack or tear at the margin of the anus that extends from the skin into the soft lining of the anus. It can affect all ages and tends to occur in women and infants. The tear, which is generally small, usually develops after stretching of the anus from passing a hard, large stool. It is associated with constipation, multiple pregnancies, and Crohn's disease. Anal intercourse increases the likelihood of a fissure. Adults usually recover in about 4 weeks, especially if the fissure is small. More severe cases may not heal without the benefit of a small operation" – Advise the patient for sitz bath – Pharmacological support: analgesics (aspirin or paracetamol), soothing creams (zinc oxide, petroleum jelly, local anesthesia), and treat constipation if any – Interventional therapy: botulinum toxin injection into the sphincter or surgical repair
Diverticular bleeding	– Explain to the patient: "Diverticular disease (also called diverticulosis) is the presence of small blind sacs or pouches called diverticula in the wall of your large bowel (colon). It is related to a lack of fiber in your diet. It rarely causes symptoms, and most people have it without knowing. A lack of fiber in the diet can cause you to experience bloating, flatulence (desire to pass wind) and abdominal pains. If infection (diverticulitis) develops, you will experience abdominal pain, usually sharp pain in the lower left half of the abdomen, nausea, and fever. These symptoms or any rectal bleeding require prompt attention by your doctor"
Colorectal cancer	– Explain to the patient: "It is the abnormal growth of large bowel lining" – Arrange for biopsy and grading to dictate management accordingly

History Taking and Management of a Patient Presenting with Hematuria

21

Abeer Al Naqbi, Kawthar Al Ameri, and Shammah Al Memari

Learning Objectives
- How to master history taking for patients presenting with hematuria?
- How to perform a focused exam for patients presenting with rectal hematuria?
- How to approach and provide management tips for patients with rectal hematuria?

Hints rule out malignancy. Repeat urinalysis when a false-positive cause is likely (after menses, 4–6 weeks, after vigorous exercise (for example, running more than 10,000 m or high intensity interval training)), and 6 weeks after acute trauma.

1. Introduce yourself.
2. Establish good rapport.

A. Al Naqbi
Ambulatory Healthcare Services, Abu Dhabi, United Arab Emirates

K. Al Ameri
Ambulatory Healthcare Services, Abu Dhabi, United Arab Emirates

Faculty of Family Medicine Residency Program, Sheikh Khalifa Medical City, Abu Dhabi, United Arab Emirates

S. Al Memari (✉)
Abu Dhabi, United Arab Emirates

Table 21.1 Types of hematuria

Type	Description
Macroscopic or gross hematuria	Grossly red, smoky-brown, or cola-colored urine. It's suggestive of glomerular disease, UTI, irritation, or trauma to the meatus or perineum
Microscopic hematuria	Grossly normal and microscopically show more than or equal to 3 red blood cells per high power field
Persistent hematuria	Hematuria that is present on repeat urinalyses over a period of 1–4 weeks

3. Identify the complaint: onset, duration, character, relieving, and aggravating factors. Timing (relation to sexual activity) associated symptoms (frequency, dysuria, urgency, backache, flank or suprapubic pain, fever, vaginal discharge, dyspareunia, depression), and clues suggesting a particular diagnosis. Refer to (Table 21.1) and work out your differentials accordingly:
   (a) Urinary tract infections (UTI): concurrent pyuria and dysuria.
   (b) Post-infectious glomerulonephritis, immunoglobulin A (IgA) nephropathy, or hereditary nephritis: recent upper respiratory tract infections.
   (c) Ureteral injury by renal calculus or malignancy: presenting as unilateral flank pain which may radiate to the groin.
   (d) Bleeding disorder to anticoagulant-induced: with or without bleeding from multiple sites (it should not be assumed that hematuria alone can be explained by chronic warfarin therapy).
   (e) Endometriosis of the urinary tract: cyclic hematuria in women, that is most prominent during and shortly after menstruation.
   (f) Schistosoma haematobium or tuberculosis: if travel or residence to endemic area.
   (g) Sterile pyuria and hematuria secondary to renal tuberculosis or analgesic nephropathy.
   (h) Loin pain-hematuria syndrome (rare): persistent or recurrent flank pain.
   (i) Medication-related: rifampicin, phenytoin, nitrofurantoin.
   (j) Other diagnoses of exclusion: Exercise-induced hematuria: recent vigorous exercise or trauma in the absence of another possible cause. Transient hematuria: seen in patients under the age of 35 years with no known underlying cause.
4. Explore patient's ideas, concerns and expectations (ICE), and effect of the complaint on quality of life.
5. Explore ongoing problems: recurrent UTI or cystitis.
6. Explore past medical history: diabetes or ureteric stones.
7. Explore surgical history, including recent cystoscopy, or gynecologic procedure.
8. Question use of regular medications (especially those that are known to cause nephritis).
9. Social history: consider intimate partner abuse.
10. Family history:
   (a) Renal diseases: as in hereditary nephritis or polycystic kidney disease.
   (b) Hemolytic diseases: as in G6PD deficiency or sickle cell disease.

    (c) Coagulation disorders.
11. Examination: blood pressure, palpate kidneys and lower abdomen, vaginal examination to assess vaginitis and vaginal bleeding, rectal exam for males to assess prostate size.
12. Order required investigations:
    (a) Urine dipsticks: are as sensitive as urine sediment examination.
    (b) Urinalysis (dysmorphic red blood cells suggestive of glomerular causes) and culture.
    (c) Imaging: ultrasound, abdominal radiograph, or computed tomography (CT): for patients presenting with unilateral flank pain suggestive of obstructive nephrolithiasis.
    (d) Cystoscopy.
    (e) Prostate specific antigen if prostate cancer is probable.
    (f) Renal function test, complement levels (C3 and C4), and anti-nucleic antibodies.
13. Arrange referral to:
    (a) Nephrology or urology if needed.
    (b) Ophthalmologist if diagnosed with Alport Syndrome (to check for ocular manifestations).
14. Management and education: share differential and probable diagnosis, as well as the prognosis:
    (a) Lifestyle modification: increase fluid intake (at least 2–3 L/day) and develop the habit of voiding after intercourse.
    (b) Antibiotics if infection is suspected.
    (c) Explain renal stones to the patient, if applicable: "Kidney stones are hard lumps that your body makes from waste products in your urine, if these lumps are big enough, they can get stuck in your bladder or urinary tract. This can be very painful. You might be able to pass the stone in your urine if it is small enough, your doctor can give you medicine to help with the pain, if the stone is too big, your doctor can use a machine that breaks the stone into smaller pieces."
15. Give reading educational materials if any.
16. Discuss health maintenance and age-appropriate screening.
17. Arrange for follow up as needed.
18. Communication skills: organized approach, mixed questioning styles (open- and close-ended questions), active listening, clear language, and reflection on patient's ICE.

History Taking and Management of Anticoagulated Patient Presenting with High INR

22

Halima Al Shehhi, Kawthar Al Ameri, and Shammah Al Memari

Learning Objectives
- How to master history taking for anticoagulated patients presenting with high INR?
- How to perform a focused exam for anticoagulated patients presenting with high INR?
- How to approach and provide management tips for anticoagulated patients presenting with high INR?

Focus areas on underlying causes of high INR, special condition such as pregnancy and breast feeding and finally management based on INR level.

1. Introduce yourself.
2. Establish good rapport.

H. Al Shehhi
Ambulatory Healthcare Services, Abu Dhabi, United Arab Emirates

K. Al Ameri
Ambulatory Healthcare Services, Abu Dhabi, United Arab Emirates

Faculty of Family Medicine Residency Program, Sheikh Khalifa Medical City, Abu Dhabi, United Arab Emirates

S. Al Memari (✉)
Abu Dhabi, United Arab Emirates

© The Author(s), under exclusive license to Springer Nature Singapore Pte Ltd. 2024
S. Lari et al. (eds.), *Family Medicine OSCE: First Aid to Objective Structured Clinical Examination*, https://doi.org/10.1007/978-981-99-5530-5_22

3. Explore patient's ideas, concern (risk of future pregnancy if previous deep vein thrombosis or pulmonary embolism was during pregnancy, safety of warfarin during breast feeding, or interactions of warfarin with contraceptives), and expectations (ICE).
4. Details of therapy: reason for anticoagulation (previous deep vein thrombosis, pulmonary embolism, or prosthetic heart valve), duration since initiation of treatment, intended duration of treatment, usual dose used.
5. Identify possible causes of high international normalized ratio (INR):
   (a) Compliance: "Are you taking the medication at the same time every day?"
   (b) Signs of acute illness: fever or diarrhea.
   (c) Chronic illnesses: heart failure, chronic liver disease, malabsorption (as in patients with history of small bowel resection or chronic small bowel disease), vitamin K deficiency or clotting factors' deficiency.
   (d) Medication history: other anticoagulants as aspirin. Any drug-drug interaction: broad-spectrum antibiotic, vitamin E in large doses (more than 400 mg per day), or oral contraceptives.
   (e) Drug-food interaction: grapefruit, ginseng tea, fish oil, or garlic.
   (f) Consider falsely elevated INR if the test was collected in heparinized tube.
6. Rule out signs of bleeding at other sites: skin bruises, epistaxis, gum bleeding, hematuria, hematochezia, or headache with confusion (sign of intracranial bleeding).
7. Explore continuous problems and past medical history: obesity, varicose veins, or peptic ulcer disease as a predisposing factor for bleeding.
8. Explore surgical (prosthetic valve), family, and social history.
9. Examination:
   (a) Vitals.
   (b) Skin for bruises.
   (c) Chest for adequacy of air entry.
   (d) Lower limb for signs of deep vein thrombosis.
10. Management:
    (a) If the patient has active bleeding: maintain patient's airway, breathing, and circulation. After stabilization, arrange referral to the emergency department for the administration of fresh frozen plasma (FFP) and intravascular vitamin K, irrespective of the INR level. Additionally, ensure comprehensive management addressing the underlying cause of the elevated INR.
    (b) Measure INR and manage accordingly. Refer to (Table 22.1).
11. Safety netting: to come back if any signs of bleeding or thrombosis.
12. Give reading educational materials if any.
13. Discuss health maintenance and screening for age.
14. Arrange for follow up.
15. Communication skills: organized approach, mixed questioning styles (open- and close-ended questions), active listening, clear language, and reflection on patients ICE.

Table 22.1 Management of anticoagulated patient with high INR level

INR level	Management
Less than 5	1. Stop the next warfarin dose 2. Explain to the patient: "Risk of bleeding with this level of INR in otherwise healthy patients is very low" 3. Monitor INR in 24–48 h and adjust the warfarin dose accordingly 4. Consider reducing warfarin's maintenance dose
5–9	1. Stop 1–2 doses of warfarin or administer 1–5 mg of oral vitamin K 2. Monitor INR in 8 h and adjust the warfarin dose accordingly
10–20	1. Administer 5–10 mg of oral vitamin K 2. Refer to the hospital for admission and INR follow up in 6 h
More than 20	1. Rapid reversal of INR is indicated by administering fresh frozen plasma (FFP) and intravascular vitamin K (slow administration advised to prevent hypotension) 2. Refer to the hospital for admission and INR follow up in 6 h

Sakina Al Bloushi, Noora Al Blooshi,
and Shammah Al Memari

Learning Objectives
- How to master history taking for patients presenting with facial weakness?
- How to perform a focused exam for patients presenting with facial weakness?
- How to approach and provide management tips for patients presenting with facial weakness?

Focus areas on the list of differential diagnosis of unilateral and bilateral facial palsy presentations (refer to Table 23.1). Distinguishing between lower and upper motor neuron diseases through examination (refer to Table 23.2).

1. Introduce yourself and establish good rapport.
2. Identify the complaint (facial weakness, swelling, or asymmetry), its side, onset, duration, progression (Bell's palsy typically progresses within 12–72 h), aggravating and relieving factors, preceding symptoms (pain around the ear, altered taste, or facial numbness), and associated symptoms (difficulty speaking, dribbling, or drooling, food collecting between the cheeks and gums, dry eye, excessive tears on the affected side, hyperacusis or ear pain). Work out the differentials of unilateral facial weakness accordingly:

S. Al Bloushi · N. Al Blooshi
Ambulatory Healthcare Services, Abu Dhabi, United Arab Emirates

S. Al Memari (✉)
Abu Dhabi, United Arab Emirates

© The Author(s), under exclusive license to Springer Nature Singapore Pte Ltd. 2024
S. Lari et al. (eds.), *Family Medicine OSCE: First Aid to Objective Structured Clinical Examination*, https://doi.org/10.1007/978-981-99-5530-5_23

Table 23.1 Differential diagnosis of unilateral and bilateral facial weakness

	Unilateral facial weakness	Bilateral facial weakness
Common causes	Bell's palsy, Ramsay-Hunt syndrome, diabetes, hypertension, cholesteatoma, parotid tumor, cerebellopontine angle tumor, and intracranial lesion (such as stroke or tumor)	Guillain-Barre syndrome, myasthenia gravis, and neuro-sarcoidosis
Less common causes	Lyme disease, HIV, syphilis, sarcoidosis, Heerfordt's syndrome, Sjogren's syndrome, systemic lupus erythematosus, vasculitis, and Melkerson-Rosenthal syndrome	Meningeal carcinomatosis, neoplastic lesions in the pons, syphilis, HIV (including cryptococcal meningitis), tuberculosis meningitis, and Lyme disease

Table 23.2 Comparison of lower and upper motor neuron diseases in facial weakness

Lower motor neuron disease	Weakness of the whole side, including the upper facial muscles
Upper motor neuron disease	Weakness of the lower half of the affected side with sparing of the upper facial muscles

    (a) Facial nerve dysfunction secondary to otitis media, upper respiratory tract infection, or microvascular neuropathy in patients with diabetes or hypertension. Other causes that can appear in HIV patients include herpes zoster infection and meningeal lymphomatosis.

    (b) Trauma involving the temporal bone or stylomastoid foramen may cause damage to the facial nerve (facial trauma).

    (c) Occurring suddenly after local anesthesia for dental procedure (suggests inferior alveolar nerve block anesthesia's complication).

    (d) Occurring acutely with pain, history of vesicles involving the hard palate, or anterior two thirds of the tongue, severe otalgia and/or vertigo (suggests Ramsay-hunt syndrome).

    (e) Combination of facial nerve palsy, anterior uveitis (which can cause eye pain), mild blurring of vision, photosensitivity, and enlargement of the parotid gland (suggests Heerfordt's syndrome).

    (f) History of tick bite in an endemic region, rash, arthritis, vertigo, or hearing loss (suggests Lyme disease).

    (g) Prolonged, steadily progressive weakness (suggests tumor compressing the facial nerve (such as a parotid tumor)).

    (h) Weakness that occurs over days to weeks (suggests cholesteatoma).

    (i) Loss of facial sensation in Trigeminal dermatomes or gradual ipsilateral hearing loss (that is eighth cranial nerve involvement) (suggests cerebellopontine angle tumor).

    (j) Recurrent facial nerve palsy, with swelling of the face, oral mucosa, gums, and lips (suggests Melkerson-Rosenthal syndrome).

3. Explore patient's ideas concerns and expectation (ICE).

4. Effect of complaint on quality of life: can cause psychological symptoms and social isolation.

5. Past medical history: previous bell's palsy, diabetes mellitus, hypertension, Sjogren's syndrome, systemic lupus erythematosus, or vasculitis.
6. Current medications and allergies history.
7. Family history: Bell's palsy (in some patients Bell's palsy may run in the family with reports of autosomal dominant inheritance).
8. Social history: marital state, smoking, alcohol and substance abuse, unprotected sexual intercourse, current employment.
9. Examination: as indicated by symptoms:
   (a) Vitals.
   (b) Look for vesicles in the external auditory meatus and palate (herpes or varicella vesicles).
   (c) Palpate parotid gland and mastoid process.
   (d) Otoscope ear exam: looking for signs of otitis media or cholesteatoma.
   (e) Cranial nerve examination especially facial nerve to differentiate between upper and lower motor neuron lesions.
   (f) Full neurological examination in all patients to determine whether there is an alternative cause to explain the symptom. Pronator drift has a high sensitivity for predicting an upper motor neuron disease process (as in stroke).
10. Investigations:
   (a) Blood sugar.
   (b) Neuro imaging urgently (within 2 weeks) using brain Magnetic Resonance Imaging (MRI) or Computed Tomography (CT) scan if MRI is contraindicated for patients with: sub-acute onset of facial weakness, progressive neurological symptoms lasting for more than 3 weeks, recurrent, ipsilateral facial paralysis, segmental facial weakness, or those with no signs of recovery after 3 months.
11. Arrange referral to:
   (a) Emergency department if acute stroke is suspected. Stabilize the patient meanwhile (refer to "Chap. 26: Stroke" for further details).
   (b) Ophthalmology if the cornea remains exposed after attempting to close the eyelid (urgent).
   (c) Neurology if there is bilateral or recurrent Bell's palsy.
   (d) ENT if the paralysis shows no improvement after 1 month or there is suspicion of a serious underlying diagnosis like cholesteatoma, parotid tumor, or malignant otitis externa.
   (e) Plastic surgeon with special interest in facial reconstructive surgery if there is residual paralysis after 6–9 months, particularly if this paralysis is complete.
12. Management and education for Bell's Palsy (refer to Table 23.3).
13. Give reading educational material if any.
14. Discuss health maintenance and screening for age.
15. Arrange for frequent follow up (expect signs of improvement by 1 month and full recovery by 6 months).

Table 23.3 Management Strategies for Bell's Palsy

Eye care	– Regular ophthalmic lubricants: preservative-free teardrops during the daytime and viscous ointment is preferred overnight. – Appose eyelids overnight with microporous tape
Medications	– Corticosteroids (within or less than 72 h of onset, to achieve full recovery) *: Options include Prednisolone 25 mg twice daily for 10 days or Prednisolone 60 mg daily for 5 days followed by a daily reduction in dose of 10 mg (for a total treatment time of 10 days). May be considered within or less than 72 h of onset, in conjunction of corticosteroids, provide 7% increase in recovery of facial function. *Prescribing corticosteroids to pregnant women is controversial and poorly studied. Consider reaching out for specialist's opinion* – Consider offering combination of corticosteroid and antiviral therapy in sever cases. Dose of valacyclovir (1g 3 time daily for 7 days) or acyclovir (400mg 5times a day for 10 days)
Physical and occupational therapy	Educate the patient: "Facial massage and exercise can maintain facial muscles tone and bulk and may help prevent permanent contractures specifically if symptoms persist for more than 4–6 weeks"

16. Safety netting and reflection on patient's ICE: advice the patient to come back in case of worsening of symptoms, encountering new neurological defects such as slurred speech or weakness of extremities, progressive redness or pain of the eye at the affected side (possible exposure keratitis).

17. Communication skills: organized approach, mixed questioning style (open- and close-ended questions), active listening, clear language, and reflection on patient's ICE.

History Taking and Management of a Patient Presenting for Premarital Screening

24

Dana Al Marzooqi
and Shammah Al Memari

Learning Objectives
- How to evaluate patients undergoing premarital screening?
- How to approach a patients requires a repeat sample in the premarital screening process?
- What are the different confirmatory tests relevant to premarital screening?
- What opportunistic advice can be delivered as part of premarital screening?

Hints Tailor the premarital screening advise according to the medicolegal requirements of the country that you practice in (the chapter is designed in line with the regulations of the United Arab Emirates), consideration of notifying the regulator about infectious cases identified, cultural acceptability of counseling the couple-to-be together or individually, and the importance of taking second opinion when in doubt in regards of interpretation of any of the component of the screening, and the fact that the medical visit is to assist patient towards autonomous decision-making rather than preventing any from going forward.

D. Al Marzooqi
Sheikh Khalifa Medical City, Abu Dhabi, United Arab Emirates

S. Al Memari (✉)
Abu Dhabi, United Arab Emirates

© The Author(s), under exclusive license to Springer Nature Singapore Pte
Ltd. 2024
S. Lari et al. (eds.), *Family Medicine OSCE: First Aid to Objective Structured Clinical Examination*, https://doi.org/10.1007/978-981-99-5530-5_24

89

24.1   Initial Visit

1. Introduce yourself and establish a good rapport.
2. Ask:
   (a) Explore patient's ideas, concerns and expectations (ICE).
   (b) Marital history: marriage order (first or second), consanguinity (none, first, second, or third degree), status of previous marriage (single or multiple partners), previous kids (number and health status).
   (c) Past medical and drug history: any chronic diseases or injectables' use.
   (d) Past surgical and procedural history: including tattoo or blood transfusions.
   (e) Other risk factors: high risk occupation (medical or dental fields), history of needle-stick injury, or having multiple sexual partners.
   (f) Family history of chronic diseases or congenitally abnormal children.
3. Advise: explain to the patient that:
   (a) Premarital screening is a legally required assessment that tests the couple-to-be as they plan to get married for complete blood count, blood group, Rhesus type, common genetic blood disorders (Sickle cell anemia, Thalassemia, and other hemoglobinopathies), common infectious diseases (Hepatitis B, Hepatitis C, Syphilis, and Human Immunodeficiency Virus (HIV)), and immunity against Rubella virus for females.
   (b) It aims at determining the odds of transmitting the above mentioned diseases to the spouse or children and providing the couple-to-be with options that help them plan for a healthy family.
   (c) It does not test against all diseases and therefore does not guarantee having normal children.
   (d) Although the results typically get back within 3–5 days, we at times need to repeat some tests for clarification or confirmation. Therefore, it is best not to plan the wedding before 2 weeks from the initial visit.
4. Assess:
   (a) Obtain vitals and examine the patient as clinically indicated by the history obtained.
   (b) Answer any questions and check your level of understanding.
5. Assist:
   (a) Order the premarital screening package (as detailed above).
   (b) Provide follow up appointment.
   (c) Consider referring patient for genetic screening and counseling if indicated by history.

24.2   Follow-Up Visit (Refer to Tables 24.1, 24.2, and 24.3)

Always have a glance on the results before calling in the patients to be sure that the setting is ready for breaking any bad news if needed. Moreover, whenever a partner has an abnormal result, try your best to interview them alone first instead of having both partners together.

Table 24.1 Tips for calling the patients in for second sample

• Once you receive the lab feedback with a possibly abnormal result, call in the patient for a second sample.
• Use tactful language to explain before ordering the confirmatory test:
(a) "It is not uncommon for patients doing premarital screening to need to provide a second sample. This is often needed for clarification or confirmation and does not necessarily mean that you have an abnormality."
(b) "The initial tests done in premarital screening are usually non-specific and can possibly be false-positive. We hence do not depend on a single result and can better assist you after the second sample is tested."
(c) If the patient still insists to know the abnormality, you can gently clarify: "The current test in question is "X." Yet, we cannot reach a conclusion without repeating the test on a new blood sample. We then will be able to discuss the results together accordingly."
(d) Consider adding the following if you find it appropriate, in a non-judgmental tone: "Do you have any idea if that can be possible?"

1. Greet the patient and follow up on the established rapport.
2. Explain the results in simple language, starting with the normal and then any abnormality or non-compatible items. Utilize breaking bad news skills as needed.
3. Assess: check your level of understanding and answer any questions.
4. Assist: "Let us share a plan which is suitable for helping you."
   (a) Manage the patient if he or she has any abnormality in reference to Table 24.4.
   (b) Provide opportunistic advice as appropriate, this can include preconception counseling (recommending females to take folic acid, ideally 3 months, prior to pregnancy), family planning, human-papilloma virus's vaccine (if a female, 9–45 years, was found not to have completed a series in her lifetime), and referral to premarital or couple counseling.
   (c) Fill in the certificate form, release, and sign it.
   (d) Provide follow up appointment if needed.

Table 24.2 Hemoglobin analysis test's interpretation

Partner 2	Partner 1							
	Normal Hb	α-Thal	β-Thal	Hb-S	Hb-C	Hb-E	Hb-D[a]	Other significant Hb
Normal Hb	Normal	α Thal carrier	*β-Thal carrier*	*S carrier*	*C carrier*	*E carrier*	*D carrier*	
α-Thal	α Thal carrier	α Thal carrier or **diseased**	*α and β-Thal carrier*	*α-Thal and S carrier*	*α-Thal and C carrier*	*α-Thal and E carrier*	*α-Thal and D carrier*	**αThal-Hb L**
β-Thal	*β-Thal carrier*	*α and β-Thal carrier*	**βThal-βThal**	**S-βThal**	**C-βThal**	**E-βThal**	**D-βThal**	**βThal-Lepore**[b]
Hb-S	*S carrier*	*α-Thal and S carrier*	**S-βThal**	**SS**	**SC**	*E and S carrier*	**SD**	**SO**[c]
Hb-C	*C carrier*	*α-Thal and C carrier*	**C-βThal**	**SC**	**CC**	*E and C carrier*	*D and C carrier*	
Hb-E	*E carrier*	*α-Thal and E carrier*	**E-βThal**	*E and S carrier*	*C and E carrier*	**EE**	*E and D carrier*	
Hb-D[a]	*D carrier*	*α-Thal and D carrier*	**D-βThal**	**SD**	*C and D carrier*	*E and D carrier*	**DD**	
Other significant Hb		**αThal-Hb L**	**βThal-Lepore**[b]	**SO**[c]				**OO**[c] **Lepore-Lepore**[b] **Hb J-Hb J Hb G-Hb G**[d] **Hb H-Hb Hope**

Key: *Hb* Hemoglobin, *BThal* Beta Thalasemia, **Bold: Diseased**

[a] Also known as Hb D Punjab or Hb D Los Angeles

[b] Also known as Hb Lepore Washington, Lepore Boston, Lepore Baltimore, or Lepore Hollandia

[c] Also known as Hb O-Arab or Hb Egypt

[d] Also known as Hemoglobin G-Philadelphia

Table 24.3 Interpreting infectious diseases' tests

Screening test	Syphilis (Enzyme Immunoassay (EIA))	Hepatitis B infection (Hepatitis B surface Antigen)	Hepatitis C infection (Hepatitis C antibodies)	HIV infection (HIV antigen/antibody test)
Causes of false positive result	• Acute or chronic viral or febrile illness • Recent immunization or blood transfusion • Pregnancy • Autoimmune or connective tissue disease • IV drug abuse • Lab error	• Transient reactivity to Hepatitis B vaccine • Autoimmune or connective tissue disease • Kidney failure • Lab error	• Acute or chronic viral or febrile illness • Autoimmune or connective tissue disease • Lab error	• Participants of HIV vaccination studies • Autoimmune, or connective tissue disease • Lab error
Confirmatory test	• VDRL • TPHA • RPR	• Full Hepatitis B panel • Hepatitis B PCR	• Hepatitis C PCR	• HIV1/HIV2 antibody test (Futher confiration can be obtained by PCR)
Risk of transmission to partner with unprotected intercourse	• Primary, secondary, and early latent stages are considered infectious, with an estimated risk of transmission per partner of 51–64%	• 40% transmission rates to non-immune partners • Vaccination reduce that risk significantly but does not protect 100%	• Long-term monogamous partner's risk is 0–0.6% per year (increasing with anal intercourse)	• Up to 2% for receptive vaginal sex, that is 1 transmission per 50 exposures, (increasing to 20% for receptive anal sex)
Disease specific management	• Latent Syphilis: treat with 3 doses of weekly Penicillin G Benzathine 2.4 million unit intramuscularly or Doxycycline 100 mg orally twice daily for 2 weeks • Consider repeating the titer after 3 months to document treatment efficacy, looking for four folds decrease or more	– Check partner's immune status and provide vaccination if needed – Consider immunizing the patient against Hepatitis A – Consider doing ultrasound of liver • Refer to hepatology clinic	– Consider immunizing the patient against Hepatitis A and B – Consider doing ultrasound of liver – Consider referral to hepatologist	– Consider doing HIV PCR and CD3/CD4 level – Refer to infectious disease clinic

Table 24.4 Managing patient with abnormal results

Abnormality	Management
Anemia	• Offer dietary advise and iron supplements
Inadequate rubella antibodies	• **Low titer**, defined as IgG[a] of less than 10 IU/mL: provide patient with Measles-Mumps-Rubella (MMR) vaccine (consider completing a full series, 2 doses, 1 month apart, if patient does not recall having had the MMR series ever) • **Equivocal titer,** defined as IgG[a] of 10–15 IU/mL: counsel her either to take an MMR booster versus repeat the level in 1 month and deciding accordingly
Rhesus blood type incompatibility	• Explain to them that this incompatibility is not a contraindication for marriage but a matter that needs precautions • The problem occurs when a female with rhesus negative blood type is exposed to a rhesus positive blood type, such as when she has bleeding or delivery of a rhesus positive baby. In that case, her body develops immune response that may lead to miscarriage, hydrops fetalis, or still birth • Describe the need for anti-D immunoglobulin injections to prevent sensitization or production of antibodies, by neutralizing any positive antigens that may have reached the female's blood stream. The antibodies are provided at 28th and 34th week of pregnancy. An additional dose is provided within 72 h of delivery of a rhesus positive baby
Hemoglobinopathy	• Explain to the patient the abnormal finding, the odds of having affected or carrier offspring in each pregnancy (all are inherited through autosomal recessive mode which necessitates that the mutation gets inherited from both parents for a child to be affected, otherwise, if only a single mutated gene is acquired, then the offspring is carrier). • Elaborate that hemoglobinopathies causes blood hemolysis leading to different clinical pictures, including regular fever or pain, failure to thrive, hepatosplenomegaly, and delayed puberty, that necessitate regular blood transfusions and admissions. The only curative therapy currently available is stem cell transplant*. • Obtain his or her permission to disclose that information to the other partner and get the consent form signed. If patient does not want to do so, or is non-decisive yet, explain that we cannot proceed with the release of certificate, but can put it on hold until he or she is ready to proceed. • Explain to the partner the items in the first point. • Provide reading materials. • Consider referring the patient or partner to hematologist or geneticist for further care. • If couple-to-be insist on proceeding with the marriage that is likely to produce affected offspring despite advice, offer connecting the partners with families of affected children to better understand the condition, and explain to them the role of assisted reproductive technologies, like in vitro fertilization, in having healthy kids

(continued)

Table 24.4 (continued)

Abnormality	Management
Infectious disease	• Explain to the patient the abnormal finding, the diagnosis, treatment options (in the table above), and risk for transmission to the partner and offspring • Screen for other sexually transmitted diseases, including chlamydia and gonorrhea • Obtain his or her permission to disclose that information to the other partner and get the consent form signed. If patient does not want to do so, or is non-decisive yet, explain that we cannot proceed with the release of certificate, but can put it on hold until he or she is ready to proceed • Explain to the partner the items in the first point • Educate to the couple, either together or individually about the precautions that need to be followed to reduce the risk of transmission to the other partner and children (if affected female) if curative treatment is not obtained. This includes abstinence of sexual activity, and safe sex (using male condom). Couple have the option to opt for assisted fertilization techniques (as in in vitro-fertilization) to have healthy uninfected children • Provide reading materials • Refer patient to specialist (hepatology, infectious, or venereal disease specialist) and health educator for further care

[a] Immunoglobulin: IgG
[*] Gene therapy have been recently approved for the treatment of sickle cell disease

History Taking and Management of a Patient Presenting with Sexual Dysfunction

25

Shaima Lari and Shammah Al Memari

Learning Objectives
- How to master history taking for patients peresenting with sexual dysfunction?
- How to perform a focused exam for patients presenting with sexual dysfunction?
- How to approach and provide management tips for patients presenting with sexual dysfunction?

Focus areas include excluding depression and correct misconceptions about normal sexual cycle or effects of chronic conditions and aging on the sexual health.

---

1. Introduce yourself and establish good rapport.
2. Identify the complaint:
   (a) Start sensitively: "I understand that talking about sexual problems can be uncomfortable for you. However, I need to ask you few questions to be able to help you." "I assure you that I will maintain your confidentiality all through."

S. Lari
Sheikh Shakhbout Medical City, Abu Dhabi, United Arab Emirates

S. Al Memari (✉)
Abu Dhabi, United Arab Emirates

© The Author(s), under exclusive license to Springer Nature Singapore Pte Ltd. 2024
S. Lari et al. (eds.), *Family Medicine OSCE: First Aid to Objective Structured Clinical Examination*, https://doi.org/10.1007/978-981-99-5530-5_25

(b) Clarify the complaint (for example. "What do you mean by weakness?") and repeat it in clear, scientific terms (for example, "I see, so you have difficulty developing penile erection long enough to complete penetration").

(c) Onset, duration, and timing: "Have you always had this problem or is it recent?" A recent onset suggests psychogenic etiology while a lifelong problem might be organic. "Does the problem happen all the time or only sometimes?" Generalized or situational (related to the partner or the place).

(d) Any relieving or aggravating factors.

3. Explore the patient's ideas, concerns and expectations (ICE):
   (a) Fears, peer, or family pressure.
   (b) Explore the partner's opinion about the same problem too.
   (c) "Do you think there is a solution?"
   (d) "How motivated are you to solve this problem?"
   (e) "Any specific treatment you have in mind?"
   (f) "Is your partner motivated to solve this problem with you?"

4. Understand the sexual activity.
   (a) Explore the source of their sexual background and literacy: *"Patients come from different* backgrounds with different sexual beliefs. Where did you get yours from?"
   (b) Frequency: "How often do you have sexual intercourse per week?"
   (c) Initiation: "Who usually initiates the process, your partner or yourself?"
   (d) Earlier experience (masturbation or previous partners).
   (e) "Can you please describe your sexual activity to me": explore the patient's and partner's sexual cycle: Desire: "Do you or your partner feel like you want to have sex?" Arousal: female "Do you have vaginal lubrication?" male "Do you have a penile erection that is long enough to complete penetration?" Orgasm: (female "Do you reach a point of maximum happiness or develop vaginal contractions?" male "Do you ejaculate?"). If it does not occur with the current activity, ask if it occurs with masturbation. Resolution.

5. Explore past history:
   (a) If a female, ask about her menses, contraception use, and last pap smear result.
   (b) History of previous Sexually Transmitted Infection (STI).
   (c) Diabetes mellitus, hypertension, coronary artery disease, asthma, arthritis, or menopause.
   (d) Operations, obstetric, and gynecological problems.
   (e) Depression, sleep, mood, and appetite.
   (f) Immunization history: including hepatitis B and human papilloma virus vaccines.

6. Question regular use of medications: Viagra, testosterone, oral contraceptive pills.

7. Social and family history:
   (a) "How long have you been married?" "Have you been living together?"
   (b) "How do you describe your intimate relationship with your partner?"
   (c) "Do you have any children? How many?"

    (d) Alcohol, smoking, extra-marital affairs, relationships before marriage.

    (e) High risk behaviors: "History of using injectable drugs?" or "Any sexual partners from high-risk areas?"

    (f) Occupation and job satisfaction.

    (g) Family, financial problems.

8. Examination: as indicated by the history.

9. Order required investigations: as indicated by the history.

10. Arrange referral: if an underlying condition requires.

11. Management and education: share differential diagnosis and prognosis.

    (a) Male's sexual dysfunction, refer to (Table 25.1)

    (b) Female's sexual dysfunction, refer to (Table 25.2)

12. Give reading educational materials if any.

13. Discuss health maintenance and age-appropriate screening.

14. Arrange for follow-up.

15. Communication skills: organized approach, mixed questioning styles (open- and closeended questions), active listening, clear language, and reflection on the patient's ICE.

Table 25.1 Management of male's sexual dysfunction

Etiology by type	Management
Desire disorders	Treat by CBT and sensate focus
Arousal and orgasmic disorders: considered organic if no anatomical problems and noticed normal morning erection	Premature ejaculation: treat by squeeze technique, CBT, and sensate focus
Others	Treat psychological and systemic diseases

Table 25.2 Management of female's sexual dysfunction

Etiology by type	Management
Desire disorders: either hypoactive sexual desire dysfunction (non-responsive) or aversion disorder (avoidance)	Treatment includes: advise partners to add intimacy, perform foreplay, eliminate routine, and communicate about sex
Pain disorders: 1. Superficial dyspareunia: pain with attempted penetration, caused by anatomical abnormality or irritation	Investigated by screening for infections and performing anatomical studies. Treatment includes relaxation, Cognitive Behavioral Therapy (CBT), and sensate focus
2. Deep dyspareunia: pain with thrusting or fast penile movement in the vagina, caused by irritable bowel syndrome or adhesions	Treatment of underlying condition
Arousal disorder: manifests as absence of vaginal lubrication or intermediate dyspareunia	Treatment includes using vaginal lubricants, CBT, and sensate focus
Orgasmic disorders	Fantasizing, Kegel exercises, CBT, and sensate focus

History Taking and Management of a Presenting with Stroke

26

Kawthar Al Ameri and Shammah Al Memari

Learning Objectives
- How to master history taking for patients presenting with stroke?
- How to perform a focused exam for patients presenting with stroke?
- How to approach and provide management tips for patients presenting with stroke?

Focus areas on the differential diagnosis of acute ischemic stroke encompass identifying conditions such as hemorrhagic stroke (intracerebral hemorrhage), subarachnoid or subdural hemorrhage, seizure with postictal paralysis, migraine with hemiparesis or other aura, syncope, hypoglycemia, hypertensive encephalopathy, and conversion disorder.

1. Introduce yourself and establish a good rapport.
2. Identify the complaint:
   (a) Presenting symptoms: Refer to (Table 26.1).
   (b) Onset and duration: try to elicit the exact time of onset of symptoms. If the symptoms were unwitnessed, identify when the last time was the patient seen well.

K. Al Ameri
Ambulatory Healthcare Services, Abu Dhabi, United Arab Emirates

Faculty of Family Medicine Residency Program, Sheikh Khalifa Medical City, Abu Dhabi, United Arab Emirates

S. Al Memari (✉)
Abu Dhabi, United Arab Emirates

© The Author(s), under exclusive license to Springer Nature Singapore Pte Ltd. 2024
S. Lari et al. (eds.), *Family Medicine OSCE: First Aid to Objective Structured Clinical Examination*, https://doi.org/10.1007/978-981-99-5530-5_26

Table 26.1 Clinical manifestation of stroke

• Facial or limb weakness, usually hemiparesis	• Loss of vision (hemianopia or monocular) or diplopia
• Sensory loss in one or more extremities	• Ataxia (truncal or limb)
• Sudden change in mental status: confusion, delirium, lethargy, stupor, or coma	• Dysarthria: slurred speech
• Aphasia: incoherent speech, lack of speech output, or difficulty understanding speech	• Vertigo, nausea and vomiting, or headache

(c) Character: worsening, improving or same since onset, and any fluctuation in severity.

(d) Any prior episodes: history of previous diagnosed stroke or unattended symptoms.

(e) Ongoing medical illnesses: coronary artery disease, congestive heart failure, valvular heart disease, atrial fibrillation, obstructive sleep apnea, hypertension, diabetes, or hyperlipidemia.

(f) Assess for risk factors: provoking stress, active or past smoking, alcohol, recreational drug use, or other less common risk factors (migraine, oral contraceptive agents, hormone replacement therapy, antiphospholipid antibody syndrome, infection, and cancer).

3. Work out your differentials accordingly (refer to "Chap. 3: Headache" for further differentials of headache), differentiating between ischemic and hemorrhagic stroke:

(a) **Ischemic stroke: Stepwise deterioration or progressive weakness that follows a single vessel pattern.**

(b) **Hemorrhagic stroke**: **Progressive neurological deterioration that may not follow a single vessel pattern,** commonly presenting with **thunderclap headache**, nausea, vomiting, and decreased level of alertness, with or without risk factors (history of head trauma, or brain tumor, patient on anticoagulation, known case of bleeding disorder, or vascular malformation).

4. Examination:

(a) Initial prompt examination checking for vitals (airway, breathing, circulation (pulse and blood pressure)), facial drop, speech difficulties, arm weakness, or pronator drift.

(b) Full examination (after stabilization, initial management, calling for ambulance, and activating stroke protocol): Neck: check for neck stiffness (suggests subarachnoid hemorrhage) and auscultate for carotid bruits. Lungs: auscultate for signs of aspiration pneumonia or congestive heart failure. Heart: auscultate for irregular rhythm (suggests atrial fibrillation which can be source of embolism) or murmurs (suggest valvular heart disease). Full neurological exam (refer to "Chap. 69: Cranial Nerves Examination" for further details). Classify the findings according to the most likely affected artery. Refer to (Table 26.2).

5. Management:

(a) Assess level of consciousness and ensure adequate airway, breathing, and circulation.

(b) Activate the stroke protocol and arrange for transfer to a hospital with a stroke unit.

Table 26.2 Artery-specific neurological findings in patients presenting with stroke

Affected artery	Findings
Large- to medium-sized arteries	– *Dominant* middle cerebral artery (MCA): dominant face and limbs (arms more than legs) weakness and sensory loss, *with aphasia* (expressive, receptive, or both) and possible hemianopia. – *Nondominant* MCA: nondominant face and limbs (arms more than legs) weakness and sensory loss, with *hemineglect*, and possible hemianopia. – Anterior cerebral artery (ACA): contralateral leg weakness and sensory loss. – Internal carotid artery: combination of contralateral MCA and ACA. – Basilar artery: **"locked-in syndrome"**: nausea, vomiting, diplopia; acute loss of consciousness, quadriparesis, or quadriplegia. – Posterior cerebral artery: unilateral hemianopia; blindness, with anosognosia if bilateral (Anton syndrome). – Posterior inferior cerebellar artery: vertigo, nystagmus, ataxia, Wallenberg syndrome (lateral medullary), resulting in ipsilateral loss of pinprick and temperature on the face and contralateral loss of pinprick and temperature on the body, along with ipsilateral Horner syndrome and ipsilateral palatal weakness with resulting dysphagia, dysarthria
Small arteries: *	– Ischemic lesion in the internal capsule or pons: pure motor hemiparesis or ataxia that is out of proportion to the hemiparesis. – Ischemic lesion of the thalamus: pure hemisensory loss. – Ischemic lesion involving both the thalamus and internal capsule: sensorimotor stroke. – Multiple localizations, typically involving the pons: Dysarthria–clumsy hand syndrome: facial weakness, dysarthria, and mild clumsiness and weakness of the hand

*In cases of small artery stroke, patients may present with lacunar syndrome, which typically spares cortical signs such as language or judgment

(c) Start the assessment towards identifying if patient is a candidate for thrombolytic or fibrinolytic therapy (timeframe is less than 4 h): Consider initial blood work up: complete blood count, coagulation profile, urea and electrolytes, troponin, glucose, as well as blood typing and crossmatch. ECG (helps in identifying arrhythmia which can be a cause). Computerized tomography (CT) scan to differentiate between ischemic and hemorrhagic stroke.

(d) Consider aspirin if patient is not a candidate for thrombolytic or fibrinolytic therapy: stroke or significant head trauma in the last 3 months, history of intracranial hemorrhage, elevated blood pressure, active internal bleeding, or a blood glucose concentration less than 50 mg per deciliter.

(e) Consider involving the family.

(f) Further management (after stabilization): Stroke work-up: transthoracic and transesophageal echocardiography, Carotid ultrasound, and Holter monitor. Involve multi-disciplinary rehabilitation team: speech and language therapy, occupational therapy, physiotherapy, psychology, and social worker.

6. Give reading educational materials if any.

7. Arrange for follow-up.

8. Communication skills: organized approach, mixed questioning styles (open- and close-ended questions), active listening, clear language, and reflection on patient's ideas concerns and expectation (ICE).

Sumiya Taheri and Shammah Al Memari

Learning Objectives
- How to master history taking for patients presenting with wrist pain?
- How to perform a focused exam for patients presenting with wrist pain?
- How to approach and provide management tips for patients presenting with wrist pain?

Focus areas on ulnar sided wrist pain (tendinopathy of extensor carpi ulnaris, triangular fibrocartilage complex injury), radial side wrist pain (scaphoid fracture, Scapholunate instability, de Quervain tendinopathy, Carpal metacarpal osteoarthritis, Radiocarpal arthritis), volar sided wrist pain (Carpal tunnel syndrome, Hook of the hamate fracture, ulnar neuropathy (Guyon's canal syndrome)), dorsal side wrist pain (Ganglion cyst, Carpal boss, Kienböck disease (avascular necrosis) of the lunate, Intersection syndrome).

1. Introduce yourself and establish good rapport with the patient.
2. Identify the complaint (wrist pain): presence of pain and referred pain, location, duration, onset, relieving and aggravating factors, timing (daytime, nighttime, cyclic, or nocturnal pain), profile (same, improving, and worsening) and association with activity, and prior episodes, previous episodes.

S. Taheri
Ambulatory Healthcare Services, Abu Dhabi, United Arab Emirates

S. Al Memari (✉)
Abu Dhabi, United Arab Emirates

© The Author(s), under exclusive license to Springer Nature Singapore Pte
Ltd. 2024
S. Lari et al. (eds.), *Family Medicine OSCE: First Aid to Objective Structured
Clinical Examination*, https://doi.org/10.1007/978-981-99-5530-5_27

(a) Clarify the symptom: "Which time of the day is the symptoms worse?", "Does it wake you up from sleep at night?", "Have you injured your hand?", "Have you noticed any small swelling/mass around your wrist?", "Any decreased movement of the wrist joint?", "Any pain while moving your thumb and/or reduced grip?"

(b) Associated symptoms: fever, joint stiffness, joint swelling, numbness, tingling, weakness, wasting (note the site and pattern if any), or change of fingers' color (white, blue, or red).

(c) Ongoing problems and past medical history: wrist problem, history of Carpal tunnel syndrome in the opposite wrist, arthritis, diabetes, thyroid disease, current pregnancy (if female patient).

(d) Family history: connective tissue disease (SLE, Scleroderma), Raynaud's phenomena, carpal tunnel syndrome.

(e) Social history: occupational history (working in cold weather or with vibrating tools), smoking, alcohol, and illicit drugs.

(f) Medication history: beta blockers, oral contraceptive pills (if female).

3. Explore patient's ideas, concerns and expectations (ICE), as well as the effect of the problem in the quality of life.

4. Examination:

(a) Vitals including pulse in upper limbs and blood pressure in both arms.

(b) Skin: rash, erythema, warmth, and discoloration.

(c) Hand and wrist examination (refer to Table 27.1 for a quick reminder. Otherwise review "Chap. 81. Wrist and Hand Examination" for further details)

5. Order required investigations:

(a) Complete blood count, erythrocyte sedimentation rate (ESR), C-reactive protein (CRP), thyroid function test, fasting glucose, HbA1c, and rheumatological screening.

(b) Nerve conduction studies or electromyography (EMG).

6. Management and education:

(a) Carpal tunnel syndrome: conservative approach: weight loss, avoid overuse of wrist, and utilize wrist splint. Pharmacological management: steroid injection. Surgical management (needed urgently if patient has thenar muscle wasting). Explain to the patient "Surgeon will cut the tendon and release the pressure."

Table 27.1 Focused hand and wrist examination in a patient presenting with wrist pain

Observe	Muscle wasting, swelling at styloid process (suggests de Quervain tenosynovitis), ganglion cyst (nodule cyst that transilluminate, tender, immobile, underlying skin have no change), or triphasic change of the finger color (white, blue, red) under cold temperature of emotional stress (Reynaud's phenomena)
Palpate	Tenderness especially at the anatomic snuffbox (suggests scaphoid fracture)
Check	Sensation and power including thumb abduction
Test	1. Phalen's test and tinsels test (positive in carpal tunnel syndrome). 2. Fleckenstein test (positive in de Quervain tenosynovitis)

    (b) Reynaud's phenomena: conservative approach: keep hands warm by wearing gloves, avoid triggers like cold weather, smoking cessation, exercise, and consideration of change of occupation. Pharmacological management: Nifedipine, alpha blockers, ACE inhibitors, selective serotonin reuptake inhibitors (SSRI), and analgesics. Surgical management: sympathectomy for severe cases.

    (c) De Quervain tenosynovitis: conservative approach: avoid load and excessive activity on the affected hand and utilize home exercise regimes. Pharmacological management: oral NSAIDS with or without splinting or steroid injection. Surgical management: aims at releasing the first extensor compartment.

7. Give reading educational materials if any.
8. Discuss health maintenance and screening for age.
9. Arrange for follow up and referral as needed.
10. Communication skills: organized approach, mixed questioning styles (open- and close-ended questions), active listening, clear language, and reflection on patient's ICE.

History Taking and Management of a Patient Presenting for Preoperative Assessment

28

Noora Al Blooshi and Shammah Al Memari

Learning Objectives
- How to master preoperative history taking?
- How to perform a focused exam in the preoperative assessment visit?
- How to approach and provide management tips for a patient undergoing surgery?

Focus areas on details about the surgery type, its duration, the type of anesthesia, the patient's medical condition and control, as well as the medication protocol before the surgery.

1. Introduce yourself.
2. Establish a good rapport.
3. Identify the chief complaint: "Patient came for preoperative assessment."
4. Assess preoperative risk:
   (a) Details of surgery: date, type, and length.
   (b) Patient activity level and exercise tolerance: "Do you usually get chest pain or breathlessness when you climb up two flights of stairs at normal speed?"

N. Al Blooshi
Ambulatory Healthcare Services, Abu Dhabi, United Arab Emirates

S. Al Memari (✉)
Abu Dhabi, United Arab Emirates

5. Ongoing problems:
   (a) Medical history including any recent admission or change of management: stroke, epilepsy, dementia, delirium, hypertension, angina (heat attack), myocardial infarction, heart failure, asthma, chronic obstructive pulmonary disease, obstructive sleep apnea, joint stiffness, arthritis of neck or jaw, diabetes, thyroid disease, gastroesophageal reflux, liver, or kidney disease.
   (b) Surgical history: "If you have been put to sleep for an operation were there any anesthetic problems?"
   (c) Medication history: antihypertensive, antiplatelet (Aspiria, non-steroidal anti-inflammatory drugs), anticoagulants (heparin, warfarin, or novel oral anticoagulants (NOACs)), hypoglycemics (insulin or oral), statins (reduces perioperative all-cause morbidity and mortality), niacin (may worsen allergies by increasing histamine. Consider stopping them 2 weeks prior to surgery), combined oral contraceptives (double the risk of deep vein thrombosis. Consider stopping them 4 weeks prior to surgery and advice use of alternative contraceptive method), steroids, herbal medications, or any over the counter medication.
   (d) Allergies.
   (e) Social history: smoking, alcohol, and illicit drugs use.
   (f) Family history: explore: "Has anyone in your family (blood relatives) had a problem following an anesthetic?"
6. Explore patient's ideas, concerns and expectations (ICE), effect on patient's life and relation to wife and family.
7. Physical examination:
   (a) Vitals and measurements. Calculate BMI (check for obesity).
   (b) Airway assessment: using Mallampati score. Check dentation.
   (c) Cardiac and pulmonary examination: check for aortic stenosis, elevated jugular venous pressure (JVP), pulmonary edema, and third heart sound (high surgical risk).
8. Investigations:
   (a) Complete blood count in all patients undergoing major and all those who are more than or equal to 65 years old: to rule out anemia and thrombocytopenia.
   (b) Urea, electrolytes, and creatinine in patients who have history of renal or cardiac disease, or those who are more than 50 years of age.
   (c) Sickle cell disease if patient with family history.
   (d) Electrocardiogram (ECG) in patients who have history of renal or cardiac disease or those who are more than 60 years of age.
   (e) Chest X-ray in patients who are more than 60 years of age.
9. Management and education:
   (a) Advise for pre-operative fasting as it is important to minimize the aspiration risk: water and chewing gum can be continued up to 2 h before induction of anesthesia. Whereas, food and milk containing drinks can be continued up to 6 h before induction of anesthesia.
   (b) Medications management: refer to Table 28.1.
10. Communication skills: Ensure organized approach, mixed questioning style (open- and close-ended questions), active listening, clear language, and reflection on patient's ICE.

Table 28.1 Medication modification guidelines prior to surgery

Type of therapy	Alteration required
Hormonal therapy	Stop 4 weeks prior to surgery
Herbal medication	Stop 2 weeks before surgery
Antiplatelet	Clopidogrel stopped 7 days before surgery or neuraxial intervention
Warfarin	Last dose 6 days before the procedure
Heparin	Stop 4 h before neuraxial block
Diabetes medications and ACEI-inhibitors	Stop on the day of surgery
Steroids	If patient is on regular dose (more than 5 mg) consider need of *increased* dose during the perioperative period
NOACs	Depends on dose and renal clearance

History Taking and Management of a Patient Presenting with Leg Pain During Physical Activity "Claudication"

Kawthar Al Ameri and Shammah Al Memari

Learning Objectives
- How to master history taking for patients experiencing leg pain when walking?
- How to perform a focused exam for patients experiencing leg pain when walking?
- How to approach and provide management tips for patients experiencing leg pain when walking?

Focus areas on understanding the difference in definition of various peripheral artery diseases and conditions: Intermittent claudication is reproducible muscular pain with ambulation that is relieved with rest due to peripheral arterial disease, while chronic limb-threatening ischemia is a clinical syndrome that is defined by the presence of peripheral artery disease in combination with rest pain, gangrene, or a lower limb ulceration for more than 2 weeks, Leriche syndrome being intermittent claudication in the buttocks, pale, cold legs, sexual impotence, and absent femoral pulses.

K. Al Ameri
Ambulatory Healthcare Services, Abu Dhabi, United Arab Emirates

Faculty of Family Medicine Residency Program, Sheikh Khalifa Medical City, Abu Dhabi, United Arab Emirates

S. Al Memari (✉)
Abu Dhabi, United Arab Emirates

1. Introduce yourself.
2. Establish a good rapport.
3. Identify patient complaint: site, radiation (feet, legs, thigh, or buttocks), onset, duration, character (squeezing or aching pain), relieving and aggravating factors (rest, movement, walking up a steep hill, or a flight of stairs), associated symptoms (cool skin, skin discoloration, open wounds, gangrene, and numbness) and risk factors of peripheral artery disease:
   (a) Age more than or equal to 70 years.
   (b) Age 50–69 years with a history of smoking or diabetes.
   (c) Age 40–49 with diabetes and at least one other risk factor for atherosclerosis.
   (d) Known atherosclerosis at other sites (like coronary, carotid, or renal artery disease).
4. Medications: anti-platelet, ACE-Inhibitors, or statins.
5. Explore patient's ideas, concerns and expectations (ICE), as well as the effect of the symptom on the quality of life.
6. Explore ongoing problems, past medical and surgical histories: diabetes, hypertension, hypercholesterolemia, peripheral neuropathy, obesity, arthritis, or chronic kidney disease.
7. Social history: smoking or alcohol use.
8. Family history: cardiovascular disease.
9. Examination:
   (a) Look at the bilateral legs for swelling, skin lesions, discoloration, ulceration, amputation, or varicose veins.
   (b) Feel for cold or warm skin or baker cyst.
   (c) Measure the calf muscle diameter for any difference.
   (d) Palpate for distal peripheral pulses: dorsalis pedis, posterior tibial, popliteal, and femoral (femoral pulse is absent in 25% of cases).
10. Order required investigations as indicated:
    (a) Ankle-brachial index (ABI): refer to management for details of interpretation.
    (b) Segmental arterial pressure to define occlusion site.
    (c) Treadmill testing: reassuring if patient walks for more than 5 min.
    (d) Duplex arterial ultrasound: significant if occlusion is more than 50%.
11. Screen for depression.
12. Management and education:
    (a) Educate: "Ischemic symptoms result when there is an imbalance between the supply and demand for blood flow. Those with peripheral arterial disease who continue to smoke or have diabetes or renal insufficiency, can progress rapidly and unpredictably."
    (b) Utilize a multidisciplinary approach involving the primary care provider, podiatrist, vascular, and plastic surgeons.
    (c) Treat based on ABI reading. Refer to Table 29.1 for details.

Table 29.1 Treatment of peripheral artery disease based on ABI reading

ABI reading	Management
Less than 0.3	Treat as limb threatening ischemia (Emergent referral)
From 0.3 to 1.0	1. Modify risk factors: • Lifestyle modification: diet and exercise (standard walking, walking on treadmill, or using stair steps 3–5 times per week for 30 min per time then to increase by 5 min until achieving 50 min per session). • Smoking cessation program. • Antiplatelet therapy: Aspirin 81–325 mg orally daily (or Clopidogrel 75 mg daily). • Optimize diabetes and hyperlipidemia management. • Revise antihypertensives if any: consider switching to Ramapril 10 mg daily as it increases walking time for extra 4 min over 6 months. 2. If no improvement, then add Cilostazol (Pletal) for 3 months (100 mg twice daily or 50 mg twice daily if patient is also on calcium channel blocker. Note that it is contraindicated in patients congestive heart failure). 3. Refer to vascular surgery if no response in 3 months
More than 1.0	Consider alternative diagnosis

13. Arrange referral as indicated:
    (a) Emergency department if patient has acute limb ischemia.
    (b) Urgently to vascular surgeon: if patient is refractory to therapy or has been diagnosed with chronic limb-threatening ischemia (pain at rest, gangrene, or non-healing ulcer) as both have high risk of limb loss.
    (c) Dietician to support in weight loss.
14. Give reading educational materials if any.
15. Discuss health maintenance and screening for age.
16. Arrange for follow up.
17. Communication skills: organized approach, mixed questioning styles (open- and close-ended questions), active listening, clear language, and reflection on patient's ICE.

History Taking and Management of a Patient Presenting with Sudden Loss of Vision

30

Sumiya Taheri and Shammah Al Memari

Learning Objectives
- How to master history taking for patients presenting with sudden loss of vision?
- How to perform a focused exam for patients presenting with sudden loss of vision?
- How to approach and provide management tips for patients presenting with sudden loss of vision?

Focus areas on retinal diseases (retinal detachment, retinal artery or vein occlusion), optic neuropathies (optic neuritis, giant cell arteritis, stroke, acute angle-closure glaucoma, cerebral mass like meningioma, or pituitary adenoma), neuro-retinitis due to infectious (cat scratch disease) or inflammatory causes (sarcoidosis, Behcet disease, polyarteritis nodosa). Other causes (vitreous hemorrhage/detachment, age related macular degeneration (AMD), eye trauma (hyphema, corneal abrasion), functional or psychogenic vision loss).

1. Introduce yourself and establish good rapport.
2. Identify the complaint:
   (a) Onset (sudden, gradual), duration.

S. Taheri
Ambulatory Healthcare Services, Abu Dhabi, United Arab Emirates

S. Al Memari (✉)
Abu Dhabi, United Arab Emirates

© The Author(s), under exclusive license to Springer Nature Singapore Pte Ltd. 2024
S. Lari et al. (eds.), *Family Medicine OSCE: First Aid to Objective Structured Clinical Examination*, https://doi.org/10.1007/978-981-99-5530-5_30

117

Table 30.1 Vision loss differential diagnosis

Clinical presentation		Probable diagnosis
Vision loss with eye pain		Optic neuritis, acute primary angle-closure glaucoma, and giant cell arteritis
Vision loss without eye pain		Retinal diseases
Vision loss with reduction in visual field (scotoma)	Floating scotoma	Vitreous pathology
	Fixed scotoma	Corneal, retinal, optic nerve, or neurologic damage
Vision loss with **color desaturation**		Optic neuropathy

    (b) Quality (complete or partial) and laterality: unilateral: Acute monocular vision loss suggests presence of damage to the visual pathway anterior to the optic chiasm. Bilateral: Binocular vision loss is indicative of damage to optic chiasm or one that is occurring posterior to optic chiasm.

    (c) Progression (worsening, improving, resolved).

    (d) Associated symptoms: refer to Table 30.1 for details.

    (e) Risk factors for retinal detachment: history of cataract surgery, high myopia, recent eye trauma, personal or familial history of retinal detachment, history of connective tissue disease.

    (f) Work out your differentials accordingly: Flashing lights, floating spots, or a dark "curtain" progressing from one side of visual field (retinal detachment). Painless "shower of black dots" or red hue to vision (vitreous hemorrhage). Severe pain, haloes, conjunctival injection, nausea/vomiting, and photophobia (acute angle-closure glaucoma). Sparkling flashes of light and blind-spot enlargement (acute idiopathic blind spot enlargement syndrome (AIBES) and multiple evanescent white dot syndrome (MEWDS)).

3. Explore patient's ideas, concerns and expectations (ICE), and effect of the complaint on quality of life.

4. Explore ongoing problems and past medical history:

    (a) Multiple sclerosis (associated with optic neuritis).

    (b) Autoimmune disease (neuromyelitis optica-related optic neuritis).

    (c) Obstructive sleep apnea (risk factor for non-arteritic ischemic optic neuropathy (NAION)).

    (d) Cardiovascular risk factors: hypertension, diabetes, obesity, hyperlipidemia, carotid artery stenosis, stroke, myocardial infarction, atrial fibrillation, and left atrial enlargement.

5. Medication history:

    (a) Anticholinergics: may lead to loss of accommodation or angle-closure glaucoma.

    (b) Bisphosphonates or Rifabutin: may lead to uveitis.

    (c) Digoxin: may lead to yellow vision.

    (d) Sildenafil: may lead to blue vision or ischemic optic neuropathy.

    (e) Sulfonamides lead to myopia.

(f) Topiramate may lead to angle-closure glaucoma.

(g) Oral contraceptives may cause ischemic, retinal, or optic nerve events.

6. Social history: marital status, smoking, alcohol, illicit drug use.

7. Family history cardiovascular and ocular diseases.

8. Examination:

(a) Vital signs: including blood pressure.

(b) Eye examination: refer to Table 30.2 for quick summary, otherwise, refer to "Chap. 71: Eye Examination."

9. Order required investigations:

(a) Initial work-up: complete blood count (CBC) and chemistry panel. Request Erythrocyte Sedimentation Rate (ESR) and C-reactive Protein (CRP) tests if there is suspicion of giant cell arteritis, particularly if the patient presents with additional risk factors such as age over 50 years, night sweats, weight loss, jaw or tongue claudication, and proximal muscle pain or weakness. Coagulation studies: prothrombin time, international normalized ratio (INR), and activated partial thromboplastin time (aPTT). Fasting lipid panel, fasting glucose, and HbA1c to assess risk of atherosclerotic vascular disease.

(b) Further work-up: consider temporal artery biopsy or by ultrasound of temporal and other cranial arteries (if suspecting giant cell arteritis). Consider additional blood and cerebrospinal fluid testing if suspecting infectious, inflammatory, or neoplastic etiologies. Consider stroke work-up if suspecting stroke.

10. Management: refer to Table 30.3.

11. Arrange referral and follow-up as needed.

12. Give reading educational materials if any.

13. Discuss health maintenance and screening for age.

14. Communication skills: organized approach, mixed questioning styles (open- and close-ended questions), active listening, clear language, and reflection on patient's ICE.

Table 30.2 Focused eye examination for a patient presenting with sudden loss of vision

Examination	Assessment technique
Inspection	Look for proptosis, chemosis, conjunctival injection, ptosis, anisocoria, erythema, tearing, and light sensitivity
Visual acuity assessment	Using Snellen charts or Jaeger reading cards
Visual field assessment	Using confrontation test
Color vision assessment	Using pseudoisochromatic plate (PIP)
Special ocular examinations	Dilated fundus examination.
	Amsler grid (if suspecting macular degeneration)
Neurological examination	Assess for muscle weakness and facial droop if stroke is suspected

Table 30.3 Management strategies for sudden loss of vision

Diagnosis	Recommended management
Acute vision loss	• **An emergency** • **Patient should be seen and evaluated by an ophthalmologist as soon as possible**
Giant cell arteritis	• Corticosteroid therapy: dose equivalent to prednisolone 40–60 mg per day as soon as a clinical diagnosis of temporal arteritis is made or suspected. **Do not** delay until the diagnosis is confirmed by biopsy or imaging
Optic neuritis	• Disease-modifying therapy: for patients at high risk for multiple sclerosis • Note that corticosteroids (do not appear beneficial for improving long-term visual acuity)
Retinal artery occlusion	• Conservative approach: ocular massage • Pharmacological management: pentoxifylline, isosorbide dinitrate, acetazolamide, isovolumic hemodilution, carbogen inhalation, or hyperbaric oxygen • Surgical intervention: embolectomy
Retinal detachment	• Surgical intervention: scleral buckling and vitrectomy with gas tamponade
Vitreous hemorrhage	• Conservative approach: inclined bed to elevate head, avoidance of strenuous activity to allow blood to clear • Surgical interventions: vitrectomy to physically remove blood

Noora Al Blooshi and Shammah Al Memari

> **Learning Objectives**
> - How to master history taking for patients presenting with shortness of breath?
> - How to perform a focused exam for patients presenting with shortness of breath?
> - How to approach and provide management tips for patients presenting with shortness of breath?

Focus areas on respiratory causes (asthma, chronic obstructive pulmonary disease (COPD), pulmonary fibrosis, bronchiectasis, cystic fibrosis, chronic pulmonary embolism, pneumothorax, pleural effusion, pneumonia), **cardiac causes** (heart failure, ischemic heart disease, cardiomyopathy, valvular dysfunction, arrhythmias, pericarditis), or causes such as metabolic conditions (acidosis), neuromuscular disease, otorhinolaryngologic disorders, functional (anxiety, panic disorder, hyperventilation).

1. Introduce yourself and establish a good rapport.
2. Identify the complaint: onset, duration, relieving and aggravating factors, timing, course (same, improving, worsening), prior episodes, associated symptoms

N. Al Blooshi
Ambulatory Healthcare Services, Abu Dhabi, United Arab Emirates

S. Al Memari (✉)
Abu Dhabi, United Arab Emirates

© The Author(s), under exclusive license to Springer Nature Singapore Pte Ltd. 2024
S. Lari et al. (eds.), *Family Medicine OSCE: First Aid to Objective Structured Clinical Examination*, https://doi.org/10.1007/978-981-99-5530-5_31

(coughing, wheezing, chest pain, hemoptysis, severe sore throat, lower leg edema, palpitation, choking, gurgling respiration, and persistent pneumonia). Work out the differentials accordingly:

(a) Intermittent shortness of breath that is triggered by triggers like pollen, with wheezing, and history of atopy (allergies, eczema) (suggests asthma).

(b) Significant smoking history, shortness of breath with exertion, wheezing, decreased breath sounds, barrel chest, prolonged expiration (suggests COPD).

(c) Shortness of breath with exertion, clubbing and crackles on exam (suggests interstitial lung disease).

(d) Sedentary lifestyle, leg fatigue associated with exertion (suggests deconditioning secondary to obesity).

(e) Pallor and fatigue (suggests anemia).

(f) Shortness of breath, chest pain, recurrent deep vein thrombosis, hypoxemia, cough, fever, and hemoptysis (suggests pulmonary embolism).

(g) Night sweats, malaise, weight loss, and hemoptysis (suggests tuberculosis).

(h) Orthopnea, paroxysmal nocturnal dyspnea, pedal edema, jugular venous distention, and rales on the exam (suggests heart failure).

3. Explore patient's ideas concerns and expectation (ICE) as well as the effect of the symptom on the quality of life.

4. Explore ongoing problems: hypertension, diabetes, coronary artery diseases, valve disease, COPD, obstructive sleep apnea, gastroesophageal reflux disease, autoimmune disease, rheumatologically disease, malignancy, trauma, pregnancy, and history of thromboembolism.

5. Drug history: topiramate, amiodarone, nitrofurantoin, digoxin, calcium channel blockers, beta blockers, and methotrexate.

6. Social history: sedentary lifestyle, smoking history including history of e-cigarette or vape use, alcohol intake, illicit drug use, history of recent travel or diving.

7. Family history: asthma, pulmonary hypertension, interstitial lung disease, and neuromuscular disease.

8. Examination:

(a) General: Vitals, respiratory rate, ability to speak, and any audible stridor (suggests upper airway obstruction). Pulses paradoxus (suggests COPD, asthma, or cardiac tamponade). Visible use of accessory muscles and asses mental status.

(b) Hand: Cyanosis clubbing (suggests bronchiectasis, idiopathic pulmonary fibrosis, lung cancer, and cyanotic heart disease).

(c) Neck: Jugular venous distention (suggest left-sided heart failure or corpulmonale). Thyroid enlargement (thyroid dysfunction may cause congestive heart failure (CHF)). Trachea position: normally is in the midline.

(d) Heart examination: Decreased or distant heart sounds (suggest pericardial effusion, obesity or hyperinflation from emphysema).

(e) Respiratory examination: Palpate to look for subcutaneous emphysema and crepitus. Percuss: for dullness (suggests consolidation) or hyper-resonance (suggest pneumothorax). Listen for wheezes.

(f) Abdomen examination: Look for hepatomegaly, ascites, or hepatojugular reflux (suggests CHF).

(g) Lower limb examination: Look for edema and signs of deep vein thrombosis.

9. Order required investigations: Pulse oximetry, blood work up (complete blood count with deferential, metabolic profile (glucose, electrolyte, renal function, blood urea and nitrogen, phosphate, and calcium), thyroid stimulating hormone, B-type Natriuretic Peptide (BNP) and pro-BNP), Chest X-ray, electrocardiogram (ECG), and Spirometry.

10. Arrange referral as needed.

11. Management and education: Share differential diagnosis and prognosis.

12. Give reading educational materials if any.

13. Discuss health maintenance and screening for age.

14. Arrange for follow-up.

15. Communication skills: organized approach, mixed questioning styles (open- and close-ended questions), active listening, clear language, and reflection on patient's ICE.

Part II

History-Taking and Management: Pediatrics

History Taking and Management of a Child Presenting with Short Stature

Shaima Lari and Shammah Al Memari

Learning Objectives
- How to master history taking for children presenting with short stature?
- How to perform a focused exam for children presenting with short stature?
- How to approach and provide management tips for children presenting with short stature?

Focus areas on (listing the differential using the mnemonic: A B C D E F G) **A**lone (neglected infant), **B**one dysplasia (rickets, scoliosis, or mucopolysaccharidosis), **C**hromosomal (Turner, or Down syndromes) or **C**hronic ongoing disease (renal or heart failure), **D**elayed growth (failure to thrive (FTT), intrauterine growth retardation (IUGR) or constitutional growth delay), **E**ndocrine (growth hormone deficiency, Cushing or hypothyroidism), **F**amilial, or **G**astrointestinal malabsorption (celiac or Crohn's).

1. Introduce yourself.
2. Establish good rapport.
3. Identify factors that may contribute to the problem:
   (a) Prenatal: maternal health during pregnancy (diabetes, smoking, alcohol use), gestational duration, and history of Intrauterine growth restriction (IUGR).

S. Lari
Sheikh Shakhbout Medical City, Abu Dhabi, United Arab Emirates

S. Al Memari (✉)
Abu Dhabi, United Arab Emirates

© The Author(s), under exclusive license to Springer Nature Singapore Pte Ltd. 2024
S. Lari et al. (eds.), *Family Medicine OSCE: First Aid to Objective Structured Clinical Examination*, https://doi.org/10.1007/978-981-99-5530-5_32

    (b) Growth pattern: height and weight at and after birth, any pubertal changes?

    (c) Underlying disease: bone disease, cartilage disease, diarrhea, hypothyroidism, chronic cough (cystic fibrosis), thalassemia, or growth hormone deficiency.

    (d) Familial: parental height, age at menarche, age at pubertal growth spurt, or similar condition among siblings.

4. Explore parents' and patients' ideas, concerns and expectations (ICE), as well as the effect of the symptom on the quality of life.

5. Review of systems: energy level, sleep pattern, headache, visual disturbance, vomiting, abdominal pain, polyuria, polydipsia, and oliguria.

6. Explore other ongoing problems, if any, and ensure up to date vaccination schedule.

7. Question regular use of medications:

    (a) Medications that directly affect growth: steroids or levothyroxine.

    (b) Treatment of chronic conditions that can predispose to growth delay: sick cell disease, heart failure, or renal failure.

8. Social and family history: exclude neglect, poor care, stress related to peer pressure or bullying at school, alcohol, and smoking.

9. Examination:

    (a) General exam: start first with checking child's measurements: weight and height plotted on the growth chart, upper to lower body segment ratio, arm span, and tanner pubertal staging. Examine for body dysmorphic features associated with Turner Syndrome, such as a webbed neck, and for dwarfism, characterized by shortened limbs in comparison to the trunk.

    (b) Determining mid parental high (in cm): boys: (father's height + mother's height + 13)/2 and girls: (father's height + mother's height − 13)/2).

    (c) Determining growth velocity or height-velocity (HV): refer to Table 32.1 for further details.

    (d) Bone age. Using left wrist and hand X-rays.

10. Arrange referral: if patient has:

    (a) Suspected chromosomal abnormality or growth hormone deficiency.

    (b) Undiagnosed or uncontrolled chronic underlying disease.

    (c) Consider referral if growth velocity less than 5 cm/year, height is more than 3 standard deviations below the mean of age, IUGR did not catch up with the growth chart by 2 years, bone age is 2 standards deviation below the chronologic age, or if there is no signs of puberty at the age of 13 for girls and 14 for boys.

Table 32.1 Normal acceptable height velocity range for children from 2 years to puberty

Age	Growth velocity
Age 2–4 years	5.5–9 cm/year (2.2–3.5 in./year)
Age 4–6 years	5–8.5 cm/year (2–3.3 in./year)
Age 6 years to puberty	• 4–6 cm/year for boys (1.6–2.4 in./year) • 4.5–6.5 cm/year for girls (1.8–2.6 in./year)

11. Order required investigations:
    (a) Complete blood count (anemia), comprehensive metabolic panel and urinalysis (hepatic and renal diseases), inflammatory markers such C-reactive protein (inflammatory bowel diseases), and thyroid stimulating hormone (TSH).
    (b) Bone age: determined by left wrist and hand X-rays.
    (c) Further testing: Insulin-like growth factor 1 (if suspecting growth hormone deficiency), tissue transglutaminase antibodies and total IgA (if suspecting celiac diseases), and karyotyping (if suspecting syndromic cause).
12. Management and education: share differential diagnosis and prognosis.
    (a) Explain to parents the differences between familial and constitutional delay regarding the nature and expected outcome.
13. Give reading educational materials, if any.
14. Discuss health maintenance and screening for age.
15. Arrange for follow-up.
16. Communication skills: organized approach, mixed questioning styles (open- and close-ended questions), active listening, clear language, and reflection on parents' ICE.

History Taking and Management of a Child Presenting with Failure to Thrive

33

Eiman Al Murar and Shammah Al Memari

Learning Objectives
- How to master history taking for children presenting with failure to thrive?
- How to perform a focused exam for children presenting with failure to thrive?
- How to approach and provide management tips for children presenting with failure to thrive?

Focus areas
- *Inadequate caloric intake*: feeding problem (as in poor sucking and swallowing), breastfeeding difficulties, difficulty transitioning to solid foods, insufficient breast or formula milk consumption, excessive juice consumption, and parental avoidance of high-calorie foods. Explore family factors like financial issues or child neglect or abuse.
- *Inadequate caloric absorption*: disorders causing frequent emesis (like metabolic disorders and food insensitivities) or malabsorption (like celiac disease, cystic fibrosis, chronic diarrhea, or protein-losing enteropathy).
- *Excessive caloric expenditure*: chronic medical conditions like congenital heart disease, chronic pulmonary disease, or hyperthyroidism.

E. Al Murar
Ambulatory Healthcare Services, Abu Dhabi, United Arab Emirates

S. Al Memari (✉)
Abu Dhabi, United Arab Emirates

© The Author(s), under exclusive license to Springer Nature Singapore Pte Ltd. 2024
S. Lari et al. (eds.), *Family Medicine OSCE: First Aid to Objective Structured Clinical Examination*, https://doi.org/10.1007/978-981-99-5530-5_33

131

1. Introduce yourself and establish good rapport.
2. Explore parents' ideas, concerns and expectations (ICE).
3. Identify the complaint:
    (a) Maternal medical history: maternal age at the child's pregnancy, gravidity, parity, abortions, pregnancy history (including a detailed history of weight gain, substance, cigarette or alcohol consumption, nutrition and unusual nutritional practices, or any perinatal complications (bleeding, infections, fever, peripartum depression).
    (b) Neonatal history: gestational age at birth, intrauterine growth restriction (IUGR), Apgar score, birth weight, length and head circumference with percentiles, neonatal course, any complications (including sepsis, jaundice, feeding intolerance), review any newborn screens (example: phenylketonuria (PKU) or other inborn errors of metabolism).
    (c) Associated symptoms: weight loss, diarrhea, vomiting, dysphagia, snoring, sleep apnea, recurrent infections, signs of immune deficiency, symptoms and signs of malabsorption, central nervous system abnormalities, or developmental delay.
    (d) Further medical history: ongoing diseases, immunizations, allergies, and medications.
    (e) Detailed history of food intake from infancy through the current period: refer to Table 33.1
4. Social and family history:
    (a) Familial growth patterns.
    (b) Family history of cystic fibrosis, inflammatory bowel disease, celiac disease, or psychiatric diseases.
    (c) Psychosocial risk factors:
5. Head-to-toe examination:
    (a) General exam: vital signs. General appearance and hygiene. Child's activity, affect, and interactions with parents or caregivers. Watch for **adverse**

Table 33.1 Elements of food intake history of a child presenting with failure to thrive

Early life milk intake	1. Proportion of breast and formula milk 2. Note any intolerance
Introduction of solid food	1. Age at introduction 2. Method of introduction 3. Any intolerance or allergies
Current feeding behaviors	1. Sucking, chewing, or swallowing difficulty 2. Appropriateness of type, frequency, and timing of meals 3. Limited food preferences (picky eater)
Caregivers' knowledge, attitude, and practices	1. Nutrition and feeding knowledge. Consumption of vitamins and other supplements 2. Religious or cultural beliefs about food and any unusual diets that may be inappropriate for a child 3. Basic needs that support preparation of food by the caregiver (example: clean water, housing or shelter, cooking facility, refrigeration, cooking knowledge)

Box 33.1 Psychosocial Risk Factors for Failure to Thrive in Pediatric Patients
- Low educational level of parents or caregivers
- Low finances or poverty
- Impaired environment and family structure
  - Lack of support system
  - High risks for or signs of maternal postpartum depression
  - Family substance abuse or addiction

behaviors: **gaze avoidance, arching, hypertonicity, refusal to attach or respond appropriately, and unusual body movements.** Measurements: weight, height, body mass index, and head circumference. Plot them on the growth chart for better interpretation. Failure to thrive is confirmed if weight is persistently below the fifth percentile for sex and corrected age.
  (b) Skin and hair: poor hair texture or amount, rashes, birthmarks, and **signs of intentional or unintentional trauma (like bruises, burns, or scars).**
  (c) Head: frontal bossing, fontanel size and patency, and dysmorphia.
  (d) Eyes: dysmorphia, ptosis, sunset sign, abnormal palpebral fissures, pallor, trauma, cataract, optic nerve hypoplasia, fundi for evidence of chorioretinitis (suggests toxoplasmosis, rubella, cytomegalovirus, and herpes simplex infection (TORCH)).
  (e) Ears: size, shape, position, and signs of acute or chronic infections in external or middle ear.
  (f) Mouth: Palate deformity, submucosal cleft, teeth, caries, glossitis, mucous membrane hydration or lesions, thrush, bleeding, unusual odors in the breath.
  (g) Neck: webbed-shaped masses, enlarged tender lymph nodes, and thyroid abnormalities.
  (h) Chest: breath sounds, cardiac examination for murmurs, cardiomegaly, or arrhythmias.
  (i) Abdomen: organomegaly, masses, bowel sounds, and umbilical healing in the infant.
  (j) Genitalia: malformations, ambiguity, signs of trauma.
  (k) Extremities (including nails, joints, spine, and back): muscle development and quality of muscle mass, range of motion, edema, or digital malformations.
  (l) Neurologic function: cranial nerves, reflexes (increased or decreased), tone, infant reflexes relative to age, gait, suck, and swallow coordination. Consider observing a feeding episode.
6. Order investigations as needed, based on history and examination:
  (a) Initial work-up: complete blood count, serum creatinine, urea and electrolytes, liver function test, thyroid function test (usually result in derangement of height more than weight), erythrocyte sedimentation rate, and urinalysis.

    (b) Consider: human immunodeficiency virus (HIV) test (if patient has recurrent unexplainable infections), sweat test (if cystic fibrosis is suspected), Quantiferon testing (if tuberculosis is suspected), stool studies (for reducing substances, odor, color, consistency, and fat content), skeletal survey for occult trauma (if physical abuse is suspected), head computed tomography (CT) scan or magnetic resonance imaging (MRI) studies (if examination reveals microcephaly, macrocephaly, congenital malformation or if abusive head trauma is a concern), bone age studies of wrists (in children who have constitutionally short stature or are extremely malnourished), and Zinc level (as it is reported to be low in malnourished infants and children).

7. Health education: explain to the parents and child the nutritional modification needed:
   (a) Eliminate empty calories from items such as soda or other high sugar drinks.
   (b) Schedule regular meals and snacks (usually three meals and two snacks per day).
   (c) Avoid grazing between meals.
   (d) Offer solids before liquids.
   (e) Consider fortifying calories with extra oils and carbohydrates.
   (f) Increase protein.
   (g) Consider vitamins and mineral supplements, especially zinc and iron.

8. Management:
   (a) Explain the differential and probable diagnosis.
   (b) Share aim of treatment: achieving and maintaining, on two occasions that are one month apart, weight and height above the 10th percentiles for age and sex.
   (c) Explain that appetite stimulants are not recommended in most cases of failure to thrive (FTT).
   (d) Share prognosis: accelerated growth should be maintained for at least 4–9 months while relapse is not uncommon.

9. Give reading educational materials if any.
10. Discuss health maintenance and screening for age.
11. Arrange for follow-up from weekly to over a few months based on the condition.
12. Consider referral if outpatient management proves ineffective after 3–4 months.
13. Communication skills: organized approach, mixed questioning styles (open- and close-ended questions), active listening, clear language, and reflection on parents' ICE.

History Taking and Management of a Child Presenting with Perianal Pruritus

34

Eiman Al Murar, Sumiya Taheri,
and Shammah Al Memari

Learning Objectives
- How to master history taking for a children presenting with anal pruritus?
- How to perform systematic physical examination for children presenting with anal pruritus?
- How to manage a child presenting with pinworm infection?

Focus areas on pin worms, candidal diaper rash, scabies, child abuse, allergic or contact dermatitis.

1. Introduce yourself and establish good rapport.
2. Identify the complaint (anal itching):
   (a) Onset, duration, and character (at day or night).
   (b) Relieving and aggravating factors (worse at night).
   (c) Risk factors for pinworms: contact with infected classmates or household member, history of previous episodes of pinworm infection? Treated? What medication and dose?
   (d) Associated symptoms: constipation, diarrhea, insomnia, irritability, restlessness, teeth grinding, dysuria, enuresis, vulvovaginitis, or abdominal pain.
   (e) Complications: infected perianal skin due to constant scratching.

E. Al Murar · S. Taheri
Ambulatory Healthcare Services, Abu Dhabi, United Arab Emirates

S. Al Memari (✉)
Abu Dhabi, United Arab Emirates

© The Author(s), under exclusive license to Springer Nature Singapore Pte
Ltd. 2024
S. Lari et al. (eds.), *Family Medicine OSCE: First Aid to Objective Structured
Clinical Examination*, https://doi.org/10.1007/978-981-99-5530-5_34

(f) Consider other differential diagnoses: Perianal abscess, scabies (if there is other area that itch), irritant contact dermatitis, child abuse (by asking sensitively: "Did you notice any behavioral changes in your child? sleep? appetite? Who takes him to school? Any other adults living in the house?").

3. Explore ongoing problems: any developmental problems or history of anemia.
4. Question regular use of medications and allergies if any.
5. Explore parent's ideas, concerns, expectations (ICE), effect of the complaint on quality of life: "How does the problem affect you and your child?". "Has the problem affected his attendance at school or day care?". "Does anyone at home suffer from similar problems?"
6. Social and family history: general hygiene measures (washing hands), eating nails in child or other family members.
7. Examination:
   (a) Vital signs.
   (b) Abdominal examination (any tenderness).
   (c) Perianal examination: itch marks, adult, or ova of pin worms.
8. Order required investigations:
   (a) Paddle test or tape test: applying an adhesive tape on the skin around anus first thing in the morning to check for ova (best within 2–3 h of sleep, before defecation, or washing the area).
   (b) Consider perineal swab or samples from under fingernails to retrieve pinworm ova.
   (c) Stool samples are not recommended as pinworms and ova are not passed in stool.
   (d) In recurrent infection, check blood count for anemia.
9. Management and education: refer to Table 34.1 for details.
10. Give reading educational materials if any.
11. Discuss health maintenance and age-appropriate screening.
12. Arrange for follow up, referral if needed.
13. Communication skills: organized approach, mixed questioning styles (open- and close- ended questions), active listening, clear language, and reflection on patient's ICE.

Table 34.1 Pinworm management approach in adults and children

Management approach	Key information
Health education	*Educate the parents and family with the following*: • Pinworms are tiny white worms that are about 1 cm long • They more commonly infect children from all socio-economic groups, especially school-aged, although they can infect adults, as they are highly communicable • Human-to-human spread is favored by close, crowded living conditions • Spread among family members is common. Hence, we ideally treat all the family or household contacts with the same treatment, at the same time • Pinworm eggs can survive on the surface of clothes, bedding, and toys for about 2–3 weeks • Pinworm infections are easily treatable, leading to the elimination of the worms • Despite being easily treatable, the highly contagious nature of pinworm infections may result in recurrence. If symptoms reappear, prompt re-treatment is advised
Hygiene practices	*Hand hygiene*: • Prioritize handwashing over medication, especially for recurrent issues • Emphasize handwashing before eating, preparing food, after toilet use, and perianal area contact *Perineal and nail care* • Thoroughly wash the perineal area and hands upon waking from sleep • Discourage fingernail biting and promote regular nail trimming • Advise children to wear tight pants, especially at night to prevent scratching *Clothing and bed linens*: • Wash all underwear and pajamas promptly at a temperature of at least 40 °C • Avoid piling clothes in a basket, as pinworm eggs can survive outside the body • Wash bed linens daily for 2 weeks for the entire family • Avoid sharing towels and wash them regularly *Toilet hygiene*: • Clean toilets daily *School collaboration*: • Instruct teachers to observe children with itching and provide education on proper toilet hygiene
Medication administration	*Children above 2 years of age and non-pregnant adults* • Two doses of mebendazole (100 g), albendazole (400 mg), or Pyrantel pamoate (11 mg/kg, maximum 1 g) in 2 weeks intervals (the first dose to kill the worms and the second dose to kill the ova (ova will hatch within 2 weeks)) • Side effects: gastrointestinal upset, abnormal liver function test, or rash
	Children below 2 years of age • Limited safety data with drugs; weight risks and benefits
	Pregnant ladies • Drug safety not studied • If significant symptoms or compromising pregnancy can use pyrantel pamoate
	All • Anti-itch ointments and creams can be applied to relieve the symptoms of itchiness.

History Taking and Management of a Child Presenting with Fever

35

Shaima Lari, Noora Al Blooshi,
and Shammah Al Memari

Learning Objectives
- How to perform a focused history and physical examination for children presenting with fever?
- How to demonstrate a good understanding of common and potential differential diagnosis for children presenting with fever?
- How to perform a focused exam for children presenting with fever?
- How to provide management for infant and children presenting with fever?

Focus areas on **infectious causes** (viral respiratory or gastrointestinal infections, bacterial infections like otitis media, pneumonia, urinary tract infections, tuberculosis, cytomegalovirus, Epstein–Barr virus, meningitis), **versus noninfectious causes** (Kawasaki disease, post vaccination fever, inflammatory bowel disease, juvenile idiopathic arthritis, systemic lupus erythematosus, lymphoma, leukemia).

1. Introduce yourself and establish a good rapport with the parents.
2. Identify the complaint:

S. Lari
Sheikh Shakhbout Medical City, Abu Dhabi, United Arab Emirates

N. Al Blooshi
Ambulatory Healthcare Services, Abu Dhabi, United Arab Emirates

S. Al Memari (✉)
Abu Dhabi, United Arab Emirates

© The Author(s), under exclusive license to Springer Nature Singapore Pte Ltd. 2024
S. Lari et al. (eds.), *Family Medicine OSCE: First Aid to Objective Structured Clinical Examination*, https://doi.org/10.1007/978-981-99-5530-5_35

(a) "What is the temperature and where was it measured?" (rectal, axillary, or tympanic).
(b) Onset, duration, and pattern.
(c) Recent regular use of medication: new medication exposure or recent antibiotic use (can mask the infection).
(d) Associated symptoms: reduced oral intake, irritability, lethargy, swollen glands, red conjunctiva, swollen eyes, dry eyes, sore throat, dental problems, mouth sores, epistaxis, flu-like symptoms, vomiting, diarrhea, abdominal pain, dysuria, urinary incontinence, flank pain, scrotal pain, bone pain, joint pain, decreased range of movement, and rash.
(e) Possible provoking factors: incidental drug ingestion, indwelling devices, recent vaccine, transfusion, surgery, travel, high-risk diet (tap water, unpasteurized dairy products, or uncooked food), history of contact with infected human or unvaccinated animals.
3. Past medical history: immunization status, previous febrile illness, or immune compromised status (using steroids, immune deficiency syndromes, or cancer).
4. Family history: immune deficiency syndromes, recurrent infection, history of periodic fever disorder or Familial Mediterranean Fever.
5. Explore parent's ideas, concerns and expectations (ICE).
6. Examination:
(a) General: general appearance (well-appearing or toxic) and vital signs.
(b) Skin: dry cracked lips, color of skin, turgor, rash, and capillary refill (normally less than 3 seconds).
(c) Eye: bilateral conjunctival injection.
(d) Neck: neck rigidity, cervical lymphadenopathy, torticollis.
(e) Ear, nose, and throat: strawberry tongue, bulging tympanic membrane, tonsillar exudate or enlargement, petechial rash on soft palate.
(f) Extremities: limb or joint swelling, refusal to bear weight.
(g) Lung and cardiac examination: tachycardia or rales.
(h) Abdomen examination: suprapubic tenderness, abdominal guarding, or rigidity.
7. Order investigation if there was no source of infection identified and if temperate above 38:
(a) Patient less than 28 days old: complete blood count (CBC) with deferential, urine analysis with culture, stool for white blood count (WBC) and culture if diarrhea present, chest X-ray, and lumbar puncture.
(b) Patient is 1–3 months old: CBC with deferential, urine analysis with culture, stool for WBC and culture if diarrhea present, Chest X-ray (if fever is 39 degrees, white blood cells is more than or equal to 20,000/mm^2, or respiratory signs are present), Lumbar puncture (if ill appearing).
(c) Patient is 3–36 months old: CBC with deferential, urine analysis with culture, stool for white blood cells and culture if diarrhea present, chest X-ray (if fever is 39°, white blood cells is more than or equal to 20,000/mm^2, or

respiratory signs are present), lumbar puncture (if neurological or meningeal signs are present).

8. Management and education: share differential diagnosis and prognosis.
   (a) Educate the patient on the following: the correct way of monitoring body temperature (rectal is the most accurate in infants and toddlers), the correct dose of antipyretic medication, and physical means of fever control. Examples of these are: wearing light clothing, taking a shower or bath in room-temperature water, and applying water compresses (made with room-temperature water) to the neck, axillae, and inguinal regions, where blood vessels are bigger, will help promote evaporation.
   (b) Patient less than 28 days old: begin empiric antibiotic treatment after cultures have been obtained : ampicillin and gentamicin, or ampicillin and cefotaxime.
   (c) Older children: manage according to the symptoms or investigation findings.
9. Arrange referral and follow up as needed:
   (a) Consider admission for all neonates and any child with no focus found.
10. Give reading educational materials if any.
11. Discuss health maintenance and screening for age.
12. Communication skills: organized approach, mixed questioning styles (open- and close- ended questions), active listening, clear language, and reflection on patient's ICE.

History Taking and Management of a Child Presenting with Skin Rash

36

Sumiya Taheri and Shammah Al Memari

Learning Objectives
- How to master history taking for a child presenting with rash?
- How to demonstrate a good understanding of common and potential differential diagnosis for children presenting with fever?
- How to perform focused exam for a child presenting with rash?
- How to provide management for children presenting with rash?

Focus areas on **infectious causes** (viral: chicken pox, erythema infectiosum, roseola infantum, measles, rubella, hand-foot-mouth disease, molluscum contagiosum, herpes simplex, pityriasis rosea. Bacterial causes: impetigo, cellulitis, scarlet fever, staphylococcus scalded skin syndrome. Fungal causes: candida, tinea. Parasitic causes: scabies, cutaneous larva migrans), versus **non-infectious causes** of rash: inflammatory (atopic dermatitis, contact dermatitis, seborrheic dermatitis, diaper dermatitis, intertrigo), drug reaction, systemic disorders (Kawasaki disease, urticaria, psoriasis, Henoch-Schonlein purpura), neonatal rashes (Melia, erythema toxicum neonatorum, neonatal acne, benign cephalic pustulosis).

S. Taheri
Ambulatory Healthcare Services, Abu Dhabi, United Arab Emirates

S. Al Memari (✉)
Abu Dhabi, United Arab Emirates

1. Introduce yourself and establish good rapport.
2. Identify the complaint (rash or eruption): site, onset, initial appearance, duration, progression (how it has evolved), exacerbating and reliving factors (prior trials of treatment), red flags (fever, inconsolability, extreme irritability, mucosal inflammation, respiratory distress, blistering, or skin sloughing), other associated symptoms (itching, stinging, tenderness, discharge, pain, fatigue, respiratory symptoms), and possible provoking factors:
   (a) Recent upper respiratory tract infection, gastroenteritis, insect bite, travel, or stress (new school, new baby at home, abuse).
   (b) History of contact.
   (c) Attendance to day care.
   (d) Exposure to new pets, medications, personal care products, or clothes.
   (e) Allergies.
   (f) History of previous similar episode and management if any.
   (g) Diarrhea or abdominal pain.
   (h) Explore secondary issues: sleep disturbance or feeling embarrassed.
3. Determine underlying health status: vaccination status, ongoing health issues, and medication history.
4. Explore parent's ideas, concerns and expectations (ICE), effect of the complaint on quality of life: "How does the problem affect you and your child? Has the problem affected his or her attendance at school or day care?"
5. Social and family history: similar complain in the family, any chronic skin conditions, or skin cancer in the family?
6. Examination:
   (a) Vital signs and general appearance of the child: assess for fever and ill looking child.
   (b) Examination of the rash (consider utilizing a Woods lamp or dermoscopy): assess morphology, color, lesion pattern (scattered, clustered, linear, or coalescing), number, distribution across affected areas, consistency, and texture. Classify accordingly (refer to Table 36.1 for details).
7. Investigations: if and only if history and physical exam was not sufficient to make a diagnosis.
8. Aim at identifying potential life threats as follows:
   (a) Complete blood count, renal function tests, and stool tests (if suspecting hemolytic uremic syndrome).
   (b) Gram stain and cultures of blood and cerebrospinal fluid (if suspecting meningococcemia).
   (c) Skin biopsy.
9. Management: refer to Table 36.2 for details.
10. Give reading educational materials if any.
11. Discuss health maintenance and age-appropriate screening.

12. Arrange for the following as needed:
    (a) Admission: if a life-threatening diagnosis is suspected or found.
    (b) Referral: if diagnosis is not clear or rash is refractory to treatment.
    (c) Follow up: in 1–2 weeks.
13. Communication skills: organized approach, mixed questioning styles (open and close ended questions), active listening, clear language, and reflection on patient's ICE.

Table 36.1 Appearance of common rashes in children

Probable diagnosis	Morphology
Chicken pox	Polymorphic rash including macules and papules that evolve to form clear vesicles, looks like **dew drop on a rose petal**
Erythema infectiosum	Initial "*slapped cheek*" rash, often with circumoral pallor, followed by erythematous maculopapular rash on trunk which spreads to limbs
Roseola infantum	Light pink discrete, irregular, circular or elliptical macules, or papules that **blanch under pressure**
Measles	Red maculopapular rash, typically beginning on the head and spreading downward. Small bluish-white lesions on buccal mucosa (*Koplik spots*) may be present during prodrome of fever, cough, coryza, and conjunctivitis
Hand-foot-mouth disease	Maculopapular or vesicular rash on palms or soles. Typically associated with painful oral lesions and fever
Pityriasis rosea	Round to oval rose-colored scaling patches, 5–10 mm in diameter, with long axes of lesions oriented along cleavage lines (**Christmas tree appearance**)
Impetigo	Vesicles, pustules, and honey-colored crust
Scarlet fever	Red, finely papular rash with "*sandpaper*" texture, typically on trunk and then spreading to extremities
Staphylococcus scalded skin Syndrome (SSSS)	Widespread sandpaper-like erythema, large bullae, and eroded, red, moist, "varnish-like" areas of denuded skin
Candida	Bright red patches, often with small **collarettes,** plus **satellite** lesions
Scabies	Small *burrows*, papules, and vesicles, usually pruritic. Usually located on *interdigital web spaces*, flexor wrists, axillae, areolae, umbilicus, genitals, knees, and ankles. Infants may have lesions on palms, soles, and head
Atopic dermatitis	Erythematous papules, excoriations, scaling, **lichenification**
Seborrheic dermatitis or cradle cap	Yellowish, white, or off-white patches with greasy scales on scalp
Milia	White or yellow 1–2 mm papules on nose, chin, cheeks, and forehead
Erythema toxicum neonatorum	Tiny 2–3 mm, yellow or white macules and papules on erythematous base that may evolve into pustules

Table 36.2 Management of common skin rashes in children

Diagnosis		Management

Viral exanthems		• Usually, self-limiting
		• Support by symptomatic management
		  – Paracetamol for fever, headaches, aches, and pains
		  – Soothing creams and emollients for pruritis
		  – Oral antihistamines for pruritus

Bacterial rashes	Impetigo	• Topical antibiotics: Mupirocin 2% ointment (3 times daily for 5–7 days) or Fusidic acid 2% cream (3 times daily until healed or up to 14 days) • Oral antibiotics (if there are numerous lesions or ulceration): oral cephalexin (25–50 mg/kg/day in 3–4 divided doses) for empiric therapy in children
	Staphylococcal scalded skin infection (SSSS)	• Pain control • Wound care (consider intensive or burn unit care for patients with extensive skin involvement) • Intravenous hydration to compensate for fluid loss, which may be profound • Antibiotic therapy for SSSS should be directed at *Staphylococcus aureus*

Fungal rashes	Candida infections	• Candida diaper dermatitis
		  – Nystatin, miconazole, or ketoconazole applied topically twice daily to affected areas
		  – Advise to start or restart the habit of applying barrier preparations like zinc oxide
		• Oral thrush
		  – Nystatin oral suspension
		  – Consider concomitant treatment of maternal breast area

	Tinea (corporis, capitus, cruris, pedis, onychomycosis)	• Topical antifungals (usually sufficient): apply to the lesion and 2 cm surrounding normal skin 1–2 times daily for about 14 days or 1 week after lesion disappears. Clotrimazole 1% twice daily for 4 weeks, econazole 1% once daily for 2 weeks, or ketoconazole 2% cream once daily for 2 weeks • Oral antifungals: consider if extensive infection: Griseofulvin for 2–4 weeks (FDA approved for tinea corporis in adults and children who are more than or equal to 2 years old)
Parasitic infestations	Scabies	• Topical permethrin 5% is for patients more than or equal to 2 months of age • To be applied by the patient and all household or close contacts who are more than or equal to 2 months of age, even if they are asymptomatic • Should be applied to all skin surfaces from the neck to toes (with special attention to groin and interdigital webs). To be kept for 8–14 h and then washed off. Nails should be clipped short and artificial nails should be avoided. This application should be repeated in 1 week

(continued)

Table 36.2   (continued)

Diagnosis		Management
Auto-immune rashes	Atopic dermatitis	• Daily bathing and showering should be limited to about 5 min • Use moisturizers (emollients) generously, including application soon after bathing. Avoid fragrances or dyes in moisturizers as they may be irritating • Use topical corticosteroids on flaring areas and as maintenance therapy for patients with recurrent flares
	Kawasaki disease	• Intravenous immunoglobulins (IVIG) as soon as the diagnosis is made and within the first 10 days of illness • Moderate or high dose of aspirin (30–50 or 80–100 mg/kg/day) for 14 days or until afebrile for 2–3 days. Switch thereafter to low-dose aspirin (3–5 mg/kg/day) and continue until the absence of coronary artery abnormalities are confirmed (6–8 weeks after the start of illness)
	Henoch- Schonlein purpura	• Self-limited disease • Supportive management (usually all that the patient needs, especially if patient has normal kidney functions): nutrition, hydration, and electrolyte balance • Consider intravenous fluids and pain killers for patients with severe pain or vomiting

History Taking and Management of a Child Presenting with Ear Pain

37

Shaima Lari, Buthaina Al Maskari,
and Shammah Al Memari

Learning Objectives
- How to master history taking for children presenting with earache?
- How to demonstrate a good understanding of common causes of earache?
- How to provide management of common causes of earache?

Focus areas includes common causes such as cerumen impaction otitis externa (fungal, bacterial, acute, or chronic), otitis media (with or without tympanic membrane perforation), or foreign body.

1. Introduce yourself and establish good rapport.
2. Identify the complaint:
   (a) Site, onset, duration, timing, character, relieving and aggravating factors, radiation, triggers (recent upper respiratory tract infection, fever, disturbed sleep, swimming, trauma).
   (b) If recurrent: check frequency, associated hearing or speech impairment.

S. Lari
Sheikh Shakhbout Medical City, Abu Dhabi, United Arab Emirates

B. Al Maskari
Ambulatory Healthcare Services, Abu Dhabi, United Arab Emirates

S. Al Memari (✉)
Abu Dhabi, United Arab Emirates

    (c) Associated symptoms: ear discharge, ear itching, hearing loss, dental problems, dermatitis, psoriasis, excessive cleaning, fingernail injury, and recent trauma to the ear.

3. Explore child's vaccination status and any ongoing problems: Down syndrome, immunocompromised state, asthma, malnutrition, learning difficulties, or failure to thrive.
4. Question regular use of medications: long term antibiotics.
5. Explore patient's or parent's ideas, concerns and expectations (ICE).
6. Social and family history: child neglect, developmental circumstances, smoking in adults.
7. Examination: refer to "Chap. 72" for further details.
8. Order required investigations: ear swab for culture and audiometry to assess for hearing loss.
9. Management: refer to Table 37.1 for details.
10. Arrange referral:
    (a) Urgently if the patient has a foreign body with injury to the tympanic membrane or middle ear, especially if the foreign body is in direct contact with the tympanic membrane or involves button batteries.
    (b) Routinely if patient has recurrent or chronic symptoms (needs myringotomy), complications (like hearing loss or learning difficulties), or malignant otitis externa.
11. Give reading educational materials if any.
12. Discuss health maintenance and age-appropriate screening.
13. Arrange for follow up.
14. Communication skills: organized approach, mixed questioning styles (open- and close-ended questions), active listening, clear language, and reflection on patients ICE.

Table 37.1 Management of ear pain in children

Diagnosis		Management
Cerumen impaction		• If asymptomatic, do not interfere as cerumen is a protective material • Options for removal include: cerumenolytics agents, manual removal, or suctioning
Otitis media		• Oral antibiotic: first line being Amoxicillin (80–90 mg/kg in two equally divided doses, 12 hours apart) for 7–10 days • Regular antipyretics and analgesics as Paracetamol or Ibuprofen
Otitis externa (advice swimming avoidance)	Bacterial	• Prescribe topical antibiotic drops for 7 days such as: ciprofloxacin-dexamethasone otic preparations
	Fungal	• Antifungal ear drops such as clotrimazole otic solution
Foreign body		• Attempt removal by forceps under direct visualization if and only if patient is cooperative

History Taking and Management of a Neonate Presenting with Jaundice

38

Shammah Al Memari

Learning Objectives
- How to master history taking for a neonate presenting with jaundice?
- How to perform a focused exam for a neonate presenting with jaundice?
- How to approach and manage a neonate presenting with jaundice?

For adults presenting with jaundice, please refer to Chap. 19 titled "History Taking and Management for Adults presenting with Jaundice" for detailed guidance.

Focus areas include major causes such as physiological jaundice, conjugated hyperbilirubinemia (biliary obstruction such as neonatal cholestasis, biliary atresia), inherited hemolytic anemias (hereditary spherocytosis and elliptocytosis), iso-immune-mediated hemolysis (blood group or rhesus incompatibility), erythrocyte enzymatic defects (glucose-6-phosphate dehydrogenase deficiency, pyruvate kinase deficiency, and congenital erythropoietic porphyria), or impaired bilirubin conjugation (Gilbert syndrome, Crigler Najjar syndrome).

S. Al Memari (✉)
Abu Dhabi, United Arab Emirates

© The Author(s), under exclusive license to Springer Nature Singapore Pte Ltd. 2024
S. Lari et al. (eds.), *Family Medicine OSCE: First Aid to Objective Structured Clinical Examination*, https://doi.org/10.1007/978-981-99-5530-5_38

151

1. Introduce yourself and establish a good rapport with the parents.
2. Identify the complaint (icterus):
   (a) Onset, timing, duration, relieving and aggravating factors, course (same, improving, and worsening), and prior episodes.
   (b) Associated symptoms: fever, decreased activity, poor feeding, recurrent vomiting, abdominal pain, easy bruisability, bleeding, dark urine, or pale stool.
   (c) Potential provoking factors: recent travel, exposure to ill persons or contaminated food, or animals.
3. Medical history:
   (a) Perinatal history: maternal illness during pregnancy (hepatitis, sexually transmitted diseases, or any other infection), anomaly scan results, gestational age at delivery (premature or full term), blood and rhesus type.
   (b) Current feeds: fully breastfeed infant or taking formula (which type of formula)?
   (c) Diagnosed diseases: chronic hemolysis, cystic fibrosis, or hepatocellular disease.
   (d) Medication history: paracetamol, antibiotics (macrolides and augmentin), anticonvulsant, anti-tuberculosis medication.
4. Explore parents' ideas, concerns and expectations (ICE).
5. Family and social history: autoimmune diseases, genetic disease, or infantile death.
6. Examination:
   (a) General: growth, nutritional, developmental, and mental status (active or fatigued).
   (b) Neck: cervical lymphadenopathy (suggests Epstein–Barr virus infection).
   (c) Skin and eye: pallor (suggests anemia), yellowish discoloration, bruising, bleeding, or rash.
   (d) Cardiovascular exam: tachycardia (suggests anemia).
   (e) Abdomen exam: rule out hepatosplenomegaly, masses, or ascites.
   (f) Neurological examination: muscle tone and deep tendon reflexes.
7. Order required investigations:
   (a) Initial testing: complete blood count, reticulocyte count, blood smear, liver function test (including direct, total bilirubin level, gamma-glutamyl transferase (GGT)), coagulation profile, lactate dehydrogenase (LDH), and haptoglobin.
   (b) Other tests to consider: hemoglobinopathy, autoimmune hemolytic screen, G6PD level, viral hepatitis screen, autoimmune hepatitis screen, cystic fibrosis, metabolic studies, ceruloplasmin level, 24 urinary copper excretion, and liver biopsy.
   (c) Ultrasound imaging to exclude other causes of obstruction.

8. Management and education: share differential, and potential diagnosis, manage accordingly:
   (a) Screen newborns of 35 weeks' gestational age or greater using total serum bilirubin or transcutaneous bilirubin at 24 to 48 hours of life or before hospital discharge.
   (b) Determine the need to initiate phototherapy or exchange transfusion based on the nomogram thresholds for both treatments, considering gestational age and other parameters.
   (c) Manage other patients according to the cause. Refer to Table 38.1 for details.
   (d) Reassure if physiological jaundice is identified.
9. Give reading educational materials if any.
10. Arrange for follow-up.
11. Communication skills: organized approach, mixed questioning styles (open- and close-ended questions), active listening, clear language, and reflection on parents' ICE.

Table 38.1 Management of neonatal jaundice according to the diagnosis

Probable diagnosis	Management
Viral hepatitis	– Reassure the parents that it is mostly self-limiting condition – Provide fluid and nutritional support – Monitor liver function test – Refer to infectious disease subspecialist or hepatologist if liver enzymes are not improving
Autoimmune hepatitis	– Advise to treat even if asymptomatic – Refer to immunologist or hepatologist – Schedule hepatitis A and B vaccines
Galactosemia	– Advise restricting dietary galactose intake with lactose-free formula and life-long elimination of dairy product sources of lactose and galactose for all types of galactosemia – Offer admission if patient has metabolic derangement – Refer to metabolic diseases' subspecialist
Biliary atresia	– Provide aggressive nutritional support – Refer to surgery for consideration of Kasai procedure or liver transplant

History Taking and Management of a Child Presenting with a Limp

Eman Al Hayayi, Noora Al Blooshi,
and Shammah Al Memari

Learning Objectives
- How to master history taking for a limping child?
- How to perform a focused exam for a limping child?
- How to approach and provide management tips for children with limp?

Focus areas
- **Bone conditions** (osteoblastoma, osteoid osteoma, clubfoot, congenital short femur, developmental dysplasia of the hip, Legg-Calve-Perthes disease (LCPD), slipped capital femoral epiphysis (SCFE), osteomyelitis, limb length discrepancy, Ewing sarcoma, leukemia, osteochondritis dissecans, stress fracture, fracture).
- **Intraarticular conditions** (hemarthrosis, septic arthritis, acute rheumatic fever, reactive arthritis, transient synovitis, juvenile rheumatoid arthritis (JIA)).
- **Neuromuscular conditions** (cerebral palsy, muscular dystrophy).
- **Soft tissue conditions** (Osgood Schlatter disease, Sever's disease, myositis, sprains, and strains).
- **Spinal conditions** (diskitis and spinal cord tumor).

E. Al Hayayi · N. Al Blooshi
Ambulatory Healthcare Services, Abu Dhabi, United Arab Emirates

S. Al Memari (✉)
Abu Dhabi, United Arab Emirates

© The Author(s), under exclusive license to Springer Nature Singapore Pte Ltd. 2024
S. Lari et al. (eds.), *Family Medicine OSCE: First Aid to Objective Structured Clinical Examination*, https://doi.org/10.1007/978-981-99-5530-5_39

1. Introduce yourself and establish a good rapport with the mother or father.
2. Identify the complaint (limping): affected limb, presence of pain (in same limb or referred), onset, duration, timing (diurnal, nocturnal, or cyclic), course (same, improving, or worsening), any previous episodes, relieving and aggravating factors (worse or improved with movement), possible provoking factors (recent infection (upper respiratory tract, gastrointestinal, or urinary)), or trauma (fracture, foreign body, or soft tissue injury), associated symptoms and red flags. Work-out the differentials accordingly (refer to Table 39.1 for details).
3. Further medical history:
   (a) Immunization status.
   (b) Ongoing diseases: history of sickle cell disease, hemophilia, or endocrine disorder (hypothyroid, panhypopituitarism, and hypogonadism).
   (c) Medication history: recent antibiotic use (penicillin, amoxicillin, or trimethoprim-sulfamethoxazole) or intramuscular vaccination.
   (d) Dietary history: Exclusively breastfed vs formula-fed (which type of formula).
4. Explore parent's ideas, concerns and expectations (ICE).
5. Social history: recent travel or history of tick bite, high risk sexual behavior and drug use.
6. Family history: connective tissue disease, developmental dysplasia of the hip, sickle cell disease, or hemophilia.
7. Examination:
   (a) General: check weight, height, and vital signs.
   (b) Skin: asses for rash, erythema, warmth, and discoloration.
   (c) Back examination: look for scoliosis or pilonidal area abnormalities.
   (d) Extremities: refer to Table 39.2 for details
8. Order required investigations:
   (a) Initial work-up: complete blood count, erythrocyte sedimentation rate, C-reactive protein, thyroid function test, and metabolic panel.

Table 39.1 Differential diagnosis of a limping child

Sign and symptoms		Probable diagnosis
Fever, night sweats, fatigue, rash, weight loss, anorexia, easy bruising with joint restriction, or swelling		Septic arthritis, JIA, systemic lupus erythematosus, leukemia, or acute rheumatic fever
Swelling or morning stiffness	For less than 6 weeks	Reactive arthritis
	For more than 6 weeks	JIA or post-streptococcal reactive arthritis
Pain limited to hip or anterior thigh or knee	Less than 3 years old	Developmental dysplasia of the hip
	2–10 years old with short stature	LCPD
	More than 10 years old	SCFE (typically overweight teenager), or transient synovitis

Table 39.2 Focused examination of lower extremities in a child complaining of limping

Look	• Symmetry • Foot position • Gait • Range of motion • Footwear
Measure	• Leg-length (measured from anterior iliac spine to medial malleolus)
Palpate	• Swelling • Mass
Examine	• Sensation • Reflexes

   (b) X-ray in Frog-leg position or bilateral anterior-posterior images: (look for deformity of femoral head in LCPD and displacement of femoral head in SCFE).

   (c) Further investigations if indicated: blood test (including serum growth hormone and blood smear), bone scan, joint ultrasound with or without aspiration, or MRI of the hip.

9. Management and education: share differential diagnosis and prognosis.

   (a) Limping child with normal imaging: analgesics (NSAIDs), reassurance and out-patient follow up.

   (b) Toddler's fracture (even if it is suspected, but imaging is negative): short leg cast, splint or walker boot. If pain persists, repeat imaging in 7–10 days.

   (c) Slipped capital femoral epiphysis (*SCFE*): Advise to avoid weight bearing. Surgical fixation: **almost unavoidable to prevent avascular necrosis** (consider prophylactic intervention for the other hip).

   (d) Legg-Calve-Perthes disease (*LCPD*): primarily treated with conservative approach using analgesics, mobilization, and monitoring. Surgical intervention can be used when indicated (femoral osteotomy).

10. Refer as needed: physiotherapy, rheumatology, orthopedics, or oncology.

11. Give reading educational materials if any.

12. Discuss health maintenance and screening for age.

13. Arrange for follow up.

14. Communication skills: organized approach, mixed questioning styles (open- and close-ended questions), active listening, clear language, and reflection on patient's ICE.

History Taking and Management of a Child Presenting with Cough

40

Noora Al Blooshi and Shammah Al Memari

Learning Objectives
- How to master the history of taking of a child presenting with cough?
- How to demonstrate good understanding of differential diagnosis of cough in children?
- How to provide management and treatment of child presenting with cough?

For adults with cough, please refer to Chap. 6, titled: history taking and management of patients presenting with cough.

Focus areas on reactive airway disease, asthma, upper or lower respiratory tract infections such as bronchiolitis, foreign body in the respiratory tract, aspiration, somatic cough syndrome, or tic cough.

1. Introduce yourself and establish good rapport with the patient and the parents.
2. Identify the complaint (cough):
   (a) Onset, duration, timing, course (same, improving, or worsening), and prior episodes.
   (b) Nature (wet or dry) and quality (barking, croupy, paroxysmal, and staccato).

N. Al Blooshi
Ambulatory Healthcare Services, Abu Dhabi, United Arab Emirates

S. Al Memari (✉)
Abu Dhabi, United Arab Emirates

(c) Possible provoking factors: preceding feeds, swallowing, exercise, exposure to cold air, allergens, nonspecific irritants, emotional stress. Recent travel. History of contact.

(d) Relieving and aggravating factors.

(e) Red flags: sudden onset, onset during feeding, reduced level of consciousness, oral intake or urinary output, failure to thrive, cyanosis, hemoptysis, or night sweats.

(f) Associated symptoms: shortness of breath, tachypnea, drooling, difficulty swallowing or speaking, dysphagia, stridor, wheeze, croup, retracted muscle of ribs (using accessory muscles).

(g) Work-out the differential accordingly: refer to Table 40.1 for details.

3. Further medical history:

(a) Past medical history: neonatal history of infection, prematurity, atopic dermatitis, recurrent ear or nose infection, response to antibiotics and bronchodilators.

(b) Medication history: use of over-the-counter cough medication.

(c) Immunization status of the child.

(d) Social history: exposure to cigarette smoke, recent pet in the house, living condition, attending daycare or preschool.

4. Family history: respiratory diseases, history of atopy, and cystic fibrosis.

5. Explore parent's ideas, concerns and expectations (ICE).

6. Examination:

(a) General: vital signs, measurements plotted on growth chart and developmental review.

(b) Skin and extremities: evidence of atopic dermatitis, clubbing, or cyanosis.

(c) Ear, nose, and throat exam: external ear canal for foreign bodies or wax impaction, tympanic membrane for fluids or sign of infection, nose for polyps, halitosis, throat for tonsillar enlargement or exudate.

(d) Chest examination: Look for deformities, use of accessory muscles, or signs of hyperinflation. Assess breathing: any wheeze, stridor, or diminished breath sounds.

(e) Cardiac examination: heart sounds, murmurs, and dextrocardia.

Table 40.1 Differential diagnosis of infant with cough

Probable diagnosis	Characteristics of cough
Viral infection	Cough with a runny nose, sore ear or throat, fever, or irritability
Foreign body inhalation	Cough that starts suddenly after episode of choking or with unilateral wheeze
Asthma	Cough with wheeze and breathlessness
Pulmonary tuberculosis	Cough with hemoptysis, night sweats, weight loss, exposure to high-risk individuals, or travel to endemic areas
Laryngomalacia	Cough, stridor, wheeze, and recurrent respiratory infection
Cystic fibrosis	Cough with gastrointestinal symptoms

7. Order required investigations:
   (a) Initial testing: complete blood count with differential, electrolytes, chest X-ray, Gram stain and culture.
   (b) Further testing if indicated: Immunoglobulin E level if atopy is suspected (non-specific), antigen test for Bordetella pertussis, sweat chloride test for cystic fibrosis, Mantoux or Quantiferon test for tuberculosis, and PH monitoring if gastroesophageal reflux disease is suspected in children with chronic cough (more than 4 weeks duration) without a cause.
8. Arrange referral to:
   (a) Emergency department if a foreign body is suspected.
   (b) Pulmonary if unclear diagnosis or uncontrolled asthma.
9. Management and education: share differential and probable diagnosis, as well as prognosis:
   (a) Conservative management: Remove or reduce environmental triggers. For acute bronchitis: assess hydration, oxygen saturation >90, nasal suctioning. Limited evidence on the use of nebulized normal saline and medication such as bronchodilators, racemic epinephrine, steroids, and antiviral or immunoglobulin therapy.
   (b) Consider trial of asthma treatment if patient has risk factors for asthma.
   (c) Consider **antibiotic** if patient has productive cough or if **pneumonia** is suspected and consider further investigation and chest X-ray if cough lasted more than 8 week.
10. Give reading educational materials if any.
11. Discuss health maintenance and screening for age.
12. Arrange for follow-up.
13. Communication skills: organized approach, mixed questioning styles (open- and close-ended questions), active listening, clear language, and reflection on patient's ICE.

History Taking and Management of a Patient Presenting with Infantile Colic

41

Abeer Al Naqbi, Buthaina Al Maskari, and Shammah Al Memari

Learning Objectives
- How to master history taking for an infant presenting with colic?
- How to perform a focused exam for an infant presenting with colic?
- How to approach and provide management tips for infant presenting with colic?

Focus areas includes infantile colic characteristics (Wessel's Criteria), intussusception, strangulated bowel in view of umbilical hernia, cow milk allergy, parental anxiety, maternal depression, or infant abuse.

1. Introduce yourself and establish a good rapport.
2. Identify the complaint:
    (a) Onset: age when the problem first started, how long has the problem been there, and time of the day that episodes usually happen.
    (b) Duration: length of the crying episodes.
    (c) Infant's behavior otherwise: active baby or lethargic.
    (d) Aggravating and relieving factors.

A. Al Naqbi · B. Al Maskari
Ambulatory Healthcare Services, Abu Dhabi, United Arab Emirates

S. Al Memari (✉)
Abu Dhabi, United Arab Emirates

© The Author(s), under exclusive license to Springer Nature Singapore Pte Ltd. 2024
S. Lari et al. (eds.), *Family Medicine OSCE: First Aid to Objective Structured Clinical Examination*, https://doi.org/10.1007/978-981-99-5530-5_41

  (e) Associated symptoms: urine or stool abnormalities, blood in urine or stool, fever, irritability, skin rash, shortness of breath, cyanosis, apnea, vomiting, change in appetite, poor weight gain or weight loss.
3. Work out if the baby fits the Wessel criteria (rule of 3):
  (a) Child is less than 3 months of age.
  (b) Colic episodes last (cumulative) more than 3 hours per day.
  (c) Occurs more than 3 days per week.
  (d) Persists more than 3 weeks.
4. Rule out organic reasons: hair tourniquet around fingers or toes, constipation, anal fissure, or signs of otitis media.
5. Rule out red flags:
  (a) Sudden crying, projectile vomiting, absence of bowel motion, rectal bleeding, and red currant jelly stool (suggests intussusception or intestinal malrotation or pyloric stenosis).
  (b) Signs of testicular torsion.
  (c) Signs of intracranial bleeding (shaken baby syndrome).
6. Explore parent's ideas, concerns and expectations (ICE).
7. Understand family dynamics:
  (a) How do parents deal with the colic?
  (b) Availability of family support, especially if young mother or first child.
8. Verify the child's developmental milestones and that vaccinations are up to date.
9. Past medical history: prenatal, natal, and postnatal periods: any previous medical illnesses or hospital admissions.
10. Examination:
  (a) Check weight, height, and plot them on the growth chart.
  (b) Assessing general appearance and level of distress.
  (c) Look for signs of organic causes: fever, ear infection, pulse for tachycardia, hand for hair tourniquet, abdomen for umbilical hernia.
  (d) Hernia, distension or tenderness, and genitalia for testicular torsion.
11. Order required investigations as indicated by the history and physical examination (infantile colic is a diagnosis of exclusion).
12. Management and education:
  (a) Describe the condition to the parents and caregivers: explain that the cause is unknown. Reassure them that colic passes by the age of 3–5 months. Acknowledge their feelings of frustration, exhaustion, and guilt.
  (b) Consider potentially soothing measures: Five **S**: harmless and potentially helpful, **s**waddling, **s**ide or **s**tomach position, **s**hushing sounds or "white noise," **s**winging, and **s**ucking (breast feeding or pacifier). Changing the type of formula or bottle used for formula-fed children might help. Maternal diet modification might be helpful too. Generally avoiding foods that cause gas can help. Explain that medications do not help.
13. Give reading educational materials if any.
14. Discuss health maintenance and screening for age.
15. Arrange for follow-up and referral if needed.
16. Communication skills: organized approach, mixed questioning styles (open- and close-ended questions), active listening, clear language, and reflection on patient's ICE.

History Taking and Management of a Child Presenting with Enuresis

42

Reem Al Mansoori, Buthaina Al Maskari, and Shammah Al Memari

Learning Objectives
- How to master history taking for a child presenting with enuresis?
- How to perform a focused exam for a child presenting with enuresis?
- How to approach and provide management tips for a child presenting with enuresis?

Hints Enuresis is not diagnosed in children younger than 5 years. Diagnostic and Statistical Manual of Mental Disorders (DSM) IV criteria to diagnose enuresis: 5 years old or above child with enuresis 3 times per week or more for 3 months or more. Recurrence after at least 6 months of urinary continence suggests secondary enuresis. Differential diagnosis includes urinary tract infection (UTI), bladder dysfunction, constipation, diabetes, hyperthyroidism, diabetes insipidus, obstructive sleep apnea, seizure disorder, psychological stress, and sexual abuse.

R. Al Mansoori · B. Al Maskari
Ambulatory Healthcare Services, Abu Dhabi, United Arab Emirates

S. Al Memari (✉)
Abu Dhabi, United Arab Emirates

1. Introduce yourself and establish good rapport.
2. Identify the complaint by explaining to the patient, "First, I need to ask you a few questions to evaluate the problem."
   (a) "How old is the child?"
   (b) "Since when he or she is bed wetting?" (duration).
   (c) "How often?" (Diurnal, nocturnal, or both).
   (d) "With or without encopresis?"
   (e) "Ever attained continence? If yes, then for how long?" (Primary or secondary).
   (f) "Now I will ask you a few questions to check if there is any specific cause that we can treat": Frequency or burning micturition (suggests urinary tract infection). Constipation. Limp, swallowing difficulty, or seizures (suggest neurological problems). Polyuria or polydipsia (suggest diabetes mellitus). Snoring or apnea (suggest adenoid or tonsillar hypertrophy).
3. Rule out red flags: dysuria, straining to urinate, combined diurnal and nocturnal enuresis, genital or rectal pain or discharge, or child abuse (ask gently: "psychological disturbances are present in one third of patients with secondary enuresis. Do you think something of this sort could have happened to your child? Any new adult or baby at home? Who takes care of him? Who takes him to school? How is his school performance?").
4. Explore ongoing problems: chronic medical or behavioral problems.
5. Question regular use of medications such as diuretics.
6. Social history: stressful events (newborn, new housemaid, parental conflict).
7. Family history of diabetes or enuresis ("Enuresis is more common in patients with a family history. If one parent was affected, the child has 40–50% risk. If both were affected, it rises to 70%. If a sibling is affected the risk increases as well").
8. Explore patient's and parent's ideas, concerns and expectations (ICE), as well as the effect of the complaint on the quality of life.
9. Examination:
   (a) Vitals and measurements: plot them on growth chart.
   (b) Ear, nose, and throat examination: look for adeno-tonsillar hypertrophy.
   (c) Abdominal examination: look for signs of constipation, abdominal mass, or costovertebral angle tenderness.
   (d) Genitalia: any hypospadias, epispadias, meatal stenosis, labial adhesions, or signs of vulvovaginitis.
   (e) Rectal examination: look for perianal excoriation, evaluate perianal sensation and rectal sphincter tone.
   (f) Focused back and neurological evaluation: including gait, muscle tone, strength, and any lumbosacral abnormalities (hair tuft).
10. Order investigations as indicated:
    (a) Urinalysis and culture.
    (b) Complete blood count, glucose level, and thyroid stimulating hormone.

    (c) Renal and bladder ultrasound.

    (d) Voiding cystourethrography.

    (e) Urodynamic studies.

11. Management and education: share diagnosis and prognosis:

    (a) Reassure family in case of primary enuresis: "Enuresis is a common problem. 15% of 5 years old children have it. However, 15% of those suffering from the problem grow out of it each year so that by age of 14 years only 1–2% still have it."

    (b) Treat any coexisting conditions: like constipation or sleep disorders.

    (c) Conservative approach: Lifestyle modification: attempt voiding 4–7 times a day as well as before going to bed and restrict fluid intake in the evening. Bed alarm with or without star chart. Keeping a record: fluid-intake diary, micturition-defecation diary, or frequency-volume chart) as it helps assessing constipation and enuresis severity, as well as monitoring treatment response. Consider motivational interviewing therapy for selected patients.

    (d) Pharmacological management: Desmopressin.

12. Give reading educational materials if any.

13. Discuss health maintenance and screening for age.

14. Arrange for follow-up and referral as needed.

15. Communication skills: organized approach, mixed questioning styles (open- and close-ended questions), active listening, clear language, and reflection on patient's ICE.

History Taking and Management of a Female Presenting with Hirsutism

43

Buthaina Al Maskari and Shammah Al Memari

Learning Objectives
- How to master history taking for a patient presenting with hirsutism?
- How to perform a focused exam for a patient presenting with hirsutism?
- How to approach and provide management tips for a patient presenting with hirsutism?

Focus areas include polycystic ovarian syndrome (PCOS), ovarian or adrenal tumors, virilization, and Cushing syndrome.

1. Introduce yourself and establish a good rapport.
2. Identify the complaint: onset (age and any provoking factors), duration, progression (same, worsening, or improving), modality and frequency of practiced (waxing, threading, laser), site (upper lip, chin, chest, abdomen, or buttocks), and associated symptoms. Work out the differentials accordingly (refer to Table 43.1 for details).

B. Al Maskari
Ambulatory Healthcare Services, Abu Dhabi, United Arab Emirates

S. Al Memari (✉)
Abu Dhabi, United Arab Emirates

© The Author(s), under exclusive license to Springer Nature Singapore Pte Ltd. 2024
S. Lari et al. (eds.), *Family Medicine OSCE: First Aid to Objective Structured Clinical Examination*, https://doi.org/10.1007/978-981-99-5530-5_43

Table 43.1 Common causes of hirsutism and their clinical features

Disease	Clinical features
Adrenal or ovarian tumors	Temporal baldness, clitoromegaly, breast atrophy, deepening of the voice, and obesity
PCOS	Acne, truncal obesity, amenorrhea or oligomenorrhea, and androgenetic alopecia
Cushing syndrome	Moon face, buffalo hump, purple striae, central obesity, easily bruises, depression, menstrual irregularity and thin hair
Prolactinoma	Galactorrhea, headache, and visual disturbances

3. Explore the patient's, and parent's ideas, concerns and expectations (ICE) and the effect of the complaint on quality of life.
4. Menstrual history: age of menarche, regularity, last menstrual period, and infertility.
5. Explore ongoing problems: medical and surgical history.
6. Question regular use of medications: steroids, androgens, Danazol (used to treat endometritis), phenytoin, minoxidil, diazoxides, and cyclosporine.
7. Social and family history: family history of hirsutism or ovarian tumors.
8. Examination:
   (a) Vitals and measurement (including body mass index).
   (b) Signs of virilization: deepening of the voice, temporal or crown balding, increased muscle mass, or evidence of clitoromegaly.
   (c) Skin: look for any acne, acanthosis nigricans, or stria, define hirsutism pattern and grade
   (d) Abdominal and pelvic exam: any mass?
9. Order required investigations:
   (a) Initial testing: total testosterone level.
   (b) Further testing is indicated when hirsutism is associated with other symptoms as follows: if patient has amenorrhea or oligomenorrhea, check beta-human chorionic gonadotropin (B-hCG), prolactin, follicle stimulating hormone, luteinizing hormone, thyroid stimulating hormone and early morning 17 hydroxyprogesterone level, while if there are signs of Cushing's syndrome, or acromegaly, check 24-hour urinary excretion of free cortisol, late-night salivary cortisol, or low-dose dexamethasone level.

Table 43.2 Management of hirsutism

Management approach	Intervention
Conservative	Photo-epilation-based hair removal: laser therapy, intense pulsed light, or electrolysis
Pharmacotherapy	Topical Eflornithine (Vaniqa) cream twice daily (slows new hair growth)
Oral (first line)	Combined oral contraceptive pills
Oral (second line)	Antiandrogen (spironolactone)

    (c) Imaging: US of the pelvis followed by CT scan: as further workup of severe hyperandrogenemia (to exclude ovarian or adrenal androgen secreting tumor).

10. Management and education: refer to Table 43.2 for details.
11. Arrange referral as needed to:
    (a) Endocrine if signs of virilization noted.
    (b) Gynecology for further treatment of PCOS.
    (c) Dermatology or cosmetology for conservative management.
12. Give reading educational materials if any.
13. Discuss health maintenance and age-appropriate screening.
14. Arrange for follow-up.
15. Communication skills: organized approach, mixed questioning styles (open- and close-ended questions), active listening, clear language, and reflection on patient's ICE.

History Taking and Management of a Female Presenting with a Breast Mass

44

Abeer Al Naqbi, Noora Al Blooshi, and Shammah Al Memari

Learning Objectives
- How to master history taking for a patient presenting with breast mass?
- How to perform a focused exam for a patient presenting with breast mass?
- How to approach and provide management tips for a patient presenting with breast mass?

Hint Carcinoma is more likely to present at peri-menopausal stage, whereas fibroadenoma is more common in young women.

1. Introduce yourself and establish a good rapport.
2. Explore patient's ideas concerns and expectation (ICE).
3. Identify the complaint:
   (a) Onset ("When and how did you first notice it?"), age at onset, and duration since then.
   (b) Any change in size over time or in relation to the menstrual cycle (fibroadenosis may produce a painful, lumpy breast prior to menstruation).
   (c) Associated symptoms: redness, fever, discharge, or pain (commonest causes infection (as in acute mastitis or breast abscess), and fibroadenosis

A. Al Naqbi · N. Al Blooshi
Ambulatory Healthcare Services, Abu Dhabi, United Arab Emirates

S. Al Memari (✉)
Abu Dhabi, United Arab Emirates

© The Author(s), under exclusive license to Springer Nature Singapore Pte Ltd. 2024
S. Lari et al. (eds.), *Family Medicine OSCE: First Aid to Objective Structured Clinical Examination*, https://doi.org/10.1007/978-981-99-5530-5_44

175

(cyclical or acyclic). Uncommon causes include carcinoma or Tietze's disease (idiopathic costochondritis, usually in the second rib).
   (d) Predisposing events: trauma (fat necrosis) or breast feeding (mastitis or abscess).
   (e) History of previous breast mass.
   (f) Any risk factors for breast cancer: advanced age, overweight or obese, high breast density, prior thoracic radiation exposure, long history of unopposed estrogen (menarche before 12 years of age, menopause after 55 years of age, and nulli-parity or age older than 35 years at first delivery), breast cancer genes mutation (BRCA1 or BRCA2), first degree relative with breast or ovarian cancer.
4. Past medical and surgical history: previous breast mass, atypical hyperplasia, or lobular carcinoma in situ, one prior breast biopsy (regardless of results), personal history of breast or ovarian cancer.
5. Medication history: history of hormone therapy or oral contraceptives' use.
6. Social history: smoking or alcohol consumption (more than one drink per day).
7. Examination (ideally performed the week after menses, as breast tissue is least engorged):
   (a) Inspect: breasts for asymmetry, obvious masses, skin changes (such as dimpling, inflammation, rashes), or nipple abnormalities (such as discharge or retraction).
   (b) Palpate while patient is supine and her arms overhead (a commonly described method for clinical breast examination emphasizes using the pads of the middle three fingers, moving in dime sized circular motions while applying light, medium, and deep pressure at each point along a vertical strip pattern): starting with breast tissue including the nipple areolar complex, then squeeze the nipple gently to elicit any discharge, followed by the axillae, supraclavicular area, chest wall, and abdomen (for hepatomegaly).
   (c) For any mass, describe its: size, location (quadrant), consistency (hard, firm, or soft), borders (discrete or ill-defined), mobility (mobile or fixed), and overlying skin changes. Refer to Table 44.1 to assist you in classifying it accordingly.
8. Order required investigations:
   (a) Diagnostic mammography.
   (b) Ultrasound.
   (c) BRCA gene mutation test if indicated (refer to Table 44.2 for details).

Table 44.1 Interpreting the characteristics of a breast mass

Diagnosis	Description
Carcinoma or non-infective	Hard, poorly defined margin with or without evidence of tethering
Fluctuant fibrocystic	Hard, discrete lump, fluctuant
Fibroadenoma	Hard, discrete lump, solid with smooth surface
Soft lipoma or lax cyst	Soft, mobile, and painless

Table 44.2 Indications for BRCA gene mutation testing in patients presenting with breast lumps

First degree relative:
- 2 first degree relatives with breast cancer, 1 of whom was diagnosed at age 50 or younger
- First degree relative with bilateral breast cancer

First or second degree relative:
Combination of 3 or more with having breast cancer regardless of age
Or
Combination of 2 or more with having ovarian cancer regardless of age
Or
Combination of both breast and ovarian cancer

History of breast cancer in male relative

Table 44.3 Indications for surgical referral in a patient with breast lump

1. Excisional biopsy as indicated by initial imaging

2. Patient has a history of breast cancer **With** suspicious symptoms such as
   - Unilateral symptoms
   - Nipple distortion
   - Persistent skin changes
   - Bloody discharge

3. Patient is a male (especially if 50 years old or above with a unilateral, firm subareolar mass with or without nipple distortion, or associated skin changes)

4. Patient is a female:
   - Post-menopausal or
   - 30 years old or above: If she has **discrete lump that persists after her next period or**
   - Below 30 years old: If she has:
     - A lump that is fixed and hard
     - An enlarging lump
     - Other reasons for concern such as family history

9. Management and education:
   (a) Explain to the patient: Breast lumps are very common in women and cause considerable anxiety. However, most are benign, that is, not cancerous. Some women have naturally lumpy breasts due to the nature of their breast tissue and this is usually no reason for concern. In many instances the lumps turn out to be areas of thickening of normal breast tissue. Figures from breast clinics report that the three most common causes of breast lumps are Fibrocystic disease; a mammary dysplasia (32% of the cases), Fibroadenoma, or "breast mouse" (23% of the cases): a smooth, discrete breast lump consisting of fibrous and adenomatous (glandular) tissue, cancer (22% of the cases), others: simple cysts, fat necrosis, milk (lactation) cysts, papilloma of the duct, and mammary duct ectasia.
   (b) Pharmacological management: analgesic for painful breasts, antibiotics for breast abscess or cellulitis.

10. Arrange for referral if indicated:
    (a) Referral to a breast surgeon based on the indications outlined in Table 44.3.
    (b) Referral to an interventional radiologist for fine needle aspiration in case imaging reports reveal a suspicious lesion.

11. Give reading educational materials if any.
12. Discuss health maintenance and screening for age.
13. Arrange for follow up.
14. Communication skills: organized approach, mixed questioning styles (open- and close-ended questions), active listening, and reflection on patient's ICE.

History Taking and Management of a Female Presenting with Dysuria

45

Dana Al Marzooqi, Sumiya Taheri,
and Shammah Al Memari

Learning Objectives
- How to master history taking for a female presenting with dysuria?
- How to perform a focused exam for a female presenting with dysuria?
- How to approach and provide management tips for a female presenting with dysuria?

Focus areas include *dermatologic causes* (irritant or contact dermatitis, lichen sclerosis, lichen planus, psoriasis, Bechet syndrome), *infectious causes* (cystitis, urethritis, pyelonephritis, vulvovaginitis, cervicitis, other sexually transmitted diseases), *anatomical causes* (urethral stricture or diverticulum), *drug related causes* (spermicides, topical deodorants, opioids, ketamine), *endocrine causes* (atrophic vaginitis, endometriosis), *idiopathic casues* (interstitial cystitis or bladder pain syndrome), or *neoplastic causes* (paraurethral leiomyoma, bladder, renal, vaginal, or vulvar cancer).

D. Al Marzooqi · S. Taheri
Ambulatory Healthcare Services, Abu Dhabi, United Arab Emirates

S. Al Memari (✉)
Abu Dhabi, United Arab Emirates

© The Author(s), under exclusive license to Springer Nature Singapore Pte Ltd. 2024
S. Lari et al. (eds.), *Family Medicine OSCE: First Aid to Objective Structured Clinical Examination*, https://doi.org/10.1007/978-981-99-5530-5_45

179

1. Introduce yourself.
2. Establish a good rapport.
3. Identify the complaint:
    (a) Duration, site, onset, character, timing (relation to sexual activity), radiation, relieving and aggravating factors.
    (b) Associated symptoms: frequency, urgency, incontinence, hematuria, malodorous urine and nocturia, fever, back, flank or suprapubic pain, nausea, vaginal discharge, or dyspareunia.
    (c) Risk factors: newlyweds, pregnancy, catheter use, elderly, or anatomical abnormalities.
    (d) Red flags (exclude pyelonephritis, sepsis): high grade fever, vomiting, or severe pain.
4. Explore patient's ideas, concerns and expectations (ICE), and effect of the complaint on quality of life.
5. Explore ongoing problems: past medical history (diabetes, ureteric stones), recurrent urinary tract infections, or cystitis.
6. Question about any regular use of medications.
7. Social history: marital status, risk of sexually transmitted infections, abuse, or domestic violence.
8. Family history.
9. Examination:
    (a) Vital signs (elevated temperature with pyelonephritis, elevated blood pressure with glomerulonephritis).
    (b) Abdominal examination: palpate for suprapubic tenderness, costovertebral angle tenderness, or masses.
    (c) Genital examination if indicated by history: vulvar lesions, vulvovaginal atrophy, vaginal discharge, urethral mass or tenderness, and bimanual examination.
    (d) Other examinations as indicated by history: joint effusion, conjunctivitis for reactive arthritis, and neurological symptoms for neurogenic bladder.
10. Order required investigations:
    (a) Urine dipstick or analysis: for all patients to exclude urinary tract infection.
    (b) Urine culture and sensitivity: for any patient with risk of complicated urinary tract infection (pregnant, history of recurrent urinary tract infections, urolithiasis), or no response to initial treatment.
    (c) Vaginal swabs: if vaginal discharge is reported or seen.
    (d) Imaging: indicated if patient is suffering from complicated urinary tract infection, abscess is suspected, or patient shows no improvement with therapy.
    (e) Blood tests not needed unless suspecting sepsis or compromise in renal function.

11. Management and education: analgesics, increase fluid intake, and education about healthy habits (voiding after intercourse, proper perennial washing technique, avoid use of spermicides, and vaginal douche). Refer to Table 45.1 for further treatments.
12. Arrange a referral if needed.
    (a) Refer to urology for cystoscopy if patient has persistent hematuria.
13. Give reading educational materials if any.
14. Discuss health maintenance and screening for age.
15. Arrange for follow up.
16. Communication skills: organized approach, mixed questioning styles (open- and close-ended questions), active listening, clear language, and reflection on patient's ICE.

Table 45.1 Treatment of dysuria based on diagnosis

Diagnosis		Treatment
Vulvovaginitis	Vulvovaginal candidiasis	• Intravaginal azole therapy or oral fluconazole
	Bacterial vaginosis	• Oral or intravaginal metronidazole
	Trichomoniasis	• Oral metronidazole or tinidazole
	Atrophic vaginitis	• Vaginal lubricants, vaginal estrogen, and might consider systemic estrogen therapy if vasomotor symptoms present
Dermatologic problems		• Treat according to the cause, avoid triggers, keep area moisturized
Cystitis	Acute uncomplicated cystitis	• Empiric antimicrobial agents like nitrofurantoin (100 mg twice daily for 5 days) or trimethoprim-sulfamethoxazole (160/800 mg twice daily for 3 days)
	Acute cystitis with pyelonephritis	• Assess need for hospitalization and prescribe Ciprofloxacin (500 mg orally twice daily for 5–7 days)
	Interstitial cystitis	• Stress management: such as pelvic floor relaxation exercises, meditation, local application of heat or cold • Behavioral modifications: avoidance of food triggers, regular voiding, and avoidance of activities that exacerbate symptoms • Oral or intravesicular medications: Cimetidine (400 mg twice daily) or low-dose amitriptyline (25 to 5 mg at bedtime)

History Taking and Management of a Female Presenting with Recurrent Urinary Tract Infection

46

Sakina Al Bloushi and Shammah Al Memari

Learning Objectives
- How to master history taking for a female presenting with recurrent urinary tract infection?
- How to perform a focused exam for a female presenting with recurrent urinary tract infection?
- How to approach and provide management tips for a female presenting with recurrent urinary tract infection?

Focus areas include acute pyelonephritis atrophic vaginitis, bladder cancer, cystitis, genital herpes, interstitial cystitis, irritant cystitis, sexually transmitted infections, overactive bladder, urethritis, vaginitis.

---

1. Introduce yourself and establish a good rapport.
2. Identify the complaint:
   (a) Onset, duration, frequency, and risk factors (new or multiple sexual partners or frequent sexual activity).
   (b) Associated symptoms: fever, nausea, vomiting, abdominal pain, hematuria, vaginal discharge, relation to sexual activity, use of spermicide.

S. Al Bloushi
Ambulatory Healthcare Services, Abu Dhabi, United Arab Emirates

S. Al Memari (✉)
Abu Dhabi, United Arab Emirates

© The Author(s), under exclusive license to Springer Nature Singapore Pte Ltd. 2024
S. Lari et al. (eds.), *Family Medicine OSCE: First Aid to Objective Structured Clinical Examination*, https://doi.org/10.1007/978-981-99-5530-5_46

183

(c) Elaboration on previous episodes: frequency, previous treatment duration, previous investigation, and pelvic infections frequency, pelvic infections, previous investigations and treatment type and duration.

3. Explore the patient's ideas concerns and expectations (ICE), and the effect on the quality of life?
4. Ask about medical and surgical history: chronic diseases: diabetes, renal disorder (congenital, polycystic kidney, vesicoureteral reflux, stones), incontinence, neurological disorder, pelvic procedures, immunosuppressant medications use.
5. Ask about medication history.
6. Ask about family history: maternal history of urinary tract infection.
7. Ask about social history marital status, partner's view on her symptoms, smoking, and alcohol use.
8. Examination:
   (a) Vital signs: fever or signs of dehydration.
   (b) Abdomen: exclude suprapubic or costovertebral angle tenderness. Refer to "Chapter 76: Abdominal Examination" for further details.
   (c) Pelvis: signs of vaginitis and cervical motion tenderness (suggests pelvic inflammatory disease).
9. Order investigation as indicated:
   (a) Renal function test and glucose level to exclude diabetes.
   (b) Urinalysis and culture.
   (c) X-ray kidney, ureter, and bladder (KUB) to rule out anatomical or structural abnormality.
10. Management of recurrent urinary tract infection (**recurrent infection defined as 2 or more episodes in 6 months or 3 or more episodes in 1 year**):
    (a) Educate patients about risk factors of recurrence: frequent sexual activity, new sexual partners, and spermicide usage.
    (b) Start empiric antibiotics if new attack: nitrofurantoin (100 mg twice daily for 5 days), trimethoprim-sulfamethoxazole (160/800 mg for 3 days), a fluoroquinolone, or ciprofloxacin.
    (c) Discuss preventive measures elaborated in Table 46.1.
    (d) Give reading educational materials if any.
11. Discuss health maintenance and screening for age.
12. Arrange for follow-up in 2 to 3 days or earlier if fever, nausea, or vomiting.
13. Communication skills: organized approach, mixed questioning styles (open- and close-ended questions), active listening, clear language, and reflection on patients' ICE.

Table 46.1 Management approach for recurrent UTI in women

Management approach	Intervention
Lifestyle modifications	– Increased fluid intake – Develop the habit of postcoital voiding and avoid delayed voiding – Use cotton undergarments – Follow a wiping pattern from the front to the back passage
Other non-pharmacological factors	– Cranberry products: They seem to notably reduce the recurrence of symptomatic cystitis, although there is no clear evidence about dosage or duration of use
Prophylactic antibiotics	*Continuous prophylaxis* – Indicated if the patient has had two urinary tract infections in the previous year – Options include Nitrofurantoin (50–100 mg) daily for 6–12 month, trimethoprim-sulfamethoxazole (40/200mg daily or three times per week for 6–12 months)
	Postcoital prophylaxis – Preferable in women with urinary tract infections temporally related to intercourse – Options include Nitrofurantoin (100mg once), trimethoprim-sulfamethoxazole (40/200mg or 80/400 mg once)

History Taking and Management of a Female Presenting with Vaginal Discharge

47

Khuloud Al Hammadi, Kawthar Al Ameri,
and Shammah Al Memari

Learning Objectives
- How to master history taking for females presenting with vaginal discharge?
- How to perform a focused exam for females presenting with vaginal discharge?
- How to approach and provide management tips for females presenting with vaginal discharge?

Focus areas on
- *Infectious causes:* candida infection, bacterial vaginosis, trichomonas vaginalis, chlamydia and gonorrhea, pelvic inflammatory disease (PID).
- *Non-infectious causes:* vaginal atrophy, irritants, and allergens.

K. Al Hammadi
Sheikh Khalifa Medical City, Abu Dhabi, United Arab Emirates

K. Al Ameri
Ambulatory Healthcare Services, Abu Dhabi, United Arab Emirates

Faculty of Family Medicine Residency Program, Sheikh Khalifa Medical City, Abu Dhabi, United Arab Emirates

S. Al Memari (✉)
Abu Dhabi, United Arab Emirates

1. Introduce yourself.
2. Establish a good rapport.
3. Identify patient complaint: onset, duration, description (amount, color, appearance, odor, and consistency), relation to menstrual cycle (normal mid-cycle discharge is sticky like mucous), stage of pregnancy, intercourse, or possible exposure to an allergen (vaginal douches, soap, bubble bath, spermicidal foam jelly or creams, use of tampons, pessaries, or condoms). Work out your differentials accordingly:
    (a) **Candida** (thrush) most common: white, thick, lumpy, **cheese like** or curd-like discharge.
    (b) *Bacterial vaginosis*: milky or off-white discharge, *fishy odor,* burning, or itching.
    (c) *Trichomonas vaginalis*: copious, **frothy, greenish-yellow discharge, offensive odor**, vulvar congestion, erythema with pruritus vulvae.
    (d) *Chlamydia or Gonorrhea*: asymptomatic or *purulent* vaginal discharge, pelvic pain (PID), and joint pain.
    (e) Associated symptoms: dysuria (suggests urinary tract infection), pruritus, abdominal and pelvic pain (suggests irritable bowel syndrome, constipation, endometriosis), dyspareunia, fever, or skin rash (suggests toxic shock syndrome: staphylococcus infection due to tampons use), altered bleeding pattern (suggests side effect of hormonal method of contraception).
4. Menstrual history: including last menstrual period.
5. Sexual history: single or multiple partners, symptoms in partner, possible exposure to sexually transmitted infections (STI).
6. Past medical history: diabetes or frequent urinary tract infections.
7. Medications history: contraceptives, steroids, antifungals, and antibiotics.
8. Social and family history: smoking or alcohol use.
9. Explore the patient's ideas concerns and expectations (ICE), and effect of the problem (physical, social, and psychological).
10. Examination: skin, oral mucosa, abdomen, joints, genitalia (discharge characteristics, adnexal tenderness), rectum.
11. Order required investigations as indicated:
    (a) High vaginal swab for wet mount or whiff test. Refer to Table 47.1 for details of interpretation of the test.
    (b) Endocervical swab or urine test for chlamydia and gonorrhea PCR.
    (c) Investigations to rule out other causes if needed: blood sugar and urinalysis for diabetes, midstream urine for urinary tract infection, serum follicle stimulating hormone (FSH), and estradiol for estrogen deficiency (perimenopausal, inadequate hormonal replacement therapy).
12. Arrange referral if resistant to treatment or PID is diagnosed.

Table 47.1 Diagnostic findings in common infectious causes of vaginal discharge

Infection	Test	Finding
Candida	Vaginal PH	Normal
	Whiff test	Negative
	Wet mount with potassium hydroxide (KOH)	Pseudohyphae (budding yeast cells)
Bacterial vaginosis	Vaginal PH	More than 4.5
	Whiff test	*Positive*
	Wet mount with potassium hydroxide (KOH)	*Clue cells* (epithelial cells coated with coccobacilli)
Trichomonas vaginalis	Vaginal PH	More (5–6)
	Whiff test	Variable
	Wet mount with potassium hydroxide (KOH)	More than 10 white blood cells per high-power field (WBC HPF) and motile trichomonas

13. Management and education (avoid empiric therapy):
    (a) Candida: Topical azole therapy intra-vaginally for 7days or oral fluconazole for complicated cases.
    (b) Bacterial vaginosis: Metronidazole (Flagyl) 500 mg twice daily for 7 days (avoid concomitant use with *alcohol if within 24 hours* (alert patient about interaction causing headache, flushing, vomiting, and psychotic symptoms) *or disulfiram if within 2 weeks*). (avoid using metronidazole with alcohol and disulfiram (if taken concomitantly it will cause side effect such as flushing, vomiting and psychotic symptoms).
    (c) Trichomonas vaginalis (treat sexual partner): Metronidazole 500 twice daily for 7 days or 2 g single dose.
    (d) Chlamydia (treat sexual partner and treat for Gonorrhea concomitantly): Azithromycin 1 g single oral dose or Doxycycline 100 mg twice daily for 7 days.
    (e) Gonorrhea (treat for Chlamydia concomitantly): single dose of ceftriaxone 250 mg intramuscular (IM) plus single oral dose.
    (f) Advice on wearing cotton underwear, pad changing, wash cotton underwear with hot water.
    (g) Consider referral if patient has red flags: failure of initial treatment, pelvic pain, or persistent systematic symptoms (fever, nausea, or vomiting).
14. Give reading educational materials if any.
15. Discuss health maintenance and screening for age.
16. Arrange for follow-up.
17. Communication skills: organized approach, mixed questioning styles (open- and close- ended questions), active listening, clear language, and reflection on patient's ICE.

History Taking and Management of a Female Presenting with Infertility

48

Kawthar Al Ameri, Sumiya Taheri,
and Shammah Al Memari

Learning Objectives
- How to master history taking for females presenting with infertility?
- How to perform a focused exam for females presenting with infertility?
- How to approach and provide management tips for females presenting with infertility?

Focus areas
- *Ovulatory dysfunction* (up to 25% of the cases): polycystic ovarian syndrome (PCOS), obesity, intense exercise, chemotherapy/radiotherapy, thyroid dysfunction, smoking, diminished ovarian reserve, primary ovarian insufficiency, or endocrine disorders (hyperprolactinemia, pituitary tumors, hypothalamic amenorrhea).
- *Tubal factors* (up to 20% of the cases): pelvic inflammatory disease (PID), tubal obstruction, peri-tubal adhesions, ectopic pregnancy, or pelvic surgery.
- *Cervical, uterine, or peritoneal disorders* (up to 13% of the cases): congenital malformations, leiomyoma, endometriosis, endometrial polyps, or luteal phase deficiency.
- *Idiopathic* (up to 28% of the cases).

K. Al Ameri
Ambulatory Healthcare Services, Abu Dhabi, United Arab Emirates

Faculty of Family Medicine Residency Program, Sheikh Khalifa Medical City, Abu Dhabi, United Arab Emirates

S. Taheri
Ambulatory Healthcare Services, Abu Dhabi, United Arab Emirates

S. Al Memari (✉)
Abu Dhabi, United Arab Emirates

191

S. Lari et al. (eds.), *Family Medicine OSCE: First Aid to Objective Structured Clinical Examination*, https://doi.org/10.1007/978-981-99-5530-5_48

1. Introduce yourself.
2. Establish good rapport.
3. Identify the complaint: duration (differentiate between primary and secondary infertility), prior infertility treatment, red flags (delayed puberty, visual disturbances, or virilization), and other associated symptoms (refer to Table 48.1 for details).
4. Menstrual and gynecologic history: age at menarche, date of last menstrual period (LMP), frequency, duration, flow (heavy or light), associated pain, spotting between periods, vasomotor symptoms, history of amenorrhea, secondary dysmenorrhea (endometriosis), pelvic inflammatory disease, or sexually transmitted diseases.
5. Sexual history: desire, coital frequency, use of vaginal lubricants, timing of sexual activity in relation to cycle, and pain with coitus.
6. Obstetric history:
   (a) Previous pregnancies and deliveries.
   (b) Miscarriages, induced abortions, dilatation, and curettage (Asherman's syndrome).
   (c) Postpartum infections and bleeding (Sheehan syndrome).
7. Explore patient's ideas, concerns and expectations (ICE).
8. Past medical history: diabetes, cystic fibrosis, Crohn's disease, tuberculosis, sarcoidosis, malignancy, chemotherapy, or radiotherapy.
9. Medication history: oral contraceptive pills (OCP), anti-hypertensive medications, or anti-pyschotics.
10. Social history: martial relationship and duration of marriage, occupation, stressful events, marital conflicts, domestic violence, job instability, smoking, alcohol, or drug abuse.
11. Information about the husband:
    (a) Age and occupation (exposure to toxin, radiation).
    (b) History of previous marriage, children, and age of the youngest child.
    (c) Past medical history of mumps infection, varicocele, or undescended testis.

Table 48.1 Associated symptoms with female infertility and corresponding probable diagnoses

Associated symptoms	Probable diagnosis
Breast changes (including galactorrhea)	Prolactinemia
Hot flushes, changes in sexual desire, nervousness, palpitations	Premature ovarian failure
Facial hair, acne, obesity, deepening of voice	PCOS
Feeling bloated, increase abdominal size	Ovarian tumor
Obesity, cold intolerance, and constipation	Hypothyroidism
Diarrhea, hot intolerance, tremor, and sweating	Hyperthyroidism
Stress, diet, weight loss, and excessive exercise	Eating disorder or depression

Table 48.2 Time frame criteria for initiating female infertility evaluation

Criteria	Time to start evaluation
Women with an obvious cause for infertility or subfertility	Immediately
Woman 40 years old or more	
Woman 36 to 39 years old	After 6 months of frequent unprotected intercourse
Women with predisposing factors for infertility	
Women 35 year or younger without known risk factors for infertility	After 1 year of frequent unprotected sexual intercourse

12. Family history: mother and sisters' age of menarche and menopause, menstrual dysfunction, infertility, diabetes mellitus, autoimmune diseases, or chromosomal abnormalities.
13. Examination:
    (d) Vitals and measurements: including height, weight, and body mass index.
    (e) General appearance: dysmorphic features (as in Kallmann or Turner syndrome).
    (f) Visual acuity and visual field (in suspected prolactinoma).
    (g) Skin: hirsutism, acne, vitiligo (suggests autoimmune disease).
    (h) Neck: thyroid mass or enlargement (suggests thyroid disease).
    (i) Chest: any breast enlargement or galactorrhea?
    (j) Abdomen: assess for mass, organomegaly, distention, tenderness, ascites, or surgical scars.
    (k) Pelvis: size and shape of clitoris, vaginal or cervical abnormality, masses or discharge, size, shape, mobility, position of uterus, adnexal masses, or tenderness.
14. Order required investigations if any: refer to tables 48.2 and 48.3.
15. Management and education: share diagnosis and prognosis using simple language.
16. Give reading educational materials if any.
17. Arrange referral as indicated to gynecological or fertility clinic.
18. Discuss health maintenance and screening for age: pap smear, mammogram.
19. Arrange for follow up.
20. Communication skills: organized approach, mixed questioning styles (open and close ended questions), active listening, clear language, and reflection on patients' ICE.

Table 48.3 Females' infertility workup

Patient	Test	Additional comment
All	Partner's semen analysis	Always start with it
With suspected ovarian disorders	Midluteal serum progesterone	More than 6 ng per mL on day 21 of a 28-day menstrual cycle indicates ovulation and normal corpus luteal progesterone production
	Urinary luteinizing hormone level	For correlation with basal body temperature measurement
	- Follicle stimulating hormone - Prolactin - Thyroid stimulating hormone - Testosterone	Check levels in blood
With suspected ovarian or uterine abnormalities	Transvaginal ultrasound	
With suspected abnormalities of the endometrial cavity	Hysterosalpingogram	
With intrauterine abnormalities detected by hysterosalpingogram, such as polyps or adhesions	Hysteroscopy	
With inconclusive results on less-invasive tests	Laparoscopy	To confirm tubal or pelvic pathology

History Taking and Management of a Female Presenting with Amenorrhea

49

Kawthar Al Ameri, Buthaina Al Maskari, and Shammah Al Memari

Learning Objectives
- How to master history taking for females presenting with amenorrhea?
- How to perform a focused exam for females presenting with amenorrhea?
- How to approach and provide management tips for females presenting with amenorrhea?

Focus areas includes poly cystic ovarian syndrome (PCOS), thyroid disorders, premature ovarian failure, prolactinoma, anorexia nervosa, hypothalamic-pituitary-ovarian failure, Asherman's syndrome (uterine adhesions after dilation and curettage (D&C)), post-pill amenorrhea, or Sheehan's syndrome (pituitary necrosis following extreme blood loss).

K. Al Ameri
Ambulatory Healthcare Services, Abu Dhabi, United Arab Emirates

Faculty of Family Medicine Residency Program, Sheikh Khalifa Medical City, Abu Dhabi, United Arab Emirates

B. Al Maskari
Ambulatory Healthcare Services, Abu Dhabi, United Arab Emirates

S. Al Memari (✉)
Abu Dhabi, United Arab Emirates

© The Author(s), under exclusive license to Springer Nature Singapore Pte Ltd. 2024
S. Lari et al. (eds.), *Family Medicine OSCE: First Aid to Objective Structured Clinical Examination*, https://doi.org/10.1007/978-981-99-5530-5_49

1. Introduce yourself and establish a good rapport.
2. Identify the complaint: onset (primary or secondary amenorrhea), with detailed menstrual history: menarche, last menstrual period (LMP), frequency, duration, amount, dysmenorrhea, withdrawal bleeding (think of secondary amenorrhea).
3. Gynecologic and obstetric history: previous pregnancies, abortions, or complications.
4. Medication history:
   (a) Anti-hypertensive medications.
   (b) Some antipsychotics and antiemetic medications can increase prolactin levels.
   (c) Radiation or chemotherapy can cause pituitary dysfunction.
   (d) Gonadotropin-releasing hormone (GnRH) analogue decreases estrogen.
   (e) Danazol increases androgen.
   (f) Contraceptives (oral, injectable, implants, or intra uterine devices).
5. Red flags: delayed puberty, visual disturbance, clitoromegaly, virilization, or temporal hair loss.
6. Work out the differentials accordingly. Refer to Table 49.1 for details.
7. Explore patient's ideas, concerns and expectations (ICE), and hidden agenda (what has brought her to clinic? perhaps an unwanted pregnancy).
8. Past medical history: diabetes mellitus, cystic fibrosis, Crohn's disease, tuberculosis, sarcoidosis, pernicious anemia, myasthenia gravis, malignancy.
9. Social history: stressful events, marital conflicts, domestic violence, job instability, smoking, alcohol, or drug abuse.

Table 49.1 Differential diagnosis of amenorrhea

Causes	Clinical presentation
Physiologic causes	• Pregnancy (nausea, vomiting, frequent urination, breast fullness, and fatigue) • Breast feeding
Vaginal issues	• Imperforated hymen: Monthly dysmenorrhea with no bleeding
Ovarian issues	• Premature ovarian failure: Hot flushes, sexual desire changes, nervousness, and palpitations • Polycystic ovarian syndrome: Facial hair, acne, and obesity • Deepening of voice, clitoromegaly (suggests virilization) • Feeling bloating, increased abdominal size (suggest ovarian tumor) • History of mumps (oophoritis)
Uterine issues	• History of septic abortion, previous dilation and curettage, or other surgeries
Hypothalamic issues	• Stress from job, school, or family, dieting and weight loss, excessive exercise (eating disorders), and depression
Pituitary issues	• Prolactinoma: headache, visual disturbance, or nipple discharge. • *Sheehan's syndrome: history of significant post-partum hemorrhage*
Other endocrine disorders	• Hypothyroidism: obesity, cold intolerance, or constipation • Hyperthyroidism: diarrhea, heat intolerance, tremors, or sweating • Cushing disease: weight gain, moon face, buffalo hump, purple striae, and fragile skin • Congenital adrenal hyperplasia (CAD): early puberty and short stature

10. Family history: mother and sister's ages at menarche and menopause, menstrual dysfunction, infertility, diabetes, autoimmune diseases, or chromosomal abnormalities.
11. Examination:
    (a) General appearance (dysmorphic features: Kallmann or Turner syndrome).
    (b) Vitals and measurements (including body mass index).
    (c) Visual acuity and visual fields testing (in suspected prolactinoma).
    (d) Thyroid examination.
    (e) Tanner staging (primary amenorrhea).
    (f) Skin: acne, hirsutism (virilization).
12. Order required investigations (tailored according to history and physical examination):
    (a) Blood: complete blood count (CBC), glucose, and hormones levels of Beta-HCG, prolactin (prolactinoma), follicle stimulating hormone (FSH), and luteinizing hormone (LH), if both low (suggest hypothalamic pituitary dysfunction) while LH to FSH ratio is 3 to 1 (suggests poly cystic ovarian syndrome), consider also dehydroepiandrosterone sulfate (DEHAS), free testosterone (Hyperandrogenism), 17-hydroxylase deficiency (congenital adrenal hyperplasia), and thyroid function test.
    (b) Pelvic ultrasound (uterine congenital anomalies and poly cystic ovarian syndrome).
13. Arrange referral to gynecology or endocrinology as necessary.
14. Management and education:
    (a) Share differential diagnosis and prognosis using simple language.
    (b) Advise according to the probable diagnosis.
15. Give reading educational materials if any.
16. Discuss health maintenance and screening for age: pap smear, Human Papilloma Virus (HPV) vaccine, mammogram, colonoscopy, advice regarding weight control, proper diet, and exercise.
17. Arrange for follow up.
18. Communication skills: organized approach, mixed questioning styles (open- and close-ended questions), active listening, clear language, and reflection on patient's ICE.

History Taking and Management of a Female Presenting with Dysmenorrhea

50

Kawthar Al Ameri, Buthaina Al Maskari,
and Shammah Al Memari

Learning Objectives
- How to master history taking for females presenting with dysmenorrhea?
- How to perform a focused exam for females presenting with dysmenorrhea?
- How to approach and provide management tips for a female presenting with dysmenorrhea?

Hints *primary dysmenorrhea* occurs with the absence of underlying pathology. *Secondary dysmenorrhea* results from specific pelvic pathology such as endometriosis or adenomyosis.

K. Al Ameri
Ambulatory Healthcare Services, Abu Dhabi, United Arab Emirates

Faculty of Family Medicine Residency Program, Sheikh Khalifa Medical City,
Abu Dhabi, United Arab Emirates

B. Al Maskari
Ambulatory Healthcare Services, Abu Dhabi, United Arab Emirates

S. Al Memari (✉)
Abu Dhabi, United Arab Emirates

© The Author(s), under exclusive license to Springer Nature Singapore Pte
Ltd. 2024
S. Lari et al. (eds.), *Family Medicine OSCE: First Aid to Objective Structured
Clinical Examination*, https://doi.org/10.1007/978-981-99-5530-5_50

1. Introduce yourself.
2. Establish a good rapport.
3. Identify the complaint:
   (a) Onset of dysmenorrhea (primary dysmenorrhea starts 6–12 months after menarche), duration of pain, intensity, radiation, relation to menses, associated symptoms, secondary activity restrictions (social, sport, or absenteeism from school or work).
   (b) Risk factors: age less than 20 years, nulliparity, heavy menses, losing weight, anxiety, depression, smoking and disruption of social support.
   (c) Red flags: abnormal uterine bleeding, menorrhagia, dyspareunia, noncyclic pain, changes in intensity and duration of pain, post-coital bleeding, intermenstrual bleeding, infertility, and abnormal pelvic examination findings that suggest underlying pathology (secondary dysmenorrhea as endometriosis and adenomyosis).
4. Obstetric and gynecological history:
   (a) Age at menarche, regularity of periods, flow (heavy or light), pregnancies, miscarriages.
   (b) Diagnosed gynecological problems, polyps, fibroids, or abnormal pap smear.
   (c) Sexual activity, sexually transmitted infections.
5. Explore patient's ideas, concerns and expectations (ICE).
6. Explore ongoing problems: past medical and social history.
7. Medications and allergy history.
8. Family history: ovarian cancer, endometrial cancer.
9. Social history: marital status, smoking, alcohol, employment, and quality of life.
10. Examination: per vaginal exam (looking for vaginal discharge or pelvic tenderness) if sexually active or if suspected endometriosis.
11. Investigations: trans-vaginal ultrasonography (endometrial thickness, masses, and ovarian cysts) and complete blood count for anemia (in cases of menorrhagia).
12. Arrange referral: for endometrial biopsy or laparoscopy if uncontrolled dysmenorrhea.
13. Management and education (share differential diagnosis and reassure if primary type):
    (a) Explain to the patient: Dysmenorrhea, a medical term for menstrual cramping, refers to the pain experienced by many women just before or at the onset of their menstrual periods. This pain, resembling a dull ache, is typically felt in the abdomen, lower back, hips, or inner thighs. It can commence shortly before or at the beginning of menstruation, lasting from 1 to 3 days. The intensity of the pain might be sufficient to hinder normal activities. Dysmenorrhea is categorized into two types: Primary dysmenorrhea, associated with common menstrual cramps, and secondary dysmenorrhea, linked to a disease or condition such as infection, ovarian cysts, or endometriosis, affecting the uterine lining.

    (b) Primary dysmenorrhea: non-steroidal anti-inflammatory drugs (NSAIDS), options include Ibuprofen (400–600 mg TID) or Mefenamic acid (500 mg initially then 250 mg q6hr for 3 days) to decrease pain and menstrual flow or Tranexamic acid to decrease menstrual flow. Hormonal contraception is second line.

    (c) Endometriosis: first line treatment is with hormonal contraceptives (combined estrogen-progestin therapy oral pills, transdermal patch, or vaginal ring).

    (d) Others: topical heat, exercise, and nutritional supplementation may be beneficial but not enough evidence to support the use of yoga, acupuncture, or massage.

14. Give reading educational materials if any.
15. Discuss health maintenance and screening for age.
16. Arrange for follow up and provide safety net.
17. Communication skills: organized approach, mixed questioning styles (open- and close- ended questions), active listening, clear language, and reflection on patient's ICE.

History Taking and Management of a Female with Menorrhagia

51

Kawthar Al Ameri, Buthaina Al Maskari, and Shammah Al Memari

Learning Objectives
- How to master history taking for females presenting with menorrhagia?
- How to perform a focused exam for females presenting with menorrhagia?
- How to approach and provide management tips for females presenting with menorrhagia?

Focus areas
- Anovulatory dysfunctional bleeding: irregular or infrequent periods, with blood flow (light or heavy) caused by hyperprolactinemia, Poly Cystic Ovarian Syndrome (PSOC), and antiepileptics or atypical antipsychotics.
- Ovulatory dysfunctional bleeding: regular bleeding intervals (every 24–35 days) caused by thyroid dysfunction, coagulation defects (von Willebrand disease), endometrial polyps, and submucosal fibroids.

K. Al Ameri
Ambulatory Healthcare Services, Abu Dhabi, United Arab Emirates

Faculty of Family Medicine Residency Program, Sheikh Khalifa Medical City, Abu Dhabi, United Arab Emirates

B. Al Maskari
Ambulatory Healthcare Services, Abu Dhabi, United Arab Emirates

S. Al Memari (✉)
Abu Dhabi, United Arab Emirates

© The Author(s), under exclusive license to Springer Nature Singapore Pte Ltd. 2024
S. Lari et al. (eds.), *Family Medicine OSCE: First Aid to Objective Structured Clinical Examination*, https://doi.org/10.1007/978-981-99-5530-5_51

1. Introduce yourself.
2. Establish a good rapport.
3. Identify the complaint (menorrhagia defined as more than 80 mL of blood loss per cycle): duration of bleeding (more than 7 days), onset, relation to menses, history of passage of clots, frequency of changing pads or tampons, associated symptoms (dysmenorrhea, bleeding elsewhere from oral cavity, bruising, melena, bleeding per rectum and symptoms of anemia), and activity restriction (social, sport) or absenteeism (school or work). Any red flags: advanced age, obesity, nulliparity, infertility, dyspareunia, diabetes mellitus, family history of colon cancer (it has the same genetic predisposition with endometrial cancer), long-term unopposed estrogen therapy, or a history of tamoxifen use.
4. Obstetric and gynecological history: age at menarche and menopause (for patient herself, her mother and sisters), regularity and nature of her periods, intermenstrual bleeding, pregnancies, or miscarriages. Any diagnosed gynecological problems, polyps, fibroids, abnormal pap smear (atypia). Sexual activity and sexually transmitted infections.
5. Explore patient's ideas, concerns and expectations (ICE).
6. Explore ongoing problems: past medical (anemia, thyroid disease, coagulation disorders) and social histories.
7. Medications (hormonal contraception, antiepileptics, atypical antipsychotics, or anticoagulants) and allergy history.
8. Family history: ovarian cancer, endometrial cancer, or bleeding disorders.
9. Social history: marital status, smoking, alcohol, employment, and quality of life.
10. Examination: general (obesity or hirsutism), skin (pallor, bruising, petechiae and acne), per vaginal exam (vaginal discharge or cervical motion tenderness, enlarged uterus or ovaries) if sexually active or if suspected endometriosis.
11. Investigations:
    (a) Childbearing age: pregnancy test, complete blood count, coagulation profile, Thyroid Stimulating Hormone (TSH), and prolactin.
    (b) Postmenopausal women: transvaginal ultrasonography or endometrial biopsy.
    (c) Endometrial polyps or uterine leiomyoma: saline-infusion, sonohysterography, or sonohysteroscopy.
    (d) Endometrial biopsy indicated in (looking for precancerous lesions and adenocarcinoma): in women more than 45 years or older, women less than 45 years old with risk factors for endometrial cancer, and women with excessive bleeding unresponsive to medical therapy.
12. Arrange referral: endometrial biopsy or laparoscopy.
13. Management and education (share differential diagnosis):
    (a) Explain to the patient: Menorrhagia refers to periods that are heavier than usual or last for 7 days or more each month. This condition can cause stress and may lead to anemia. Some women experience heavy periods during the early years of menstruation or in the years preceding menopause. Menorrhagia has various causes, such as hormonal changes, blood clotting

issues, and the presence of fibroids or polyps in the uterus. The most serious potential cause is uterine cancer. In cases where no apparent cause is found, a sample of the uterus may need to be taken to check for cells that could indicate cancer. Additionally, an ultrasound might be necessary. Treatment options are diverse and include hormone pills and surgical interventions. An intrauterine device (IUD) is an alternative for those averse to pills; it contains progestin, thinning the uterine lining to reduce bleeding and can remain in the body for up to 5 years. Surgical procedures, such as those involving freezing or heating the uterus and hysterectomy (uterus removal), are available for women who no longer wish to have children.

(b) Give general advice: Keep menstrual diary. Take iron supplements. Eat a well- balanced diet. Avoid aspirin if possible (may increase the bleeding).

(c) If the patient desires future fertility and has ovulatory bleeding: Non-Steroidal Anti- Inflammatory Drugs (NSAIDS), tranexamic acid or levonorgestrel intrauterine contraceptive device or injectable progestin.

(d) If the patient desires future fertility and has anovulatory bleeding (hyperplasia): Combined Oral Contraceptive Pills (COCP) or cyclic progestin 21 days or levonorgestrel intrauterine contraceptive device.

(e) Surgical management: If patient desires fertility: myomectomy of fibroids. In case of undesired fertility: endometrial ablation or uterine artery embolization or hysterectomy (definitive).

(f) Others: thyroid dysfunction, coagulation defects (Von Willebrand disease), endometrial polyps, and submucosal fibroids.

14. Give reading educational materials if any.
15. Discuss health maintenance and screening for age.
16. Arrange for follow up, safety net and reflect patient's ICE.
17. Communication skills: organized approach, mixed questioning styles (open- and close-ended questions), active listening, clear language, and reflection on patient's ICE.

History Taking and Management of a Female Presenting with Post-menopausal Bleeding

Shaima Lari, Sumiya Taheri,
and Shammah Al Memari

Learning Objectives
- How to master history taking of post-menopause women presenting with bleeding?
- How to perform a focused exam and investigation for females presenting with postmenopausal bleeding?
- How to provide management for postmenopausal bleeding?

Focus areas include uterine (genital tract atrophy, endometrial polyps, endometrial adenocarcinoma, endometrial hyperplasia), cervical (polyps, ectropion, cervicitis, carcinoma), vulvovaginal (atrophy, condyloma, infection, trauma, carcinoma), or other causes (postmenopausal hormonal therapy, anticoagulant use, hematuria, rectal bleeding).

S. Lari
Sheikh Shakhbout Medical City, Abu Dhabi, United Arab Emirates

S. Taheri
Ambulatory Healthcare Services, Abu Dhabi, United Arab Emirates

S. Al Memari (✉)
Abu Dhabi, United Arab Emirates

© The Author(s), under exclusive license to Springer Nature Singapore Pte Ltd. 2024
S. Lari et al. (eds.), *Family Medicine OSCE: First Aid to Objective Structured Clinical Examination*, https://doi.org/10.1007/978-981-99-5530-5_52

1. Introduce yourself and establish a good rapport.
2. Identify the complaint (postmenopausal bleeding (PMB) defined as any bleeding occurring 12 months after menopause or unscheduled bleeding while taking hormonal replacement therapy (HRT):
   (a) Onset of bleeding, duration, intensity of bleeds, age at menopause, date of Last Menstrual Period (LMP), associated symptoms (abdominal pain, bowel or urinary problems, weight loss, dyspareunia, post-coital bleeding, pallor, and fatigue), aggravating factors (trauma, intercourse, intimate partner violence).
   (b) Identify risk factors for endometrial cancer: obesity, diabetes mellitus, hypertension, Chronic un-ovulatory states [Poly Cystic Ovarian Syndrome (PCOS)], nulliparity, and hereditary nonpolyposis colorectal cancer (HNPCC).
3. Obstetric and gynecological history:
   (a) Age at menarche, regularity of periods, parity, miscarriages, breast feeding, sexual activity.
   (b) Diagnosed gynecological problems: sexually transmitted infections, polyps, fibroids, abnormal pap smear.
   (c) Last pap smear and results.
4. Explore patient's ideas, concerns and expectations (ICE).
5. Explore ongoing problems: past medical and social history.
6. Question about the use of any regular medication, allergies, Hormone Replacement Therapy (HRT): duration, type, and indication.
7. Family history: family history of colon ovarian, endometrial, and/or breast cancers.
8. Social history: marital status, smoking, alcohol, employment, quality of life.
9. Examination:
   (a) Vital signs, including patient's body mass index (BMI).
   (b) Pelvic examination: inspect for vaginal, cervical, urethral or rectal sites of bleeding, palpate for uterine size and position, palpate for adnexal masses.
10. Order required investigations:
    (a) Transvaginal ultrasound or endometrial biopsy EMB as first line investigations to rule out endometrial cancer; endometrial biopsy preferred, if TVU is done first any endometrial thickness > 4 mm warrants EMB (if patient is at high risk of endometrial cancer should undergo EMB regardless of TVU findings).
    (b) All patients should have a cervical smear.
    (c) Hysteroscopy: should be considered for women with persistent uterine bleeding with benign endometrial sampling or insufficient endometrial sampling after ultrasound.
    (d) If signs and symptoms of anemia present: CBC, ferritin.
11. Arrange referral: urgent for work up for endometrial cancer.
12. Management and education: share differential diagnosis and prognosis. Refer to Table 52.1 for details.
13. Give reading educational materials if any.
14. Discuss health maintenance and screening for age.
15. Arrange for follow up.

Table 52.1 Management of females with post-menopausal bleeding

Causes	Diagnosis	Management
Uterine causes	Endometrial polyps	Removal of all polyps indicated in postmenopausal women (risk of malignancy is higher in postmenopausal women
	Endometrial hyperplasia	Progesterone therapy or hysterectomy
	Endometrial adenocarcinoma	Depends on staging but mainly total hysterectomy and bilateral salpingo-oophorectomy
Vulvovaginal causes	Vulvovaginal candidiasis	Intravaginal azole therapy or oral fluconazole
	Bacterial vaginosis	Oral or intravaginal metronidazole
	Trichomoniasis	Oral metronidazole or tinidazole
	Atrophic vaginitis	Vaginal lubricants, vaginal estrogen, might consider systemic estrogen therapy if vasomotor symptoms present
Cervical causes	Polyps	Should be removed if they are symptomatic (bleeding, excessive discharge), large (≥3 cm), or appear atypical
	Abnormal cervical smear	The approach to treating cervical cancer is tailored based on the patient's age and the specific type of abnormality
Other causes of bleeding identified		Treat the identified cause with medication. if bleeding disorder refer to hematology

History Taking and Management of a Female Presenting with Urinary Tract Infection

53

Buthaina Al Maskari and Shammah Al Memari

Learning Objectives
- How to master history taking for females presenting with urinary incontinence?
- How to perform a focused exam for females presenting with incontinence?
- How to approach and provide management tips for females presenting with incontinence?

Focus areas include stress vs urge vs overflow incontinence. Any recurrent urinary tract infections or pelvic masses.

1. Introduce yourself.
2. Establish a good rapport.
3. Identify the complaint:
   (a) Onset (gradual or rapid).
   (b) Duration.
   (c) Frequency and progression (worsening, improving, or unchanged).
   (d) Timing (day or night).
   (e) Relieving or aggravating factors.

B. Al Maskari
Ambulatory Healthcare Services, Abu Dhabi, United Arab Emirates

S. Al Memari (✉)
Abu Dhabi, United Arab Emirates

© The Author(s), under exclusive license to Springer Nature Singapore Pte Ltd. 2024
S. Lari et al. (eds.), *Family Medicine OSCE: First Aid to Objective Structured Clinical Examination*, https://doi.org/10.1007/978-981-99-5530-5_53

(f) Associated symptoms: coughing, sneezing, and laughing (stress incontinence), urge, frequency, cannot hold urine (urge incontinence), hesitancy, poor stream, dribbling, incompletes emptying (obstructive incontinence), a sensation of heaviness or lump vaginally (vaginal prolapse), dysuria, fever (UTI), sexual dysfunction or symptoms.

4. Explore the patient's ideas, concerns and expectations (ICE):
   (a) Ideas: "What might be the cause of your urinary issues?"
   (b) Concerns: embarrassment, social struggle, depression, quality of life.
   (c) Expectations: "How you like me to help you today?"
5. Explore continuous problems: diabetes mellitus, recurrent UTIs, benign prostatic hyperplasia, obesity, menopause, stroke, and dementia.
6. Past medical, surgical, and family histories. Social history: employment, caffeine intake, smoking, alcohol, illicit drug use.
7. Medication use: Diuretics, tricyclic antidepressants, antihistamines, benzodiazepines, anticholinergics.
8. Examination: vitals, abdominal and pelvic examination looking for pelvic floor muscle function, vaginal atrophy, pelvic masses, and prolapse in females.
9. Investigations: urinalysis and urine culture for all patients, while the diagnosis is primarily clinically based on history and examination, additional testing may be conducted to support the diagnosis. This may involve assessing kidney function in the case of urinary retention, conducting a bladder stress test, measuring postvoid residual volume via ultrasound, and performing urodynamic testing.
10. Management:
    (a) Advise patients to keep a voiding diary, lose weight if obese, reduce caffeine, have a normal fluid intake, and smoke cessation.
    (b) Pelvic floor muscle Kegel exercises, bladder training, topical vaginal estrogen if peri or post-menopausal.
    (c) For stress incontinence, devices like pessaries, medications like duloxetine, last option is surgical therapy (mid-urethral sling).
    (d) For urge incontinence, medications are in two different classes: Antimuscarinics (oxybutynin and tolterodine) and Beta-3 adrenergic agents (mirabegron and vibegron).
11. Give reading educational materials if any.
12. Discuss health maintenance and screening for age.
13. Arrange for follow-up, consider referral if not improving on treatment, or the patient has vaginal prolapse requiring surgery.
14. Communication skills: organized approach, mixed questioning styles (open- and close-ended questions), active listening, clear language, and reflection on the patient's ICE.

Part IV

History-Taking and Management: Men's Health

History Taking and Management of a Male Presenting with Dysuria

54

Dhuha Al Ameri, Kawthar Al Ameri, and Shammah Al Memari

For details on females with dysuria, please refer to Chap. 45.

Learning Objectives
- How to master history taking for male patients presenting with dysuria?
- How to perform a focused exam for male patients presenting with dysuria?
- How to approach and provide management tips for male patients presenting with dysuria?

Focus areas include Sexually transmitted disease, penile lesions, pyelonephritis, cystitis, urethritis, epididymitis or orchitis, prostatitis, neoplasm, bladder, or kidney stones.

D. Al Ameri
Ambulatory Healthcare Services, Abu Dhabi, United Arab Emirates

K. Al Ameri
Ambulatory Healthcare Services, Abu Dhabi, United Arab Emirates

Faculty of Family Medicine Residency Program, Sheikh Khalifa Medical City, Abu Dhabi, United Arab Emirates

S. Al Memari (✉)
Abu Dhabi, United Arab Emirates

© The Author(s), under exclusive license to Springer Nature Singapore Pte Ltd. 2024
S. Lari et al. (eds.), *Family Medicine OSCE: First Aid to Objective Structured Clinical Examination*, https://doi.org/10.1007/978-981-99-5530-5_54

1. Introduce yourself and establish a good rapport.
2. Ask about the main presenting complaint using open questions.
3. Explore the patient's ideas, concerns and expectations (ICE).
4. Explore details of symptoms:
   (a) Frequency and pattern.
   (b) Associated symptoms: urgency, hesitancy, fever, hematuria, abdomen or pelvic pain, nocturia, hesitancy, terminal dribbling, poor stream, incontinence, weight loss or anorexia, urethral discharge, testicular masses, or testicular pain.
   (c) Sexual dysfunction, and sexual contacts: the presence of symptoms in partners.
5. Past medical history, social and family history.
6. Home medications and allergies to antibiotics if any.
7. Examination:
   (a) Abdominal exam, palpate kidneys, inguinal adenopathy.
   (b) Genital exam: penile ulcers or discharge, scrotal swelling or tenderness(epididymitis), tender per rectum exam (prostatitis).
8. Order required investigations: urine dipstick, urine culture, urethral discharge culture if present, and serum creatinine.
9. Management: share diagnosis, prognosis, and medications: analgesic and antibiotics. Consider prophylactic antibiotics as follows:
   (a) Chlamydia coverage: Azithromycin 1 gram orally as a single dose or Doxycycline 100 mg orally twice daily for 7 days.
   (b) Gonorrhea coverage: (Ceftriaxone 1 g IM).
   (c) Recurrent symptoms with the same partner (cover Trichomonas and Ureaplasma): **drug 1:** Metronidazole 500 mg orally daily for 5 days and **drug 2:** choose one of the following: Azithromycin 500 mg orally once daily for 5 days or Doxycycline 100 mg once daily for 7 days.
10. Health education in regards of self-care and prevention: increase water intake to 2–3 liters per day, schedule frequent voiding (before sleep, after intercourse), and practice safe sex.
11. Give reading educational materials if any.
12. Discuss health maintenance and screening for age.
13. Arrange for follow-up.
14. Communication skills: organized approach, mixed questioning styles (open- and close-ended questions), active listening, clear language, and reflection on patient's ICE.

History Taking and Management of a Male Presenting with Erectile Dysfunction

55

Dhuha Al Ameri, Noora Al Blooshi,
and Shammah Al Memari

Learning Objectives
- How to master history taking for male patients presenting with erectile dysfunction?
- How to perform a focused exam for male patients presenting with erectile dysfunction?
- How to approach and provide management tips for male patients with erectile dysfunction?

Focus areas include Metabolic syndrome, cardiovascular disease, endocrine disorders (hypogonadism, hyperprolactinemia, thyroid disorders), neurologic conditions (multiple sclerosis, spinal cord injury, Parkinson's disease, stroke), obesity, Peyronie disease, psychological conditions (anxiety, depression, history of sexual abuse, marital problems, stress), sedentary lifestyle, tobacco use. The majority of impotent patients do not complain directly about impotence. The candidate needs to suspect the hidden agenda from the patient's verbal and non-verbal cues, e.g., patient may ask for vitamins or any other tonics, or he may complain of backache or psychological symptoms.

D. Al Ameri · N. Al Blooshi
Ambulatory Healthcare Services, Abu Dhabi, United Arab Emirates

S. Al Memari (✉)
Abu Dhabi, United Arab Emirates

© The Author(s), under exclusive license to Springer Nature Singapore Pte Ltd. 2024
S. Lari et al. (eds.), *Family Medicine OSCE: First Aid to Objective Structured Clinical Examination*, https://doi.org/10.1007/978-981-99-5530-5_55

217

1. Introduce yourself.
2. Establish a good rapport.
3. Details of the complaint:
   (a) Onset (gradual or sudden) and course (static or progressing) of the impotence.
   (b) Degree of dysfunction (chronic, occasional, or situational).
   (c) Early morning and nocturnal erection (present or absent).
   (d) Degree and part of sexual cycle affected: desire, arousal, orgasm.
   (e) Is there another sexual partner or wife? And is the problem the same with her?
   (f) Precipitating factors: Is the marriage stable and happy? Does the wife contribute to the problem?
   (g) Associated symptoms: Gynecomastia, loss of secondary sexual characteristics. Presence of visual or neurological symptoms. Psychosocial history: depressive symptoms.
   (h) Previous treatment for this problem.
4. Explore ongoing problems and risk factors:
   (a) History of diabetes, hypertension, dyslipidemia, renal failure, hepatic cirrhosis, neurologic disease (like multiple sclerosis), thyroid dysfunction, hypogonadism, and hyperprolactinemia.
   (b) History of pelvic trauma, pelvic surgery, or spinal cord surgery.
   (c) History of psychiatric illnesses.
   (d) History of alcohol, smoking, and intravenous drug abuse.
5. Question regular use of medications: Diuretics, antihypertensive, H2 blockers, and antidepressants. Ensure compliance with diabetic medications if any to estimate adherence to treatment and level of control.
6. Other factors:
   (a) Any new stressful event.
   (b) Home environment.
   (c) Emotional or financial problems.
   (d) Loss of job or loss of a relative.
   (e) Drug and alcohol history use if any.
7. Explore the patient's ideas, concerns and expectations (ICE), and their effect on the patient's life and relation to his wife and family.
8. Order required investigations: rule out diabetes mellitus, check morning testosterone level (level less than 12 nmol/L directs to hypogonadism), lipid profile. Consider additional investigations such as: FSH, LH, thyroid function test, and PSA.
9. Management: share a diagnosis, prognosis, and management options:
   (a) Lifestyle modification (weight loss, exercise, smoking cessation).
   (b) Phosphodiesterase type 5 inhibitors (like Sildenafil, Tadalafil, Vardenafil, and Avanafil). Contraindicated in men taking nitrates risk of hypotension. [Side effects: include headache, flushing, dyspepsia, rhinitis, back pain, and color visual disturbance].
   (c) Vacuum erection device.

    (d) Alprostadil intraurethral suppositories or intra-cavernous drug injection.

    (e) Penile prosthesis implantation.

    (f) Testosterone therapy for hypogonadism [side effects: fatigue, muscle weakness, mood changes, erythrocytosis (follow-up hematocrit) increase prostate size and elevated Prostate Specific Antigen (PSA), may worsen heart disease, migraine, and Obstructive Sleep Apnea OSA)].

10. Health education: explain:

    (a) The relation between control of diabetes mellitus and erectile dysfunction.

11. Discuss health maintenance and age-appropriate screening.

12. Arrange for follow-up.

13. Communication skills: organized approach, mixed questioning styles (open- and close-ended questions), active listening, clear language, and reflection on patient's ICE.

History Taking and Management of a Male Presenting with Infertility

56

Halima Al Shehhi and Shammah Al Memari

For information in female infertility, refer to Chap. 48.

Learning Objectives
- How to master history taking for male patients presenting with infertility?
- How to perform a focused exam for male patients presenting with infertility?
- How to approach and provide management tips for male patients with infertility?

Focus areas include History of bilateral cryptorchidism, history of chemotherapy or radiation therapy, vasectomy. Systemic disease (diabetes, upper respiratory disease). Exposure to alcohol, tobacco, or recreational drugs.

H. Al Shehhi
Ambulatory Healthcare Services, Abu Dhabi, United Arab Emirates

S. Al Memari (✉)
Abu Dhabi, United Arab Emirates

© The Author(s), under exclusive license to Springer Nature Singapore Pte Ltd. 2024
S. Lari et al. (eds.), *Family Medicine OSCE: First Aid to Objective Structured Clinical Examination*, https://doi.org/10.1007/978-981-99-5530-5_56

1. Introduce yourself and establish a good rapport.
2. Identify the complaint: current age, age at onset, length of current marriage, (Are the couple living together? Is the marriage stable and happy?), any previous marriages and any children, previous treatment for this problem if any and when was it established? and associated symptoms:
   (a) Excessive weight changes in the last 6 months (hypothalamic failure).
   (b) Anosmia and peripheral vision loss (pituitary adenoma).
   (c) Galactorrhea (prolactinoma or ingestion of hormonal supplements).
   (d) Cold intolerance, constipation, tremors, or anxiousness (thyroid disease).
   (e) Hematuria and weight loss: (bladder cancer).
   (f) Scrotal pain and swelling (hydrocele, or varicocele).
   (g) Scrotal pain and swelling with urethral discharge (sexually transmitted disease (STD)).
   (h) Low mood and loss of interest (depression).
3. Explore ongoing problems and adherence to their treatment if any: diabetes, ischemic heart disease, chronic kidney disease, hepatic failure, neurologic diseases such as multiple sclerosis, sickle cell disease, or sexually transmitted disease.
4. Past medical history including:
   (a) Pelvic trauma, pelvic surgery, or spinal cord surgery.
   (b) Childhood illness: mumps or undescended testis in specific.
   (c) Delayed or missed secondary sexual characteristics at mid-teens.
5. Question regular use of medications: antihistamine, anti-hypertensive, antipsychotic, and antidepressant agents.
6. Explore the patient's ideas, concerns, expectations (ICE), and the effects on his life relationship with his wife and family.
7. Social history:
   (a) Home environment, emotional and financial status, stress level.
   (b) Smoking, alcohol, or recreational drugs use.
   (c) Tight clothes or hot tubs use.
   (d) Occupation (any exposure to toxins or radiations).
8. Sexual history: refer to Table 56.1 for details.
9. Family history: infertility or genitourinary cancers (bladder or prostate).
10. Partner's history: age, sexual history as well as past medical and obstetric history. Inquire about previous marriages and pregnancies if any.
11. Examination:
    (a) Vitals especially blood pressure.
    (b) Weight, height, and body mass index (BMI).
    (c) General appearance: the presence of secondary sexual characteristics including male voice and male pattern hair distribution. Dysmorphic features with learning disabilities.
    (d) Eye exam including visual field.
    (e) Breast exam: any gynecomastia or galactorrhea.

Table 56.1 Causes of sexual dysfunctions in males

Causes of sexual dysfunction	Comments
Frequency of intercourse	Check adequacy
Defects in phases of the sexual cycle	
Low desire	This might be due to chronic fatigue syndrome, hypogonadism, hypothyroidism, or psychological conditions
Arousal phase-related problems	Cause premature ejaculation that might be due to anxiety, relationship problems, thyroid dysfunction, or prostatitis
Impaired quality and timing of orgasm including anorgasmia	This might be due to alcohol abuse, Cushing syndrome, thyroid dysfunction, medications (e.g., antihistamines, antipsychotics, beta-blockers, selective serotonin reuptake inhibitors, thiazides, tricyclic antidepressants), psychological causes, surgery of the pelvis or prostate
Early morning and nocturnal erection	Present or absent
Absence of ejaculation	Does he have any ejaculation? Absence of ejaculation is indicative of retrograde ejaculation or obstruction due to infection, surgery, or trauma
Pain (priapism)	This might be due to hematological disorders such as sickle cell anemia, medications, injury, ischemic diseases, or illicit drugs and alcohol

Table 56.2 Management of male infertility

Cause	Management
Obstructive azoospermia	Surgery
Gonadotrophin or gonadotrophin-releasing hormone deficiencies	Hormonal treatment (chorionic gonadotrophin *OR* chorionic gonadotrophin and follitropin alfa)
Primary hypogonadism	Clomifene *OR* chorionic gonadotrophin
High estrogen levels in combination with low testosterone	Anastrozole *OR* Anastrozole and Clomifene
Hyperprolactinemia due to pituitary adenoma	Bromocriptine *OR* Cabergoline
Presence of anti-sperm antibodies	Assisted reproductive techniques (ART)
The presence of varicocele and no other cause of infertility were detected	Surgery
Idiopathic male infertility	Hormonal treatment (follitropin alfa). May consider antioxidant such as vitamins C and E, L-carnitine, pentoxifylline, and glutathione

(f) Genital exam: any varicocele, hydrocele, hypospadias, epispadias, penile stricture, undescended testis, epididymitis, or inguinal hernia. Check for cremasteric reflex (intact reflex indicates normal thoracolumbar erection function).

(g) Per rectal examination: check for anal sphincter tone, prostate enlargement, or tenderness.

12. Order required investigations: semen analysis, follicle-stimulating hormone (FSH), luteinizing hormone (LH), complete blood count (CBC), thyroid function test, lipid profile, fasting blood sugar, prolactin, morning testosterone (peak at 8 am and trough at 8 pm), creatinine, and urine analysis. Consider testicular biopsy (in non-obstructive azoospermia) or genetic testing (like in Klinefelter syndrome) in some cases.

13. Management and education: share diagnosis, prognosis, and treatment plan:
    (a) Encourage smoking cessation.
    (b) Treat and control according to the cause: refer to Table 56.2 for details.
    (c) Consider referral for "nocturnal penile tumescence test": a device attached in the evening to detect erection with Rapid Eye Movement (REM) sleep. Its absence indicates organic pathology.

14. Discuss health maintenance and screening for age.

15. Arrange for follow-up.

16. Communication skills: organized approach, mixed questioning styles (open- and close-ended questions), active listening, clear language, and reflection on the patient's ICE.

History Taking and Management of a Male Presenting with Enlarged Breasts (Gynecomastia)

57

Sumiya Taheri and Shammah Al Memari

Learning Objectives
- How to master history taking for male patients presenting with enlarged breasts (gynecomastia)?
- How to perform a focused exam for male patients presenting with enlarged breasts (gynecomastia)?
- How to approach and provide management tips for male patients presenting with enlarged breasts (gynecomastia)?

Focus areas include Physiologic gynecomastia, medication-induced, cirrhosis, hypogonadism (primary hypogonadism: androgen insensitivity syndrome, congenital anorchia, hemochromatosis, Klinefelter syndrome, testicular torsion, testicular trauma, viral orchitis. Secondary hypogonadism: Kallmann syndrome, hypopituitarism, hyperprolactinemia, pituitary and/or hypothalamic damage from disease, surgery, or radiation), tumors (adrenal tumors, gastric carcinoma producing hCG, pituitary tumors, renal cell carcinoma producing hCG, testicular tumors), thyrotoxicosis, chronic renal insufficiency, familial gynecomastia, human immunodeficiency virus, malnutrition disorders.

S. Taheri
Ambulatory Healthcare Services, Abu Dhabi, United Arab Emirates

S. Al Memari (✉)
Abu Dhabi, United Arab Emirates

1. Introduce yourself.
2. Establish a good rapport.
3. Identify the complaint:
   (a) Ask the patient; what brought you here today (might complain of breast enlargement, breast mass, breast pain, fear of breast cancer, or embarrassment). Onset and duration of the problem.
   (a) Ask about breast symptoms: breast pain, lump, nipple discharge, nipple retraction, and skin changes. Ask if unilateral or bilateral symptoms.
   (b) Ask about hypogonadism symptoms: decreased libido, decreased strength, erectile dysfunction, fertility issues, lack of facial hair, soft voice, small genitals.
   (c) Ask about thyroid symptoms, especially thyrotoxicosis, heat intolerance, tremor, palpitations, anxiety, weight loss, diarrhea.
   (d) Ask about testicular mass, weight loss, night sweats.
   (e) Ask specifically if there are any liver diseases or renal disease.
   (f) Ask about medications, recreational drugs (marijuana, alcohol, opioids, or anabolic steroids), and exposure to estrogen (occupational, medical, dietary, accidental).
4. Explore the patient's ideas, concerns and expectations (ICE), and the effect of the complaint on the quality of life.
5. Explore ongoing problems: past medical history (liver disease, renal disease, thyroid disease, history of undescended testis or mumps).
6. Question any regular use of medications (antiandrogenic agents: cimetidine, ranitidine, methotrexate, omeprazole, spironolactone. Estrogenic agents: anabolic steroids, growth hormone, digoxin. Others: haloperidol, metoclopramide, amlodipine, finasteride).
7. Social and family history: marital status, alcohol or illicit drug use, family history of gynecomastia, breast cancer, testicular cancer, and genetic diseases.
8. Examination:
   (a) Vital signs.
   (b) General examination to look for: signs of under virilization or systemic disease (voice, facial and body hair, muscular development, and secondary sexual development). Signs of thyrotoxicosis, liver, and renal disease.
   (c) Examine the thyroid gland.
   (d) Breast examination (rule out true gynecomastia from pseudo gynecomastia (lipomastia; increased subareolar fat without enlargement of the breast glandular component) and rule out any breast masses.
   (e) Genital exam: testicular and phallus size and development of testicular masses, pubic hair development.
9. Order required investigations:
   (a) *Blood tests*: If no underlying cause can be identified, then consider hormonal tests (should be ordered by a specialist): testosterone, estradiol-17 beta, sex hormone-binding globulin, luteinizing hormone, follicle-stimulating hormone, thyroid-stimulating hormone, prolactin, human chorionic gonadotropin, alpha-fetal protein.

Liver function tests—serum glutamic oxaloacetic transaminase (SGOT), serum glutamate-pyruvate transaminase (SGPT), and albumin renal function tests—creatinine, blood urea nitrogen (BUN).
   (b) *Imaging*: consider testicular ultrasound as testicular examination alone might not detect testicular masses. Breast ultrasound and mammogram only if clinical suspicion of breast cancer.
10. Management:
   (a) Pseudogynecomastia: reassurance, advise weight loss, liposuction can be done if it is necessary and patient preference.
   (b) Physiologic gynecomastia: reassurance and watchful waiting with biannual follow-up, might resolve within 6 months to 2 years.
   (c) Medications can be used for physiologic, persistent pubertal, and idiopathic gynecomastia and best if used early: Tamoxifen or other SERMs (10–20 mg twice daily for 3–9 months, might cause constipation, diarrhea, and pruritus). Aromatase inhibitors: anastrozole (less effective than SERMs).
   (d) Discontinue any offending medications; it takes 3 months for breast tissue to regress.
   (e) Testosterone deficiency: offer testosterone treatment.
   (f) Breast cancer: diagnose with tissue biopsy and treatment accordingly (surgery, radiotherapy, chemotherapy, hormonal therapy).
11. Arrange referral if needed (usually for all causes other than physiologic or pseudo-gynecomastia).
12. Give reading educational materials if any.
13. Provide emotional support and appropriately evaluated for low self-esteem or depression.
14. Discuss health maintenance and screening for age.
15. Arrange for follow-up.
16. Communication skills: organized approach, mixed questioning styles (open- and close-ended questions), active listening, clear language, and reflection on the patient's ICE.

History Taking and Management of a Male Presenting with Difficulty Voiding

58

Sumiya Taheri and Shammah Al Memari

Learning Objectives
- How to master history taking for male patients presenting with difficulty voiding?
- How to perform a focused exam for male patients presenting with difficulty voiding?
- How to approach and provide management tips for male patients presenting with difficulty voiding?

Focus areas include Obstructive causes (benign prostatic hyperplasia, urethral stricture, primary bladder neck obstruction, bladder neck contracture, prostate cancer, meatal stenosis, bladder calculi, bladder neoplasm, fecal impaction; gastrointestinal or retroperitoneal malignancy/mass, foreign bodies, and stones), infectious and inflammatory causes (balanitis, prostatic abscess, prostatitis, acute vulvovaginitis, Guillain-Barré syndrome, periurethral abscess, transverse myelitis, tubercular cystitis, urethritis).

S. Taheri
Ambulatory Healthcare Services, Abu Dhabi, United Arab Emirates

S. Al Memari (✉)
Abu Dhabi, United Arab Emirates

© The Author(s), under exclusive license to Springer Nature Singapore Pte Ltd. 2024
S. Lari et al. (eds.), *Family Medicine OSCE: First Aid to Objective Structured Clinical Examination*, https://doi.org/10.1007/978-981-99-5530-5_58

229

1. Introduce yourself.
2. Establish good rapport.
3. Identify the complaint:
   (a) Ask the patient; what you mean by difficulty in urination. (pain, burning, straining, loss of control).
   (b) Onset, duration, timing, relieving and aggravating factors, is it getting worse? any previous history of a similar problem.
   (c) Associated urinary symptoms (frequency, urgency, dripping, incontinence, hematuria, malodorous urine, and nocturia), other associated symptoms (back, flank, or suprapubic pain, fever, nausea, dyspareunia, pelvic pressure or pain, rectal pain, pain, erythema, swelling of the foreskin and/or penis, weight loss, chronic constipation).
   (d) Ask about recent infections, history of trauma to back or pelvis, self or family history of autoimmune diseases.
   (e) Ask about risk factors, catheter use, elderly, anatomical abnormalities, recurrent sexually transmitted infections)).
   (f) Ask about any new medications (some medications that can cause urinary retention are mentioned below).
   (g) Red flags (high-grade fever, pain, anuria (complete obstruction or acute kidney injury, back pain, weight loss, symptoms started after trauma to back)).
4. Explore the patient's ideas, concerns and expectations (ICE), and the effect of the complaint on the quality of life.
5. Explore ongoing problems: past medical history (diabetes mellitus, urolithiasis, multiple sclerosis or autoimmune diseases, recurrent UTIs or STDs).
6. Question any regular use of medications Anticholinergics: atropine, scopolamine. Antidepressants: amitriptyline, Imipramine. Antihistamines: chlorpheniramine, diphenhydramine. Muscle relaxants: baclofen cyclobenzaprine)).
7. Social and family history: marital status, risk of sexually transmitted infections, abuse, alcohol or illicit drug use, any cancers, autoimmune or neurologic diseases in the family.
8. Examination:
   (a) Vital signs.
   (b) Abdominal examination: including palpation and percussion of the bladder and abdominal/pelvic organs, evaluation for flank tenderness.
   (c) Digital rectal examination in men to assess prostate size with or without nodularity and the presence or absence of rectal masses.
   (d) Complete pelvic examination.
   (e) Neurologic evaluation to assess strength, sensation, muscle tone, and reflexes relative to lower thoracic, lumbar, and sacral spinal levels.
9. Order required investigations:
   (a) Urine analysis: to rule out infections and check for blood, protein, and glucose in the urine.
   (b) Renal function: to evaluate for kidney injury.

(c) PSA: may be elevated in prostate cancer, benign prostatic hyperplasia, prostatitis, and in the setting of acute urinary retention.

(d) Serum glucose: to check for undiagnosed diabetes mellites in neurogenic bladder.

(e) Renal and bladder ultrasound: to evaluate bladder and urethral stones, hydronephrosis, and upper urinary tract disease and postvoid residual volume: usually 500–800 ml in a patient with acute urinary retention, in chronic urinary retention volume might be above 800 ml.

(f) Other imaging if suspecting specific diagnosis (MRI brain and spine, cystoscopy, urodynamic studies).

10. Management and referral: refer to Table 58.1 for details.

Table 58.1 Management of males with difficulty voiding

Diagnosis		Management
Acute urinary retention		– Might need urgent referral to urology – Stop offending medications if any and treat any infections – If suspecting any neurological condition refer to neurology for further evaluation and management – If any genitourinary infection is present treat accordingly and follow up for response
Benign prostatic hyperplasia (BPH)	Mild BPH	Watchful waiting, limit fluid intake, avoid excess alcohol and caffeine, and increase physical activity
	Moderate to severe BPH	Drug one alpha-1 blockers; alfuzosin 10 mg, tamsulosin 0.4–0.8 mg, terazosin 2–10 mg, orally once daily. Wait for 2–3 weeks to see an effect. Might cause dizziness, hypotension, or syncope. Not to be used with phosphodiesterase-5 inhibitor. Drug two 5-alpha reductase inhibitors; dutasteride 0.5 mg and finasteride 5 mg orally once daily. Recommended for men with increased risk for progression, such as those with prostate volume >40 mL and/or elevated PSA concentration (>1.4–1.6 ng/mL). Might take 3–6 months to see a response. Surgery if inadequate response to conservative management and drug treatment
Prostatitis	Acute prostatitis	Assess for the need for catheterization, start with antibiotics treatment (ciprofloxacin 500 mg orally twice daily or levofloxacin 500 mg orally once daily or co-trimoxazole 160 mg/800 mg orally twice daily). For those with a high risk of STD, co-treat for Neisseria gonorrhoeae and Chlamydia trachomatis
	Chronic prostatitis	Recurrent or ongoing bacterial infection of the prostate usually lasting >3 months. Treat with antibiotics for acute prostatitis for a longer duration of up to 12 weeks

11. Give reading educational materials if any.
12. Discuss health maintenance and screening for age.
13. Arrange for follow-up.
14. Communication skills: organized approach, mixed questioning styles (open- and close-ended questions), active listening, clear language, and reflection on the patient's ICE.

Part V

History-Taking and Management: Geriatrics

History Taking and Management of an Elderly Patient Presenting with Dementia

59

Sakina Al Bloushi and Shammah Al Memari

Learning Objectives
- How to master history taking care of patients presenting with dementia?
- How to perform a focused exam for patients presenting with dementia?
- How to approach and provide management tips for patients presenting with dementia?

Focus areas include Dementia syndromes, depression, delirium, intracranial tumor, stroke, encephalitis, vasculitis, metabolic deficiencies, chronic alcoholism, and medications. (Most patients with dementia do not present themselves; it is often a spouse or relative who brings the problem to attention).

1. Introduce yourself.
2. Establish good rapport.
3. Identify the complaint (memory loss): duration, onset, timing, profile (same, improving, or worsening), and prior episodes.

S. Al Bloushi
Ambulatory Healthcare Services, Abu Dhabi, United Arab Emirates

S. Al Memari (✉)
Abu Dhabi, United Arab Emirates

© The Author(s), under exclusive license to Springer Nature Singapore Pte Ltd. 2024
S. Lari et al. (eds.), *Family Medicine OSCE: First Aid to Objective Structured Clinical Examination*, https://doi.org/10.1007/978-981-99-5530-5_59

235

4. Ask for specific symptoms:
   (a) Forgetting keys, misplacing objects, difficulty in learning and retaining new information, performing complex tasks, solving simple problems, and expressing self, getting lost in familiar places and wandering, irritability, and apathy: (Alzheimer's disease).
   (b) Chorea, behavioral disturbance, and progressive cognitive impairment suggests Huntington's disease.
   (c) Cognitive disturbances: aphasia, apraxia, agnosia, difficulty planning or organizing tasks.
   (d) The combination of ataxia, urinary incontinence, dementia suggests normal-pressure hydrocephalus.
   (e) Visual hallucinations, parkinsonism, fluctuating alertness, falls, often Rapid Eye Movement (REM) behavior disorder: (suggest Lewy body dementia).
   (f) Stepwise deterioration in memory, motor, and sensory functions (vascular dementia).
   (g) Depressed mode and social isolation (depression).
   (h) Decreased consciousness (delirium).
   (i) History of recent fall (subdural hematoma).
5. Explore the patient's and spouse's or relative's ideas, concerns and expectations (ICE).
6. Explore ongoing problems: hypertension, DM, atherosclerosis, Parkinson's disease, vitamin B12 deficiency, and chronic alcoholism.
7. Explore safety-compromising factors, if any: driving, living alone, cooking, financial capacity, falls, wandering, and becoming lost.
8. Question regular use of medications: sedatives, antihistamines, antidepressants, narcotic analgesics, anticonvulsants, or sleeping pills.
9. Explore the history of substance abuse (IV drug or alcohol abuse) and smoking.
10. Explore family support and social status: ask specifically about the primary caregiver and arrange a meeting with the family.
11. Explore possibilities of caregiver and/or family abuse: untreated physical conditions, over or under-medication, changes in behavior in the elder, frequent arguments between the elder and the caregiver, caregiver not allowing interviewing or assessing the elder alone, history or signs of unexplained injuries, unsuitable clothing, sudden significant changes in the financial status of the elder, and unexplained genital infections.
12. Examination:
   (a) Neurological exam: look for evidence of prior stroke, gait disturbances, and sensory loss.
   (b) Mini-mental status and cognitive tests (refer to mini-mental state exam station).
13. Order required investigations: complete blood count, thyroid-stimulating hormone level, vitamin B12 level, neuroimaging (brain computed tomography or magnetic resonance imaging).
14. Management and education:

(a) Share deferential diagnosis and prognosis.
(b) Encourage participation at social gatherings with family and friends.
(c) Guide the access to social support groups or seniors' daycare centers.
(d) Encourage exercise, promoting physical activity is advisable, as there is evidence indicating that exercise enhances cognitive function and the capacity to carry out daily activities in individuals with dementia.
(e) Address the caregiver's emotions and stress.
(f) The decision to start a trial of therapy with cholinesterase inhibitors or memantine should be based on individual patient assessment (e.g., benefits versus risks).
(g) Discontinue medications causing cognitive impairment.

15. Give reading educational material if any.
16. Discuss health maintenance and screening for age.
17. Arrange for follow-up or referral to specialty clinics as indicated according to the underlying cause.
18. Communication skills: organized approach, mixed questioning styles (open- and close-ended questions), active listening, clear language, reflection on patient's ICE.

Buthaina Al Maskari and Shammah Al Memari

> **Learning Objectives**
> - How to master history taking for elderly patients presenting with a fall?
> - How to perform a focused exam for elderly patients presenting with a fall?
> - How to approach and provide management tips for elderly patients presenting with a fall?

> **Focus areas** include Mobility issues, postural hypotension, hypoglycemia, stroke or transient ischemic attack (TIA), visual impairment, urinary incontinence, osteoporosis.

1. Introduce yourself.
2. Establish good rapport.
3. Identify the complaint: onset, site (at home or outdoors, from a high level or low level), mechanism, prodromal symptoms (vision disturbances, dizziness, or loss of consciousness (LOC), ear ringing or vertigo, sweating, chest pain, joint pain or problems), relieving or aggravating factors, previous falls, any witnesses.
4. Explore the patient's ideas, concerns and expectations (ICE):
   (a) Ideas: "What could have caused you to fall?"
   (b) Concerns: falling again, serious underlying illness.

B. Al Maskari
Ambulatory Healthcare Services, Abu Dhabi, United Arab Emirates

S. Al Memari (✉)
Abu Dhabi, United Arab Emirates

© The Author(s), under exclusive license to Springer Nature Singapore Pte Ltd. 2024
S. Lari et al. (eds.), *Family Medicine OSCE: First Aid to Objective Structured Clinical Examination*, https://doi.org/10.1007/978-981-99-5530-5_60

   (c) Expectations: pain management, reducing risks, fall prevention.
5. Explore continuous problems: diabetes mellitus, osteoarthritis, urinary incontinence, visual impairment, osteoporosis, dementia, Parkinson's, and depression.
6. Past medical, surgical, and family histories. Social history: environment, home hazards, employment, smoking, alcohol, illicit drug use.
7. Medication use: Benzodiazepines, antidepressants, antihypertensives (check Beers list of medications).
8. Examination: vitals (BP sitting and standing), vision and hearing assessments, cardiovascular and neurological assessment, gait and balance problems, get up and go test, check footwear. Examine the location of the fall, looking for any open wounds, deformities, bruising, ROM, and neurovascular supply.
9. Order investigation as indicated based on history and physical exam. Lab tests could include, urea and electrolytes, HbA1c, hemoglobin, and vitamin D levels. Imaging, X-rays to rule out fracture, and brain imaging if you suspected stroke.
10. Management:
   (a) Multidisciplinary risk factor screening/intervention program, home hazard assessment, and exercises for strength and balance.
   (b) Medications review.
   (c) Supplement vitamin D through a diet rich in oily fish, fortified juices or milk, and exposure to sunlight, or consider supplementation with daily cholecalciferol at 1000 IU.
11. Give reading educational materials if any.
12. Discuss health maintenance and screening for age.
13. Arrange for follow-up, consider referral to physical therapy for strength and balance training and occupational therapy to assess home environments.
14. Communication skills: organized approach, mixed questioning styles (open- and close-ended questions), active listening, clear language, and reflection on the patient's ICE.

Buthaina Al Maskari and Shammah Al Memari

> **Learning Objectives**
> - How to master history taking for patients presenting with osteoporosis?
> - How to perform a focused exam for patients presenting with osteoporosis?
> - How to approach and provide management tips for patients with osteoporosis?

> **Focus areas** include identifying risk factors for osteoporosis and ways to prevent them.

1. Introduce yourself and establish a good rapport.
2. Ask: about patient's ideas, concerns and expectations (ICE), and detailed history:
   (a) Typically, patients presenting with osteoporosis are asymptomatic, but ask about back pain, joint pain, previous fractures especially fragility fractures (vertebral bodies, proximal humerus, distal radius, pelvis, and proximal femur), menstrual history (LMP, pregnancies and lactation, menopause).
   (b) Past medical history: hyperparathyroidism, hyperthyroidism, hypogonadism, celiac disease, inflammatory bowel disease, anorexia nervosa, rheumatoid arthritis, epilepsy, chronic kidney disease (CKD).

B. Al Maskari
Ambulatory Healthcare Services, Abu Dhabi, United Arab Emirates

S. Al Memari (✉)
Abu Dhabi, United Arab Emirates

© The Author(s), under exclusive license to Springer Nature Singapore Pte Ltd. 2024
S. Lari et al. (eds.), *Family Medicine OSCE: First Aid to Objective Structured Clinical Examination*, https://doi.org/10.1007/978-981-99-5530-5_61

    (c) Medication use: glucocorticoids, heparin, aromatase inhibitors, antiepileptic drugs, proton pump inhibitors, and medroxyprogesterone.

    (d) Past surgical history: Bariatric surgery.

    (e) Family history: Osteoporosis, hip fractures.

    (f) Social history: occupation, lifestyle (diet and exercise), smoking, alcohol, illicit drug use.

3. Health education: explain to the patient:

    (a) It is important to screen for osteoporosis and prevent it through proper interventions, as it has no symptoms but can increase your risk of fractures in case of falls which can lead to devastating outcomes.

    (b) According to the USPTF screening should begin in postmenopausal women after the age of 65 with a DEXA scan.

    (c) The preferred assessment method is the DEXA scan, a bone density test that assesses the strength of your bones. During the procedure, you will lie down on a bed, and an imaging machine will scan your spine and hips. There is no need to undress, and the test is considered "non-invasive."

4. Order and interpret the patient's DEXA scan: refer to Table 61.1 for details.

5. Management: refer to Table 61.2 for details.

6. Safety netting: "If you develop any side effects from medications, come back to discuss them."

7. Follow up: if medications were started, follow up in 2 to 4 weeks.

8. Brief assessment of underlying conditions and screening for age.

9. Give away reading material if available.

10. Communication skills: ensure organized approach, mixed questioning style (open- and close-ended questions), active listening, clear language, and reflection on the patient's ICE.

Table 61.1 Interpretation of DEXA scan

T-score	Interpretation
Spinal or hip BMD within 1.0 SD below the young adult female reference range (T- score ≥ -1.0)	Normal
Spinal or hip BMD between 1.0 and 2.5 SDs below the young adult female reference mean (T-score < -1.0 and > -2.5)	Osteopenia
Spinal or hip BMD ≥ 2.5 SDs below the young adult female reference mean (T-score ≤ -2.5)	Osteoporosis

Table 61.2 Management of patient with osteoporosis

Types	Details
Non-pharmacological therapies	Fall prevention (weight-bearing resistance and balance training)
	Exercise and physical therapy
	Dietary modification (balanced meals with calcium, protein, vegetables, and fruits)
	Vitamin D supplementation and sunlight exposure (30 min/day for 5 days a week)
	Smoking cessation and cutting down on alcohol
Pharmacological therapies	Bisphosphonates (first line, oral options include alendronate and risedronate, IV options include zoledronic acid once yearly, advice patient to take them with water and wait 30 min upright before eating or drinking, discontinue after 5 years of use)
	Raloxifene (selective estrogen receptor modulator, side effects include vasomotor symptoms, has increased risk of Venous Thromboembolism (VTE) and decreased risk of invasive breast cancer)
	Calcitonin (nasal spray, antiresorptive agent, has modest analgesic properties for those with acute or chronic vertebral fractures)
	Teriparatide (recombinant human parathyroid hormone, daily subcutaneous injection, for 2 years)
	Denosumab (human monoclonal antibody, subcutaneous injection, every 6 months for 3 years)

Buthaina Al Maskari and Shammah Al Memari

Learning Objectives
- How to master history taking for patients presenting with bilateral knee pain?
- How to perform a focused exam for patients presenting with bilateral knee pain?
- How to approach and provide management tips for patients with bilateral knee pain?

Focus areas include ruling out other causes of joint pain (septic arthritis, rheumatoid arthritis, psoriatic arthritis).

1. Introduce yourself.
2. Establish good rapport.
3. Identify the complaint: onset, location (small or large joints, number involved, symmetrical or asymmetrical), duration, character, relieving or aggravating factors (relieved by rest worse with activity in osteoarthritis (OA)), joint swelling,

B. Al Maskari
Ambulatory Healthcare Services, Abu Dhabi, United Arab Emirates

S. Al Memari (✉)
Abu Dhabi, United Arab Emirates

© The Author(s), under exclusive license to Springer Nature Singapore Pte Ltd. 2024
S. Lari et al. (eds.), *Family Medicine OSCE: First Aid to Objective Structured Clinical Examination*, https://doi.org/10.1007/978-981-99-5530-5_62

245

erythema, tenderness, stiffness (how long it lasts? <30 min in (OA), joint locking, instability, or catching. Associated symptoms (weight loss or gain, skin rash, nail changes, fever), history of trauma.

4. Explore the patient's ideas, concerns and expectations (ICE).
5. Explore continuous problems: diabetes mellitus, rheumatoid arthritis, hemochromatosis, and Wilson disease.
6. Past medical, surgical, and family histories. Social history: occupation, physical activity smoking, alcohol, illicit drug use.
7. Examination: vitals (obesity is a risk factor), skin examination, specific joint examination (look for signs of inflammation, joint redness, warmth or swelling, palpate for tenderness, look for muscle atrophy). In osteoarthritis, findings include (crepitus, bony tenderness, bony enlargement, restricted joint movement, and joint effusion without palpable warmth).
8. Order investigation as indicated based on history and physical exam. OA is a clinical diagnosis. Labs (CRP, ESR, and CBC), assessment of synovial fluid if other causes of joint pain are suspected. Imaging, X-rays will show (joint space narrowing, osteophytes, subchondral bone sclerosis, and subchondral cysts).
9. Management:
   (a) Lifestyle modification (weight loss, exercise (low impact: walking, biking, swimming), proper footwear).
   (b) Pain relief (Paracetamol and oral or topical nonsteroidal anti-inflammatory drugs (NSAIDs)).
   (c) Intra-articular corticosteroid injection.
   (d) Surgery is reserved for refractory cases.
10. Give reading educational materials if any.
11. Discuss health maintenance and screening for age.
12. Arrange for follow-up, consider referral to physical therapy for strength and balance training, and occupational therapy to asses home environments.
13. Communication skills: organized approach, mixed questioning styles (open- and close-ended questions), active listening, clear language, and reflection on the patient's ICE.

History Taking and Management of a Patient Presenting with Polypharmacy

63

Sumiya Taheri and Shammah Al Memari

Learning Objectives
- How to master history taking for elderly patients presenting with polypharmacy?
- How to perform a focused exam for elderly patients presenting with polypharmacy?
- How to approach and provide management tips for elderly patients with polypharmacy?

Focus areas include Patient medical history. Patient's social history and patient's beliefs. The use of over the counter medication and herbal medication.

---

1. Introduce yourself and establish a good rapport.
2. Ask:
   (a) The patient will not present complaining of polypharmacy, they might present with adverse drug effects or tired of taking lots of medications, physicians should always investigate medication history as part of assessing any symptoms in the geriatric population.
   (b) Ask the patient what brought them today to the clinic (new symptoms, worsening chronic illness, follow-up management of chronic conditions).

S. Taheri
Ambulatory Healthcare Services, Abu Dhabi, United Arab Emirates

S. Al Memari (✉)
Abu Dhabi, United Arab Emirates

    (c) Ask about the chronic conditions (medical and psychiatric, duration of each illness, how well controlled, and how many specialties the patient is following).

    (d) Ask about the risk factors for polypharmacy (multiple chronic conditions, lack of primary care physician, resident of long-term care facility).

    (e) Ask about detailed medication history (type, number, dose, frequency, duration, any new medications, any adverse effects).

    (f) Ask about over the counter medications use, herbals, illicit drugs, alcohol.

    (g) Ask about patient's ideas, concerns and expectations (ICE).

3. Advice:

    (a) Explain to the patient: "In simple words, polypharmacy is the use of multiple medications by the patient. The use of greater numbers of drug therapies is associated with an increased risk for an adverse drug event and an increased risk of hospital admission. Polypharmacy has also been associated with a decreased physical and cognitive capability."

    (b) Assess patient's medication needs.

    (c) Discuss and record patient medication experience including patient beliefs, attitudes, and preferences concerning drug therapy.

    (d) Identify patient medication-related problems or issues including medication appropriateness: "Is the drug indicated for the patient's condition?" "Is it the most effective alternative for the patient's condition?" "Does the drug achieve intended therapeutic goals?" "Is taking the drug associated with adverse events for the patient?" "Is the dose appropriate? (Consider the effectiveness and adverse events)" "Does the patient take the medication as intended?" "Are potentially appropriate medications omitted?"

    (e) "Brown bag assessment" (the gold standard for medication reconciliation); "patients told to bring in all medicines including over-the-counter agents and dietary supplements in a bag to each appointment." "Go through the items in the bag with the patient asking open-ended questions to determine": If anything is missing. How each medicine is taken? What each medicine is for? "If the patient is taking medicine incorrectly, investigate reasons and explain intended use in simple language."

    (f) Explain deprescribing to the patient: "It is a process of medication withdrawal with the goal of managing polypharmacy and improving outcomes. This includes a comprehensive review of the patient's medication list and systematically discontinuing or reducing the dose of all medications with an unfavorable balance of benefits and harms, as well as efforts focused on specific types of high-risk medication."

4. Assess:

    (a) Patient understanding of polypharmacy, associated risks, and impact on overall health.

    (b) Patient willingness to change and understanding of deprescribing.

5. Assist:

    (a) Develop a patient care plan with the patient and other team members that includes personalized interventions and patient-specific therapy goals including: "Patient education, changing current drug dosing, using alternative drugs, discontinuing unnecessary drugs, or adding appropriate new therapy." "Establish patient-specific therapy goals for each medical condition based on comorbidities, risk, other medications, physician or other prescriber intentions, and patient preferences." "Determine outcome measures that permit monitoring and evaluation of therapy impact at follow-up." "Determine when follow-up and monitoring should occur, considering patient clinical conditions and planned care transitions."

(b) While prescribing: "take patient-centered approach (understanding patient living situation, family dynamics)," "promote patient education to empower patient," "tailoring process of discontinuation to medications potential for immediate harm and patient needs, along with monitoring for drug discontinuation adverse effects."

6. Arrange:
(a) Regular follow-ups to determine if: "therapeutic goals are being met," "new drug-related problems have developed," "the drug is being taken," "monitor drug discontinuation adverse effects."
(b) Communication with subspecialty physicians to come up with a patient-centered plan for medication use.
(c) Education sessions for patients about polypharmacy, use of over-the-counter medications and herbals.
(d) Give reading materials.

7. Communication skills: organized approach, mixed questioning styles (open- and close-ended questions), active listening, clear language, and reflection on patients' ICE.

Part VI

History-Taking and Management: Mental Health

History Taking and Management of a Patient Presenting with Depressive Symptoms

64

Kawthar Al Ameri, Sumiya Taheri, and Shammah Al Memari

Learning Objectives
- How to master history taking for patients presenting with depression?
- How to perform a focused exam for patients presenting with depression?
- How to approach and provide management tips for patients with depression?

Hints When a patient presents with depressive symptoms, the physician should thoroughly assess for other mental and physical illnesses that may be interconnected with or coexist with depression. This includes conditions such as bipolar disorder, mood disorders (persistent depressive disorder, adjustment disorder, premenstrual dysphoric syndrome, postpartum depression, seasonal affective disorder), anxiety disorders (posttraumatic stress disorder, generalized anxiety disorder), domestic violence, abuse, insomnia, grief and bereavement, as well as medical causes (malignancy, Parkinson's, thyroid disorders, hypercalcemia, Cushing disease, sleep apnea).

K. Al Ameri
Ambulatory Healthcare Services, Abu Dhabi, United Arab Emirates

Faculty of Family Medicine Residency Program, Sheikh Khalifa Medical City, Abu Dhabi, United Arab Emirates

S. Taheri
Ambulatory Healthcare Services, Abu Dhabi, United Arab Emirates

S. Al Memari (✉)
Abu Dhabi, United Arab Emirates

© The Author(s), under exclusive license to Springer Nature Singapore Pte Ltd. 2024
S. Lari et al. (eds.), *Family Medicine OSCE: First Aid to Objective Structured Clinical Examination*, https://doi.org/10.1007/978-981-99-5530-5_64

Table 64.1 Details of symptoms of depression (mnemonic SIGME CAPS)

Symptom	Description
Sleep pattern	Trouble falling asleep or sleeping too much
Loss of Interest	Anhedonia
Guilty feelings	Feeling a failure of letting self or others down
Mood	Today and most of the days, any diurnal variation (feeling down, depressed, or hopeless)
Energy reduction	Feeling tired or having little energy
Trouble concentrating	While reading or watching television
Appetite changes	Decreased or increased
Psychomotor symptoms	Moving or speaking slowly where people could have noticed it or the opposite (restless)
Sexuality and suicide or homicide	– Loss of sexual desire – Thoughts that you would be better off dead or hurting yourself or others.

1. Introduce yourself.
2. Establish a good rapport.
3. Identify the complaint:
   (a) Onset (mean age is late 20 s), duration, symptoms of depression (use mnemonic "SIGME CAPS): refer to (Table 64.1), preceding psychiatric conditions (anxiety, panic attack, phobias), or any psychosocial stressors.
   (b) Ask about somatic symptoms: (headache, back pain, shortness of breath, abdominal pain, palpitations..., etc.)
   (c) Ask about the severity of symptoms and impairment.
   (d) Ask about the seasonality of symptoms.
   (e) In females ask relation of symptoms to the menstrual cycle, last menstrual periods, and current pregnancy.
   (f) Ask about psychotic symptoms: delusions or hallucinations.
   (g) Ask about past hypomania or mania symptoms ("Have you ever had a time where you felt happier or more energetic than usual, for no particular reason? Or have you had times when your mood was really up, euphoric, or 'on top of the world' for no particular reason?").
   (h) Ask about risk factors: older age; recent childbirth, stress, or trauma; co-existing medical conditions (diabetes, cancer, stroke, MI, and obesity); personal or family history of depression; certain medications, and female sex.
   (i) Ask about medications (steroids, some antibiotics, isotretinoin, varenicline, narcotics and benzodiazepines, finasteride).
   (j) Explore ongoing medical problems: neurological conditions including (stroke, Parkinson's disease, dementia, multiple sclerosis), malignancy, infectious disease, thyroid disease, diabetes mellitus, and cardiovascular diseases.
   (k) Ask about past or coexisting psychiatric illness.

4. Social and family history: triggers such as stressful events, marital conflicts, domestic violence, loss of a close person, or job instability. History of smoking, alcohol, or substance abuse. Is anyone with whom you would open up about this issue? Similar history in the family?

5. Explore patient's ideas, concerns, and expectations (ICE): "I can see that this is really difficult for you, have you been coping with it all? Any concerns?"

6. Examination:
   (a) Thyroid examination if hypo or hyperthyroid symptoms.
   (b) Neuro examination and cognitive assessment if suspecting dementia, multiple sclerosis, Parkinson's.
   (c) Mental status testing.

7. Investigations: Blood tests as indicated by history.
   (a) Thyroid function test.
   (b) CBC.
   (c) Liver and renal function.
   (d) Electrolytes (calcium and others).
   (e) Vitamin B12 level.
   (f) Cortisol level.
   (g) HIV testing.

8. Management and education:
   (a) Explain to the patient the diagnosis: according to DSM-5, a major criterion for diagnosis is a depressed mood most of the day, nearly every day, for a period of 2 weeks along with 4 other symptoms of depression. Elaborate on the link between the physical symptoms they have with their mood.
   (b) **Decide the best approach to managing the patient at hand. Refer to Table 64.2 for details.**
   (c) **Explain to the patient, who is in need for antidepressants, about the medications as follows**: Initially, they might experience agitation, anxiety, and increased suicidal ideation and make sure that they know when and how to ask for help. Yet, they will need to take the medications daily and avoid changing the dose in order to see improvement as it builds up over 2–3 weeks. Once stable, the medications need to be continued for 6–12 months to prevent relapse.
   (d) **Explain possible side effects as follows:** Mirtazapine (sedative, weight gain, sexual dysfunction), Tricyclic Antidepressants (TCA) (excessive sleep, weight gain, drowsiness, prolonged QT interval), Venlafaxine (severe nausea, vomiting, elevated blood pressure so avoid in hypertensive patients), Paroxetine (cause delayed ejaculation, recommended in cases with premature ejaculations), Sertraline (diarrhea, insomnia, tremulousness), Trazodone (sedative, orthostatic hypotension (avoid in elderly)), Fluoxetine: (weight loss, tremulousness), and Bupropion (agitation, lower seizure threshold (avoid in epilepsy patients))).

Table 64.2 Management approach to depression

Management approach	Indication and intervention
Lifestyle modification	(a) Offer sleep hygiene advice as appropriate: Establishment of regular sleep and wake times, avoiding eating, smoking, or alcohol use before sleep, maintaining an appropriate environment for sleep, regular physical exercise (b) Structured physical activity program: Typically, 3.45-min to 1-h sessions/week for 10–14 weeks (average is 12 weeks), programs should be group-based with support from an appropriate instructor (c) Get social support
Psychotherapy	(a) Cognitive behavioral therapy (CBT) (b) Problem-solving therapy (PST)
Pharmacotherapy (mild to moderate)	– Consider if the patient does not respond to psychotherapy; and has recurrent. depression, prior use of antidepressants, positive family history of psychiatric illness, or patient preference) – Recommended antidepressants (serotonin reuptake inhibitors, serotonin-norepinephrine reuptake inhibitors, tricyclic antidepressants or bupropion)
Pharmacotherapy (moderate to severe)	(a) Antidepressants (detailed above + Esketamine nasal spray) (b) Electroconvulsive therapy (ECT) for severe unresponsive major depression or urgent need for a response
Hospitalization	In patients at risk of homicide or suicide or those who are dependent, lack social support, or complicating medical conditions

9. Give reading educational materials if any.
10. Discuss health maintenance and screening for age.
11. Arrange Referral: psychotherapy as needed. Admission if suicidal.
12. Arrange for a follow-up in 1–2 weeks.
13. Communication skills: show empathy, organized approach, mixed questioning styles (open- and close-ended questions), active listening, clear language, and reflection on the patient's ICE.

History Taking and Management of a Patient Presenting with Anxiety

65

Dana Al Marzooqi, Buthaina Al Maskari, and Shammah Al Memari

Learning Objectives
- How to master history taking for patients presenting with anxiety?
- How to perform a focused exam for patients presenting with anxiety?
- How to approach and provide management tips for patients with anxiety?

Focus areas include Generalized anxiety disorder, panic attacks, specific phobias, depression, somatoform disease, illness anxiety disorder or trichotillomania, cardiovascular diseases, or hyperthyroidism.

---

1. Introduce yourself, establish good rapport, and encourage patient contribution.
2. Identify the anxiety (as defined by DSM IV criteria. Use the mnemonic "AND I C REST"): **A**nxious, **N**o control over the worry, **D**uration of anxiety symptoms (more than 6 months), onset (sudden or gradual) course (continuous, episodic, or diurnal variation to rule out panic attacks and phobia), relieving or aggravating factors, timing (any change in severity), associated symptoms

---

D. Al Marzooqi
Sheikh Khalifa Medical City, Abu Dhabi, United Arab Emirates

B. Al Maskari
Ambulatory Healthcare Services, Abu Dhabi, United Arab Emirates

S. Al Memari (✉)
Abu Dhabi, United Arab Emirates

© The Author(s), under exclusive license to Springer Nature Singapore Pte Ltd. 2024
S. Lari et al. (eds.), *Family Medicine OSCE: First Aid to Objective Structured Clinical Examination*, https://doi.org/10.1007/978-981-99-5530-5_65

257

(**I**rritability, **C**oncentration impairment, activity level: retarded or **R**estless, decreased **E**nergy, **S**leep disturbance, **T**ension in muscles, change in appetite or weight, palpitations, trembling, shortness of breath, fear of dying, fear of losing control, paresthesia).

3. Red flags: cardiovascular disease (palpitations, chest pain, paroxysmal nocturnal dyspnea, relation of symptoms to exercise, syncope, and irregular beats), depression (loss of interest, low mood), hyperthyroid (heat intolerance, excessive sweating).

4. Explore patient's ideas, concerns and expectations (ICE), the effect of the complaint on the quality of life, and respond to patient's cues.

5. Explore ongoing problems (symptoms of anxiety disorders):
   (a) Psychological (excessive worrying, nervous mood, irritability, disturbed sleep, or difficulty in concentration).
   (b) Neurological (dizziness, headache, twitching paresthesia, or blurring of vision).
   (c) Cardiovascular disease (palpitation or chest discomfort).
   (d) Respiratory (hyperventilation, breathing difficulty, chest tightness).
   (e) Gastrointestinal (dry mouth, nausea, difficulty swallowing, choking, abdominal distress, or diarrhea).
   (f) Urinary (frequency, urgency), menstrual disturbance, or reduced libido.
   (g) Others (muscle aches, tension, or tiredness).

6. Histories: similar problem, any other psychiatry disease (obsessive-compulsive disorder, agoraphobia, social phobia, post-traumatic stress disorder), chronic diseases, previous surgeries, medications (alcohol, drugs, benzodiazepine withdrawal, caffeine (amount), smoking history), social (identify stressors: occupation, finances, marital status) and family history (similar problem or any other psychiatric disease).

7. Management and education: share diagnosis and prognosis.
   (a) Advise on aerobic exercise, mindfulness-based stress reduction, and yoga.
   (b) Cognitive Behavioral Therapy (CBT).
   (c) Trial of short-acting anxiolytics like benzodiazepines (be aware of the risk of abuse).
   (d) Selective Serotonin Reuptake Inhibitors (SSRIs) are first-line pharmacotherapy (escitalopram, fluoxetine, paroxetine) side effects include agitation and insomnia, sexual dysfunction, and weight gain. Two to four weeks for clinical response to occur.

8. Give reading educational materials if any.

9. Discuss health maintenance and age-appropriate screening.

10. Arrange for follow-up.

11. Communication skills: organized approach, mixed questioning styles (open- and close-ended questions), active listening, clear language, and reflection on patient's ICE.

History Taking and Management of a Patient Presenting with Obsessive Compulsive Disorder (OCD)

66

Eiman Al Murar, Kawthar Al Ameri, and Shammah Al Memari

Learning Objectives
- How to master history taking for patients presenting with obsessive-compulsive disorder?
- How to perform a focused exam for patients presenting with obsessive-compulsive disorder?
- How to approach and provide management tips for patients with obsessive-compulsive disorder?

Focus areas include screening for Major depressive disorder, panic disorder, body dysmorphic disorder, generalized anxiety disorder (GAD), social phobia and simple phobia, attention deficit hyperactivity disorder (ADHD), neurodermatitis, idiopathic torticollis, substance abuse, eating disorders, hypochondriasis, or tics.

E. Al Murar
Ambulatory Healthcare Services, Abu Dhabi, United Arab Emirates

K. Al Ameri
Ambulatory Healthcare Services, Abu Dhabi, United Arab Emirates

Faculty of Family Medicine Residency Program, Sheikh Khalifa Medical City, Abu Dhabi, United Arab Emirates

S. Al Memari (✉)
Abu Dhabi, United Arab Emirates

© The Author(s), under exclusive license to Springer Nature Singapore Pte Ltd. 2024
S. Lari et al. (eds.), *Family Medicine OSCE: First Aid to Objective Structured Clinical Examination*, https://doi.org/10.1007/978-981-99-5530-5_66

259

1. Introduce yourself.
2. Establish a good rapport.
3. Identify the complaint:
   (a) "Do you suffer from repetitive distressing intrusive thoughts or images (violent or horrific scenes)? Do you repetitively do any mental acts (such as: counting or repeating words silently)? Do you respond in unresisting compulsive ways? Do you have excessive worries (doubts or superstitious beliefs) about contamination, arrangement, or safety like checking things over and over or putting objects in certain positions?"
   (b) Onset, duration, frequency, and associated symptoms.
   (c) Check for insight and recognition of the disorder: Do the thoughts make sense? Do they seem absurd? Are these thoughts yours or did someone put them in your mind? Can you resist these unenjoyable thoughts? What do you do to counteract them? Do you feel relieved after responding? How do you feel when you attempt to ignore, avoid, or suppress obsessions or neutralize them with another thought or action? Do you feel guilty if you do not do anything toward these obsessive thoughts?
   (d) Check for dysfunctional beliefs: overestimating a threat, perfectionism, uncertainty, and believing that having a forbidden thought is as bad as acting on it.
   (e) Check for severity: How does this affect your life? How long do you spend time in a certain obsession or compulsion? Mild to moderate symptoms when spending 1–3 h/day.
4. Explore the patient's ideas, concerns and expectations (ICE).
5. Exploration of ongoing problems and red flags:
   (a) Past medical history of other psychiatric disorders: schizophrenia or schizoaffective disorder, bipolar disorder, eating disorders such as anorexia nervosa and bulimia nervosa, or Tourette disorder.
   (b) Look for other psychiatric disorder patient is at risk to develop: 1.76% lifetime risk of having anxiety disorder panic disorder, social anxiety disorder, generalized anxiety disorder, or specific phobia. 2.63% lifetime risk of having mood disorder mainly depression. 3.30% lifetime risk of having a comorbid obsessive-compulsive personality.
   (c) Red flags: suicidal ideation.
   (d) Previous hospital admission.
   (e) Medication trials.
   (f) Antecedent infections, especially streptococcal and herpetic infections (some studies link these infections to OCD).
6. Question regular use of medications.
7. Social history: current or past substance abuse or dependence, any distressing life to the patient and the family, obsessive thoughts about harming self or others, fantasy sexual thoughts.
8. Family history: OCD, Tourette disorder, tics, ADHD, or other psychiatric diagnoses.

9. Examination:
   (a) Hair loss related to trichotillomania (compulsive hair pulling).
   (b) Eczematous eruptions related to excessive washing.
   (c) Excoriations related to neurodermatitis (compulsive skin picking).
10. Management and education:
   (a) Cognitive Behavioral Therapy (CBT).
   (b) Selective Serotonin Reuptake Inhibitors (SSRIs) are the first line if a patient failed CBT, or upon patient preference fluvoxamine, fluoxetine, sertraline citalopram.
   (c) Tricyclic Antidepressants (TCA) as Clomipramine.
11. Monitor the patient's course of illness and response to treatment using the Yale-Brown Obsessive-Compulsive Scale (Y-BOCS).
12. Refer to the psychiatry clinic if symptoms are severe or initial treatment failed.
13. Give reading educational materials if any.
14. Discuss health maintenance and age-appropriate screening.
15. Arrange for follow-up.
16. Communication skills: organized approach, mixed questioning styles (open- and close-ended questions), active listening, clear language.

History Taking and Management of a Patient Presenting with Insomnia

67

Kawthar Al Ameri, Buthaina Al Maskari, and Shammah Al Memari

Learning Objectives
- How to master history taking for patients presenting with insomnia?
- How to perform a focused exam for patients presenting with insomnia?
- How to approach and provide management tips for patients with insomnia?

Focus areas include possible underlying causes such as anxiety, depression, mania, schizophrenia, hyperthyroidism, and jet lag.

---

1. Introduce yourself and establish a good rapport.
2. Identify the complaint:
   (a) Onset.
   (b) Character: Sleep onset insomnia (difficulty falling asleep at the desired time, but sleep quality and quantity are good) versus sleep maintenance

---

K. Al Ameri
Ambulatory Healthcare Services, Abu Dhabi, United Arab Emirates

Faculty of Family Medicine Residency Program, Sheikh Khalifa Medical City, Abu Dhabi, United Arab Emirates

B. Al Maskari
Ambulatory Healthcare Services, Abu Dhabi, United Arab Emirates

S. Al Memari (✉)
Abu Dhabi, United Arab Emirates

© The Author(s), under exclusive license to Springer Nature Singapore Pte Ltd. 2024
S. Lari et al. (eds.), *Family Medicine OSCE: First Aid to Objective Structured Clinical Examination*, https://doi.org/10.1007/978-981-99-5530-5_67

insomnia (difficulty sleeping through the night with frequent awakening or waking up too early).

(c) Relieving and aggravating factors (time, place, surrounding environment, naps, and excess caffeine intake).

(d) Red flags (repeated sleeping attacks, breathing disturbance during sleep, excessive daytime sleepiness, and significant sleepwalking).

(e) Explore the patient's sleeping pattern, environment, and rituals if any.

3. Rule out underlying diseases:

(a) Anxiety: nervous mood, excessive worries, irritability, apprehension, difficulty concentrating, palpitations, hyperventilation, and chest pain.

(b) Depression: low mood, loss of interest, low energy, change in appetite or weight, loss of libido, feeling guilty, and suicidal thoughts.

(c) Chronic diseases: cardiovascular disease, chronic obstructive pulmonary disease (COPD), gastro esophageal reflux disease (GERD), thyroid problem, asthma, obstructive sleep apnea (OSA), or pain.

4. Drug history, smoking, or alcohol abuse: alcohol intake, caffeine, BDZ, barbiturates, antihistamine, decongestants.

5. Explore patient's ideas, concerns, and expectations (ICE), and the effect of the problem on quality of life (daytime somnolence, decreased concentration at work).

6. Rule out other sleeping disorders: parasomnia (narcolepsy or sleepwalking), restless leg syndrome, obstructive sleep apnea (have you ever woken up with shortness of breath or choking sensation?)

7. Explore ongoing problems: diabetes mellitus, hypertension, coronary artery disease (orthopnea, paroxysmal nocturnal dyspnea), COPD, GERD, urinary tract infection (UTI), erectile dysfunction, delirium, or pain of any source.

8. Question regular use of medications: antihistamines, decongestants, sedatives (Benzodiazepines or barbiturates), stimulants (Amphetamines or aminophylline).

9. Social and family history: stressful events, marital conflicts, domestic violence, job instability, smoking, caffeine, or alcohol use.

10. Order required investigations as indicated.

11. Arrange referral: urgently if red flags are present, with or without sleep lab or psychiatry if long-standing.

12. Management and education: refer to Table 67.1 for details.

13. Give reading educational materials.

14. Discuss health maintenance and screening for age.

15. Arrange for follow-up.

16. Communication skills: organized approach, mixed questioning styles (open- and close-ended questions), active listening, clear language, and reflection on patient's ICE.

Table 67.1   Management of patient with insomnia

Item		Details
Lifestyle modification		(a) Regular bedtime and rise time and avoid napping (b) Avoid watching screens (for example TV) in bed. Prepare for sleep: Turn lights off, quiet place, cool temperature, and comfortable bed (c) Avoid heavy meals before going to bed, avoid alcohol, avoid caffeine 5–6 h before bedtime, and do late-night exercise (d) Keep a 2-week sleep diary
Psychotherapy		(a) Cognitive behavioral therapy is the first-line treatment for chronic insomnia
Drugs	**Sleep onset insomnia**	(a) Melatonin (b) Z class medications like zopiclone (c) Sedating antidepressants like amitriptyline and mirtazapine (d) Off-label use medications like diphenhydramine and doxylamine
	Sleep maintenance insomnia	(a) First line options include dual orexin receptor antagonists (DORA) like daridorexant, lemborexant, and low-dose doxepin (b) Other options include the same medications for sleep onset insomnia except for melatonin

Part VII

Performing Physical Examination

Performing Neonatal Physical Examination

68

Shammah Al Memari

Learning Objectives
- How to conduct a comprehensive, systematic physical examination for newborns?

1. Introduce yourself.
2. Extend congratulations to the parents on their newborn and take permission to examine the baby.
3. Wash your hands.
4. Explain to your parents what you are going to do.
5. Measure:
   (a) Vital signs.
   (b) Growth chart including weight, length, and head circumference.
6. Comment on general appearance:
   (a) Dysmorphic features: cleft lip (Down syndrome), small jaw (Robin syndrome).
   (b) Cry: feeble, pitch.
   (c) Color: jaundice, cyanosis.
   (d) Degree of distress if any.
7. Examine the head:
   (a) Fontanelles (size, bulge).
   (b) Sutures (split, overriding).
   (c) Shape (molding).
   (d) Swellings (cephalohematoma, caput succedaneum).

S. Al Memari (✉)
Abu Dhabi, United Arab Emirates

© The Author(s), under exclusive license to Springer Nature Singapore Pte Ltd. 2024
S. Lari et al. (eds.), *Family Medicine OSCE: First Aid to Objective Structured Clinical Examination*, https://doi.org/10.1007/978-981-99-5530-5_68

8. Examine ear, nose, throat, and neck:
   (a) Visualize: palate (cleft, Epstein's pearls, gums).
   (b) Palpate: with your little finger inside the mouth (cleft palate, high arched palate in Marfan Syndrome). Tongue for tongue tie.
   (c) Ears: position, skin tags.
   (d) Neck evaluation: masses, abnormalities, range of motion.
   (e) Clavicle.
9. Examine the eyes:
   (a) Check red reflex.
   (b) Check for any discharge.
   (c) Ensure symmetrical eye movement.
10. Examine the lungs:
   (a) Auscultates bilaterally, anterior, and posterior.
   (b) Work of breathing (retractions, nasal flaring, respiratory rate, head bobbing, the use of accessory muscles).
11. Examine the cardiovascular system:
   (a) Auscultates four points on chest (apex, lower and upper left sternal borders then right upper sternal boarder).
   (b) Femoral and peripheral pulses.
12. Examine the abdomen:
   (a) Inspect for distention (obstruction), scaphoid abdomen (in diaphragmatic hernia), and comment on the umbilical stamp (bleeding, discharge).
   (b) Check liver, spleen, and kidney size.
   (c) Check the umbilical cord (if only one artery, think of renal problems).
   (d) Palpate for masses, umbilical and inguinal hernia.
   (e) Auscultate bowel sounds.
13. Examine the genitourinary system:
   (a) Male: check the **scrotum** by examining the location of the testes (comment if descended or undescended, check for hydrocele, or hernia). Examine the **penis** and check for its size, and the location of the meatus (the meatus will be located ventrally in the case of hypospadias). Examine the **anus** for patency and location.
   (b) Female: inspect the hymen and labia for hymenal tags and discharges. Look at the **clitoris** and **urethra** (observe for clitoromegaly). Examine the **anus** for patency and location.
14. Perform a neurologic exam.
   (a) Level of alertness.
   (b) Tone.
   (c) Check root, Moro, and grasp reflexes.
   (d) Ensure the newborn moves all four limbs.
15. Examine the extremities including hips.
   (a) Barlow and Ortolani tests.
   (b) Examines feet: looking for club feet.
   (c) Obvious deformities in the digits like polydactyly or syndactyly.
   (d) Check range of motion.

16. Examine the back:
    (a) Observe for Lipoma, hair tuft (spina bifida), Mongolian spot, or port wine stain.
    (b) Palpate for spinal abnormalities (spina bifida) or Scoliosis.
17. Examine the skin:
    (a) Cyanosis.
    (b) Vernix, lanugo.
    (c) Perfusion (mottling, capillary refill time).
    (d) Rashes, petechiae.
    (e) Birthmarks.
18. Thank the parents and give feedback.
19. Redress the newborn.
20. Ensure systematic approach.

Performing Cranial Nerves Physical Examination

69

Khuloud Al Hammadi and Shammah Al Memari

Learning Objectives
- How to conduct a comprehensive and systematic cranial nerve exam?

---

1. Introduce yourself.
2. Ask for his or her name and take permission to examine.
3. Wash your hands and maintain privacy.
4. Explain what you are going to do.
5. Expose the body parts to be examined appropriately.
6. Comment on patient's general appearance.
7. Perform Cranial Nerve I exam: olfactory nerve:
   (a) Ask the patient: "Did you notice any change in smell?"
   (b) Check smell using a known odor (preferably not strong), such as that of an apple.
   (c) Tell the patient "Close one nostril, can you smell this?" "Now the other one please, can you smell this?"
8. Perform Cranial Nerve II exam, or optic Nerve. Refer to Table 69.1 for details.
9. Perform Cranial nerves III, IV, and VI exam (Oculomotor, Trochlear, and Abducent).
   (a) Inspection: inspect the eye for an abnormal position (squint) or ptosis. Position the patient's head in a neutral position and fix the head. Ask the patient: "Look at my index finger, follow it with your eyes." Then ask the patient to report any

---

K. Al Hammadi
Sheikh Khalifa Medical City, Abu Dhabi, United Arab Emirates

S. Al Memari (✉)
Abu Dhabi, United Arab Emirates

Table 69.1 Examination of cranial nerve II: optic nerve

Examination	Details
Visual acuity	• Snellen chart (ideal) • If not available, you can check roughly by asking: • "Can you read this newspaper, please?" • If not able "how many fingers are in front of you?" • If not able "can you see the hand moving?" • If not able then check for light perception
Visual field	• Finger or red-headed pin confrontation test. You may ask the patient to cover his right eye and you should cover your left eye (mirror the patient). Ask the patient to look directly at you and not move his head during the test. Then face the patient and examine each eye separately from the outer aspect (three directions, 10 o'clock, 2 o'clock, and 8 o'clock)
Pupils	• Symmetry: Comment as an example: "Pupils look rounded and symmetrical" • Light reflex (direct and consensual reflexes, cranial II afferent—Cranial III efferent) • Accommodation: Response to looking at something moving toward the eye
Fundoscopy	• Red reflex (from one foot away, check for corneal or lens opacities; cataract or retinoblastoma) • Look at the optic disc (gray-optic atrophy; pale cup-glaucoma; swelling- papilledema) • Look also for retinal vessels and any lesions or spots and finally look at the macula (temporal view)
Color vision	• Ishihara plates

Table 69.2 Nystagmus assessment

Steps to assess nystagmus		Details
Define the nystagmus based on its phases	Uniphasic or pendular nystagmus	• Moves like pendulum
	Biphasic, jerky, or central nystagmus	• Slow movement of the eyes in one direction and then return in a jerky movement
Define the nystagmus based on its movement in the faster component	Vertical nystagmus	• Indicates a central nervous system (CNS) lesion
	Horizontal	• Indicates peripheral nervous system (PNS) lesion

double vision "Tell me if you see my index finger doubled (diplopia)." Move your finger in all directions (draw an H shape in the air) and ask the patient to look up and medially (inferior oblique muscle) and laterally, down, and medially (superior oblique). During examination look for nystagmus and comment on the type of nystagmus as detailed in Table 69.2.

(b) Test for convergence by asking the patient to look at a near object (note that all the following muscle: superior rectus muscle, medial rectus, inferior rectus, Inferior oblique, and levator palpebrae superior produce the convergence reflex). Refer to Table 69.3 to classify any findings according to the probable lesion based on to the nerve supply of the extra-ocular muscles.

Table 69.3 Classification of abnormalities found on cranial nerves III, IV and VI's examination

Affected nerve	Defective muscle	Examination findings when patient has nerve lesions
Trochlear nerve IV	Superior oblique muscle	• The eye will go up and out • The patient cannot move it down
Abducens nerve VI	Lateral rectus	• The eye will go down and in • Patients cannot move it laterally
Oculomotor nerve III	All other extra-ocular muscles	• The eye will go down and out, pupil dilated, ptosis

10. Perform Cranial nerve V exam: trigeminal nerve: three divisions (ophthalmic, maxillary, mandibular).
    (a) Inspect for temporal wasting and jaw deviation.
    (b) To check the sensory functions, demonstrate sensation on the patient's sternum first to ensure he knows what it should feel like (sensations to be checked at the areas supplied by the three branches while the patient is closing his or her eyes. Ask the patient to volunteer his sensation rather than wait for you to ask if he or she feels it. Remember to compare both sides) for **light touch** using a fingertip or a cotton ball and **pain** sensation using a pinprick. **Two-point discrimination.**
    (c) Check the motor function (by mandibular branch only) and ask the following questions: "Clench your teeth" (feel for masseters and temporalis muscles), "Open your mouth, stop me from closing it." Ask the patient to move their jaw to either side and apply resistance to it.
    (d) Reflexes: there are multiple reflexes you needed to assess for trigeminal nerve which includes the jaw **reflex**. The **corneal reflex**: touch the cornea with the tip of cotton by approaching the eye from the side in a way that the patient does not see the cotton tip (afferent is cranial nerve V and efferent (is VII) cranial nerve).
11. Perform Cranial nerve VII: facial nerve.
    (a) Inspection: forehead (comment on any eyelid sag), nasolabial fold (comment on any flattening), mouth corner (comment on any droop).
    (b) Movements (explain: *"I will check your muscles of facial expressions"*): see Box 69.1 to describe how to assess facial nerve through muscle movement.
    (c) Sensory: taste sensation in the anterior 2/3 of the tongue on each side: hold the tongue with gauze; touch each side of it with sugar, salt, and vinegar. Ask: *"what does it taste like?"*
12. Cranial nerve VIII: vestibulocochlear nerve:
    (a) Hearing: check Box 69.2 for hearing assessment.
    (b) Vestibular test or Dix Hallpike test.
    (c) Romberg test: Ask the patient to stand with their feet together (touching each other). Then ask the patient to close their eyes. Remain close at hand in case the patient begins to sway or fall.

13. Cranial Nerves IX and X: glossopharyngeal and vagus nerves:
    (a) Keep your mouth open, say "aaaa" and inspect uvula: central or deviated to one side.
    (b) Gag reflex: touch the back of the pharynx with a tongue depressant.
    (c) Voice: Hoarseness—nasal tone.
    (d) Test sensation in posterior 1/3 of the tongue.
    (e) Swallowing.
14. Cranial Nerve XI: Accessory Nerve innervate trapezius and sternocleidomastoid muscle.
    (a) Stand behind the patient and inspect the trapezius muscle (comment on any atrophy or fasciculations?).
    (b) Ask the patient: "Shrug your shoulders, keep them shrugged." Push down the shoulders.
    (c) Inspect sternocleidomastoid muscle bilaterally.
    (d) Ask the patient: "Turn your head to left side and then to the right." Feel for the sternocleidomastoid muscles on the side opposite to the turned head.
15. Cranial Nerve XII: Hypoglossal (motor only):
    (a) Ask the patient *"Open your mouth."* Look for tongue wasting and fasciculation "Put your tongue out." Look for tongue deviation (it deviates towards the affected side of the brain).
    (b) "Wiggle it from side to side." Look for tongue movement.
16. To complete the neurological examination mention: "I would like to examine the gait, power, and reflexes, comment on patient consciousness and orientation to time, place and person, check for neck stiffness and meningeal signs."
17. Give feedback and thank the patient.
18. Ensure a systematic approach.

Box 69.1 Assessing the Facial Nerve Through Muscle Movement
To assess the facial nerve, ask the patient for the following:
- Look up or raise your eyebrows; (look for symmetrical wrinkles on the forehead).
- Close your eyes tightly and don't let me open them.
- Blow your cheeks or whistle.
- Smile or show me your teeth.

Box 69.2 Hearing Assessment of the Vestibulocochlear Nerve

(a) Ask: "Any problems with hearing?"
(b) Rub fingers and thumb together in front of each ear in turn and ask, "Can you hear that?"
(c) Whisper test (whisper in each ear separately 1, 2, 3 while distracting the other ear by wrinkling a paper and ask the patient to repeat what you said). If impaired perform: Rinne and Weber tests.
(d) Weber's test: strike the 512 Hertz tuning fork and place it on the middle of the forehead. Ask if the patient hears it in both ears equally? If not ask, "Where is it higher right or left?"
(e) Rinne's test: strike the 512 Hz tuning fork and place it on the mastoid bone. Ask the patient if he or she can hear and instruct him or her to let you know when they do not. This is testing for Bone Conduction (BC). When no longer heard, move it in front of the hearing canal (2.5 cm from the external auditory meatus) until he or she can't hear and this tests for Air Conduction (AC) and compare the interval.
(f) Classify the patient accordingly:
   • Normal: AC more than BC (with AC intervals is twice that of BC) and Weber is equal on both sides.
   • Conductive hearing loss: BC more than AC and Weber lateralizes towards the affected ear.
   • Sensorineural hearing loss: AC more than BC and Weber Lateralizes towards the normal ear.
(g) Vestibular test or Dix Hallpike test.
(h) Romberg test: ask the patient to stand with their feet together (touching each other). Then ask the patient to close their eyes. Remain close at hand in case the patient begins to sway or fall.

Preforming Mini-Mental State Examination

70

Shaima Lari and Shammah Al Memari

> **Learning Objectives**
> - How to conduct a comprehensive and systematic mini-mental state exam?

1. Introduce your self and explain what you are going to do?
2. Perform the Standardization mini-mental status exam available in article https://pubmed.ncbi.nlm.nih.gov/9447431/. (Adopted from Molloy and Standish 1997).
3. Total score interpretation:
   (a) Normal score is more than or equal to 24 points.
   (b) Eighteen to twenty-three points are indicative of moderate dementia.
   (c) Less than or equal to 17 points is severe dementia.
4. Provide feedback by acknowledging that the results may be subject to limitations, including cultural, educational, and language factors.
5. Thank the patient and ensure systemic approach.
6. Thank the patient and ensure a systematic approach.

S. Lari
Sheikh Shakhbout Medical City, Abu Dhabi, United Arab Emirates

S. Al Memari (✉)
Abu Dhabi, United Arab Emirates

© The Author(s), under exclusive license to Springer Nature Singapore Pte Ltd. 2024
S. Lari et al. (eds.), *Family Medicine OSCE: First Aid to Objective Structured Clinical Examination*, https://doi.org/10.1007/978-981-99-5530-5_70

Preforming Eye Physical Examination

71

Abeer Al Naqbi and Shammah Al Memari

> **Learning Objectives**
> - How to conduct a comprehensive and systematic eye examination?

1. Introduce yourself.
2. Wash your hands.
3. Explain why and what you are going to do.
4. Expose the body parts to be examined appropriately and get permission to examine the patient.
5. Inspect:
    (a) Face: comment on any dermatomal rash (herpes zoster) and eyebrows: seborrheic dermatitis.
    (b) Eye position and alignment (exophthalmos or strabismus).
    (c) Eyelid: comment on any swelling (stye or chalazion), scars, discharge, xanthelasma, eyelashes (entropion or ectropion), and ptosis.
    (d) Lacrimal apparatus: look for any swollen lacrimal sac.
    (e) Sclera and conjunctiva: comment on red eye (conjunctivitis, scleritis, or episcleritis), jaundice, and pallor.
    (f) Cornea and lens: comment on any opacities (cataract).

A. Al Naqbi
Ambulatory Healthcare Services, Abu Dhabi, United Arab Emirates

S. Al Memari (✉)
Abu Dhabi, United Arab Emirates

© The Author(s), under exclusive license to Springer Nature Singapore Pte Ltd. 2024
S. Lari et al. (eds.), *Family Medicine OSCE: First Aid to Objective Structured Clinical Examination*, https://doi.org/10.1007/978-981-99-5530-5_71

    (g) Pupils: comment on size (miosis or mydriasis), shape, symmetry (anisoco-ria or unequal size of pupils), and reaction to light (direct and consensual).

    (h) Iris: comment on iris, rubeosis iridis, or iridectomy if present.

6. Palpate: remember to look at the face of the patient in case of tenderness.

    (a) Eyeball for tenderness and tension (high intraocular pressure).

    (b) Measure intraocular pressure if Tonopen is available.

7. Visual acuity: use Snellen's chart at 6 meters distance and cover the other eye properly.

8. Check color vision: use Ishihara plates.

9. Check range of motion: draw an H shape in the air, ask the patient to follow your finger, and observe extraocular eye movements (cranial nerves III, IV, and VI).

10. Visual field: confrontation test at 20–30 cm distance while covering one eye (check in all directions: nasal and temporal fields bilaterally).

11. Fundoscopy (check the machine before starting): dim the lights and ask the patient to fix his or her sight at a specific object (looking straight).

    Remember to test the right eye with the right hand and examine from the right side of the patient.

    (a) Check pupillary light reflex.

    (b) Red reflexes.

    (c) Anterior structures: comment on any vitreous floaters or cataract.

    (d) Optic disk: clarity of outline, color, elevation, and condition of the vessels (any papilledema, glaucomatous cupping, optic atrophy, arteriovenous nip-ping, or copper wiring).

    (e) Background of the retina (comment on any hemorrhages, exudates, cotton-wool patches, microaneurysms, and pigmentations).

    (f) Macula: you will find it temporal to the optic disk or ask the patient to look directly at the ophthalmoscope light; this will automatically place the mac-ula in full view (comment on any macular degeneration).

12. Give feedback and thank the patient.

13. Ensure a systematic approach.

Performing Ear Physical Examination

72

Abeer Al Naqbi and Shammah Al Memari

Learning Objectives
- How to conduct a comprehensive and systematic ear exam?

---

1. Introduce yourself.
2. Wash your hands.
3. Explain why and what you are going to do.
4. Expose the body parts to be examined appropriately and get permission to examine the patient.
5. Inspect bilaterally: Any deformity, swelling, lump or foreign body, skin changes (rash, redness, scars, keloids, epidermoid cyst), or discharge. Look behind the patient's ears for scars.
6. Palpate bilaterally:
   (a) Temperature.
   (b) Tenderness: over the auricle, tragus, mastoid bone, and any masses.
   (c) Tug test: move the auricle up and down and press on the tragus (pain indicating otitis externa).
7. Otoscopy (bilaterally, starting with the normal side): Pull the auricle upward, backward, and slightly outward for adults and downward and backward for children. Through the otoscope speculum, observe and comment on the canal

---

A. Al Naqbi
Ambulatory Healthcare Services, Abu Dhabi, United Arab Emirates

S. Al Memari (✉)
Abu Dhabi, United Arab Emirates

© The Author(s), under exclusive license to Springer Nature Singapore Pte Ltd. 2024
S. Lari et al. (eds.), *Family Medicine OSCE: First Aid to Objective Structured Clinical Examination*, https://doi.org/10.1007/978-981-99-5530-5_72

(cerumen, swelling, erythema), eardrum (erythema, budging, light reflex, tympanosclerosis, perforation, or any grommet).

8. Tympanometry if available.
9. Test hearing:
    (a) Close the other ear, whisper numbers (patient should not read the lips of examiner) or rub two fingers near to the tested ear.
    (b) Special tests (use a 512 Hertz tuning fork).
10. Perform a Rinne's test:
    (a) First place the tuning fork over the mastoid bone until no further sound is heard, then keep it near the external canal of the ear (2 cm).
    (b) Interpret as Rinne's (see Table 72.1 for further details).
11. Perform a Weber test:
    (a) The tuning fork is placed at the center of the forehead. Interpret as in Table 72.1.
12. Eye (bilateral): look for any evidence of nystagmus.
13. Dix–Hallpike maneuver: Seat the patient at the edge of the examination table, then assist him or her to lie down suddenly with the head hanging 45° backward and turned 45° to one side (once to right, once to left, and once in the middle) while keeping the eyes open. Check for the development of vertigo or nystagmus. Interpret as follows:
    (a) Severe vertigo or nystagmus of fixed direction with characteristic onset after 3–10 s, and that lessen with repetition indicating peripheral cause of vertigo.
    (b) Mild vertigo or nystagmus of variable direction with immediate onset and continuous presence with repetition indicating the central cause of vertigo.
    (c) Can be followed by Epley's maneuver as a therapeutic option for benign paroxysmal positional vertigo (BPPV) to remove debris from the semicircular canals and deposit it in the utricle where hair cells are not stimulated.
14. Give feedback and thank the patient.
15. Ensure a systematic approach.

Table 72.1 How to interpret Rinne's and Weber's tests?

Patient's condition	Test and its interpretation	
	Rinne	Weber
Normal	Air conduction (AC) more than bone conduction (BC)	If sound is heard equally on both sides
Conductive deafness	BC more than AC	Sound heard higher on the affected side
Sensory neural deafness	AC more than BC	Sound heard is higher on the normal side

Performing Thyroid Physical Examination

73

Kawthar Al Ameri and Shammah Al Memari

Learning Objectives
- How to conduct a comprehensive and systematic thyroid exam?

1. Introduce yourself.
2. Wash your hands and maintain privacy.
3. Explain what you are going to do.
4. Expose the relevant body parts for examination and take permission to examine the patient.
5. General inspection (take a step back and observe):
    (a) Obese or thin.
    (b) Greasy or brittle hair.
    (c) Depressed, pale, or irritable.
    (d) Inappropriate dressing for the current weather.
    (e) Puffy cheeks (myxoedematous facies in hypothyroidism).
6. Hand exam:
    (a) Inspect: sweaty or dry, comment on any palmar erythema, onycholysis, thyroid acropachy (clubbing), fine tremors (put a piece of paper on the patient's outstretched hands), and xanthomas.

K. Al Ameri
Ambulatory Healthcare Services, Abu Dhabi, United Arab Emirates

Faculty of Family Medicine Residency Program, Sheikh Khalifa Medical City, Abu Dhabi, United Arab Emirates

S. Al Memari (✉)
Abu Dhabi, United Arab Emirates

  (b) Palpate: radial pulse for rate and rhythm (bradycardia or atrial fibrillation or collapsing pulse).
7. Eye exam: inspect for.
  (a) Exophthalmos (observe from lateral aspect).
  (b) Evidence of pallor (anemia common in hypothyroidism).
  (c) Xanthelasma (secondary hyperlipidemia).
  (d) Periorbital edema (chemosis).
  (e) Loss of lateral 1/3 of eyebrow "Cleopatra sign".
  (f) Proptosis (protrusion of the eyeball—seen better from above).
  (g) Special tests: lid lags (delay in the drop of the upper eyelid), lid retraction (sclera visible above the cornea), and extraocular muscles movements.
8. Thyroid:
  (a) Inspection:
    • Any swelling or goiter, discoloration, discharges, pulsations, or scars.
    • Hand the patient a glass of water, ask him to take a sip and watch the thyroid movement when the patient swallows.
    • Ask the patient to protrude their tongue. Observe for the presence of any mobile cyst, such as a thyroglossal duct cyst, which is the most prevalent anterior neck mass in children and moves upward during tongue protrusion, distinguishing it from a thyroid nodule that remains stationary.
  (b) Palpate (from back using right index and middle fingers): the thyroid isthmus and lobes [comment on size, texture, if any swelling (diffuse or nodular), mobility, and tenderness]. Palpate for any lymph node enlargement.
  (c) Percuss: over the clavicles and sternum (extension for goiter).
  (d) Auscultate: bruits or thrill.
  (e) Special test: Pemberton's sign (instruct the patient to elevate both arms above the head). The sign is considered positive if the patient exhibits inspiratory stridor, facial flushing, and distended neck veins, indicative of a retrosternal goiter.
9. Leg exam:
  (a) Inspect: shins for hair distribution and any pretibial myxedema.
  (b) Check for proximal myopathy by asking the patient to stand up without the use of their hands or by asking the patient to rise from a squatting position.
  (c) Reflexes: Knee and ankle reflexes. Look for any delay in relaxation or a brisk jerking movement.
10. Finish examination by examining the cardiorespiratory system for signs of heart failure or pleural effusion in acute thyrotoxicosis.
11. Give feedback and thank the patient.
12. Ensure a systematic approach.

Preforming a Cardiovascular System Physical Examination

74

Khuloud Al Hammadi and Shammah Al Memari

Learning Objectives
- How to perform a comprehensive and systematic cardiovascular examination?

1. Introduce yourself.
2. Wash your hands.
3. Explain why and what you are going to do and expose the chest appropriately.
4. Look at the observation chart for temperature, oxygen saturation, and blood pressure (ideally check blood pressure in all four limbs, in supine and standing positions for orthostatic hypotension).
5. Inspect:
   (a) Around the bed: nitroglycerin spray (ischemic heart disease), oxygen mask or nasal cannula, and drips.
   (b) The patient: comfortable at rest, cyanosis, breathless, any syndromic features (Marfan's, Down's, Turner's), and cachexia.
   (c) Hands: clubbing (congenital cyanotic heart disease, infective endocarditis, atrial myxoma), splinter hemorrhages, Osler's node, capillary refill time, peripheral cyanosis, nicotine staining, pale palmer creases (anemia), Janeway lesions, and tendon xanthomata (hypercholesterolemia).
   (d) Check the radial pulse: Assess rate (over 15 s) and rhythm (sinus, regularly irregular or irregularly irregular). Assess for radio-radial delay (coarctation of the aorta). Check for collapsing pulse (found in aortic regurgitation).
   (e) Feel the brachial pulse: assess the character (slow rising, bounding, pulsus arterans, pulsus bisferiens).

K. Al Hammadi
Sheikh Khalifa Medical City, Abu Dhabi, United Arab Emirates

S. Al Memari (✉)
Abu Dhabi, United Arab Emirates

S. Lari et al. (eds.), *Family Medicine OSCE: First Aid to Objective Structured Clinical Examination*, https://doi.org/10.1007/978-981-99-5530-5_74

287

(f) Face: look for signs of pain (ischemic heart disease), Cushing's, and malar flush (mitral stenosis).

(g) Eyes: xanthelasma, corneal arcus, anemia, and an ophthalmoscopy (look for Roth spots and hypertensive retinopathy).

(h) Mouth: high arch palate (Marfan's), central cyanosis, and telangiectasia.

(i) Check the neck: The jugular venous pressure (a direct assessment of right atrial pressure indicating central venous pressure): Position the patient at 45° and turn his or her head slightly to the left. Look for arising column of fluid between the two heads of the sternocleidomastoid muscle if observed and feel the carotid pulse.

(j) Chest inspection: for shape (pectus excavatum and carinatum), any scars (e.g., midline sternotomy for coronary artery bypass graft surgery, left axillary scar for mitral valve replacement), or pacemaker boxes.

6. Palpate:
   (a) Feel the apex beat (usually in the fifth intercostal space in the mid-clavicular line; the angle of Louis marks the second intercostal space).
   (b) Palpate for thrills and heaves: use a Z-shaped pattern for examination.
   (c) Make sure you look at the patient for any tenderness or concern to be addressed, as well as to rule out muscular pain.

7. Percuss and auscultate:
   (a) Auscultation: Listen in inspiration to accentuate right-sided murmurs. Listen in expiration to accentuate left-sided murmurs. At the apex (mitral area); use the bell and ask the patient to roll to the left side while listening (mitral stenosis). For assessing mitral regurgitation, use the diaphragm. To auscultate the tricuspid area, place the stethoscope in the fourth intercostal space and for the pulmonary area place it in the left sternal edge in the second intercostal. Auscultate the right sternal edge in the second intercostal space for aortic area and ask the patient to lean forward (assessing for aortic regurgitation). Listen over the carotid for radiation (assessing for aortic stenosis).
   (b) Percuss and listen to the lung bases for any sign of pleural effusion (assessing for heart failure) and pulmonary edema.
   (c) Palpate for sacral edema that is indicative of right heart failure.

8. Check the abdomen:
   (a) Palpate for abdominal aortic aneurysm.
   (b) Palpate the liver. Note if it is pulsatile in case of tricuspid regurgitation, or enlarged in case of right-sided heart failure.
   (c) Hepatojugular reflex (only if JVP is high): Ask the patient to breathe from his or her mouth while you apply some pressure on the liver and sustain it for 10 s. A sustained elevation of JVP for 10 s is indicative of tricuspid regurgitation, heart failure due to other nonvalvular causes, constrictive pericarditis, cardiac tamponade, and inferior vena cava obstruction.

9. Check the lower limbs:
   (a) Palpate for peripheral pulses: check femoral (radio-femoral delay), popliteal, posterior tibial, and dorsalis pedis.
   (b) Examine for ankle edema.

10. Give feedback and thank the patient.

11. Ensure a systematic approach.

Performing Respiratory System Physical Examination

75

Reem Al Mansoori and Shammah Al Memari

Learning Objectives
- How to perform a systematic respiratory system examination on a patient?

---

1. Introduce yourself, ask for his or her name, and take permission to examine.
2. Wash your hands.
3. Explain what you are going to do.
4. Expose the body parts to be examined appropriately and take permission to examine the patient (expose chest and abdomen).
5. General examination:
   (a) Check vital signs including oxygen saturation and respiratory rate (note its rate, rhythm, depth, and type of respiration).
   (b) Stand at the end of the bed: comment on general appearance, comfort at rest, no distress, any audible wheeze or stridor, any bedside nebulizer, ventilator, or oxygen supply beside the patient.
   (c) Hand: comment on clubbing, peripheral cyanosis, nicotine stain in the heavy smoker, palmar erythema, tremors [flapping (carbon-dioxide retention) or fine (Beta2-agonist overuse)].
   (d) Face: comment on pallor, nasal flaring, air hunger, pink puffer, central cyanosis, signs of Horner syndrome (miosis, ptosis, anhidrosis).
   (e) Tongue: central cyanosis.

R. Al Mansoori
Emirates Medical Association of Family Medicine, Abu Dhabi, United Arab Emirates

S. Al Memari (✉)
Abu Dhabi, United Arab Emirates

© The Author(s), under exclusive license to Springer Nature Singapore Pte Ltd. 2024
S. Lari et al. (eds.), *Family Medicine OSCE: First Aid to Objective Structured Clinical Examination*, https://doi.org/10.1007/978-981-99-5530-5_75

289

      (f) Neck: check for raised jugular venous pressure.

      (g) Lower limb and sacrum: palpate for the presence of edema.

6. Inspect:

      (a) Shape of thorax: comment on symmetry, deformities of the chest, and barrel chests cars (lateral thoracic or central).

      (b) Breathing movements normally in a male is abdomino-thoracic and in female is thoraco-abdominal.

      (c) Comment on the use of accessory muscle.

7. Palpate:

      (a) The **trachea** for central deviation or enlarged lymph nodes.

      (b) For any **tenderness** (think of costochondritis).

      (c) The **apex** beat (comment on any displacement).

      (d) Chest expansion: Perform a chest expansion test at three levels anteriorly and posteriorly (supramammary, mammary, and inframammary). The chest expansion decreased in cases of pneumonectomy, pneumonia, pleural effusion, and pneumothorax.

      (e) Use the ulnar surface of your hand when a patient says 99 to check **tactile vocal fremitus** at the three levels mentioned above anteriorly and posteriorly. The sound is decreased in case of pneumonia or pleural effusion.

8. Percuss:

      (a) Anteriorly: at the apex of the lung, clavicle, supramammary, mammary, inframammary areas, axilla, and liver (will be pushed below the costal margin in case of lower lobe pneumonia).

      (b) Posteriorly: at the apex of the lung, intrascapular and infrascapular areas.

      (c) Comment on percussion as follows:

            • Resonance indicates normal percussion note.

            • Dullness indicates consolidation (pneumonia).

            • Stony dullness indicates pleural effusion.

            • Hyperresonance indicates pneumothorax.

9. Auscultate:

      (a) Air entry: good air entry in the normal exam, while air entry decreased in case of consolidation, pleural effusion, and pneumothorax.

      (b) Type of breathing: refer to Table 75.1 for details.

Table 75.1 Types of breathing sounds and their interpretation

Type of breathing	Characteristic	Interpretation
Vesicular	Inspiratory phase followed by a short expiratory phase, low-pitched, and soft	Normal
	With prolonged expiration	Asthma, emphysema, chronic obstructive pulmonary disease (COPD)
Bronchial breathing (usually localized)	A gap between two phases is noted and expiration is prolonged, high-pitched and loud	Consolidation

(c) Intensity: decreased air entry with pneumonia and pneumothorax.

(d) Added sound: wheezes, rhonchi, pleural rub, fine and coarse crackles.

(e) Vocal resonance or bronchophony: instruct the patient to say "99" while auscultating the lungs.
   • Normal test will be louder clearer sound.
   • Positive test will be muffled sounds.

(f) Egophony: by asking the patient to say long "E" vowel sound.
   • Normal test will be long E sound.
   • Positive test reveals an "E" to "A" transition.

(g) A normal chest auscultation denotes good air entry, vesicular breathing, with normal intensity bilaterally and no added sounds.

10. Ask the patient to sit forward and repeat inspection, palpation, percussion, and auscultation over the back.

11. Give feedback and thank the patient.

12. Ensure a systematic approach.

Performing Abdominal Physical Examination

76

Reem Al Mansoori and Shammah Al Memari

Learning Objectives
- How to perform a systematic abdominal examination on a patient?

Hint During an abdominal examination, the order of assessment is slightly different from the general rule of inspection, palpation, percussion, and auscultation. The correct order for an abdominal examination is inspection, followed by auscultation, palpation, and, finally, percussion. This is because palpation and percussion can disturb the bowel sounds, which are important to assess during auscultation. It is important to remember this order to ensure accurate assessment and diagnosis during an abdominal examination.

1. Introduce yourself, ask for his/her name, and take permission to examine.
2. Wash your hands and maintain privacy.
3. Explain what you are going to do.
4. Expose the body parts to be examined appropriately and take permission to examine the patient (ideally from the nipple to the knee).

R. Al Mansoori
Ambulatory health care services, Abu Dhabi, United Arab Emirates

S. Al Memari (✉)
Abu Dhabi, United Arab Emirates

© The Author(s), under exclusive license to Springer Nature Singapore Pte Ltd. 2024
S. Lari et al. (eds.), *Family Medicine OSCE: First Aid to Objective Structured Clinical Examination*, https://doi.org/10.1007/978-981-99-5530-5_76

5. General examination:
   (a) Vital signs.
   (b) General appearance: comfortable or in pain, connection to devices, gastric tubes, jaundice, examination pigmentation (hemochromatosis and Addison), body built [underweight (malignancy), obese (fatty liver)], hydration status, and mental status (hepatic encephalopathy, fulminant hepatitis).
   (c) Hands: Look at the nails for leukonychia (chronic liver disease), koilonychia (iron deficiency anemia), and clubbing (cirrhosis, inflammatory bowel disease). Look at the palms for palmar erythema (chronic liver disease), anemia, Dupuytren's contracture (alcoholism and diabetes), and flapping tremors (liver failure).
   (d) Arms: bruising (clotting abnormality in liver damage), scratch marks, (obstructive jaundice, biliary cirrhosis), spider nevi (cirrhosis, alcohol abuse), and arteriovenous fistula.
   (e) Eyes: sclera: pallor, jaundice, Kayser–Fleischer [brownish–greenish ring (indicating copper deposit)], and xanthelasma.
   (f) Face: parotid enlargement (parotitis, mumps).
   (g) Mouth: Check for teeth and breath [halitosis, sweet smell (fetor hepaticus)]. Check for the tongue: leukoplakia, glossitis, and macroglossia. Check angular stomatitis, aphthous ulcers, and oral thrush.
   (h) Lower limb: check for edema.
6. Inspect:
   (a) Skin: scars (site and length), rashes, caput medusa, and venous dilatation.
   (b) Contour of the central abdomen: (flat, rounded, protuberant, distended, and scaphoid).
   (c) Symmetry.
   (d) Visible pulsation (particularly aortic pulsation in the upper abdomen: indicate thin patients or aortic aneurysm) or visible peristalsis (intestinal obstruction).
   (e) Discoloration in flanks: Grey–Turner sign and Cullen's sign in acute pancreatitis.
   (f) Ask the patient to cough and check for bulging at hernial orifices.
7. Auscultate:
   (a) Bowel sound: at a point midway between the umbilicus and the anterior superior iliac spine. Describe its character (high-pitched, tinkling, rushes, rumbling).
   (b) Aortic bruits: at the mid-epigastric area.
   (c) Renal arteries bruits: at 2 cm left and right from the umbilicus.
   (d) Femoral arteries bruits: at 2 cm lateral to the inguinal ligament and midclavicular line palpate.
8. Palpate:
   (a) Superficial palpation of all quadrants (tenderness, muscular spasm, or rigidity).
   (b) Deep palpation (tenderness, rebound tenderness), masses, pulsations (abdominal aortic aneurysm), palpable bowel loops, or movement.

Table 76.1 Signs of appendicitis

Sign	Description
Rebound tenderness	At the McBurney's point (a point 2/3 from the umbilicus and 1/3 from the anterior superior iliac spine on a line joining them)
Rovsing's sign	Deep palpation of the left iliac fossa (LIF)will cause pain in the right iliac fossa (RIF)
Psoas sign	Hyperextension of hip while lying on the left lateral position or raising the hip against resistance will cause pain in RIF
Obturator sign	Flexion of the hip and knee, followed by internal rotation of hip, will cause pain in the RIF

  (c) Kidney ballottement.
  (d) Organomegaly (liver and spleen): measure liver span.
  (e) Note: remember to check costophrenic tenderness when the patient is in the sitting position.
  9. Percuss:
  (a) All over the abdomen: tender in case of peritonitis.
  (b) Liver (check the span as well, normally 10–12 cm).
  (c) Spleen.
  (d) Urinary bladder (full bladder is dull) from symphysis pubis upward.
  (e) Shifting dullness and fluids thrills (fluid wave test) for ascites.
  10. Special tests and signs (include a brief description if possible):
  (a) For obese patients: scratch test: to identify the liver span especially when palpation is difficult.
  (b) For cholecystitis: Murphy's sign. (Ask the patient to breathe out, then place your hand below the right costal margin at the mid-clavicular line. Then ask the patient to breathe in. A positive response will be if the patient stops breathing or winces with a "catch" in breath.)
  (c) For appendicitis: check Table 76.1 for signs of appendicitis.
  11. At the end of the examination: check for hernias and genitalia and per-rectal (PR) exam.
  12. Give feedback and thank the patient.
  13. Ensure a systematic approach.

Performing Neck Physical Examination

77

Shammah Al Memari

Learning Objectives
- How to perform a systematic neck examination on a patient?

1. Introduce yourself, wash your hands, and expose examined body parts appropriately.
2. Explain what you are going to do and ensure a systematic approach.
3. Inspect (from front and back):
   (a) Skin (redness, scar, discoloration).
   (b) Asymmetry: masses, torticollis (twisting of the neck to one side that results in the abnormal carriage of the head), or bone deformity.
   (c) Muscle wasting.
4. Palpate:
   (a) Temperature.
   (b) Tenderness (check by thumbs) over the clavicle, cervical rib (an extra rib that forms above the normal first rib, growing from the base of the neck just above the collarbone), cervical spines, para-spinous muscles, and supraclavicular fossa.
   (c) Thyroid and lymph nodes.
5. Auscultate: carotid artery.
6. Check the range of motion (active, passive, and resisted):
   (a) Forward flexion, extension, lateral flexion (side bending), and lateral rotation (70° each way) (twisting).

S. Al Memari (✉)
Abu Dhabi, United Arab Emirates

7. Special tests (check for neural or vascular compression sequel):
    (a) Check hands for pulses and capillary refill (any ischemia), and sensation over hypothenar muscle.
    (b) Check power distally in the limb: in the arms, assess abduction (innervated by C5) and adduction (innervated by C6, C7, and C8); at the elbow, assess flexion (innervated by C6) and extension (innervated by C7); and in the hands, ask the patient to make a fist and squeeze your fingers to assess for C8.
    (c) Atlantoaxial compression test or Spurling's test: apply an axial load to the top of the head while the neck is twisted (radicular pain in the shoulder and arm probably means cervical root irritation).
    (d) Forward flexion test: forward flex the neck with the head turned toward the side (radicular pain in the arm probably means disc impingement on a cervical nerve root irritation).
    (e) Adson's maneuver: Locate the radial pulse. Have the patient take a deep breath, extend the neck, and rotate the head toward the painful shoulder (positive if the radial pulse diminishes and probably means thoracic outlet syndrome).
    (f) Reflexes: biceps (C5), triceps (C7), and brachioradialis (C6).
8. Check one joint above and one joint below (shoulder).
9. Give feedback and thank the patient.
10. Ensure a systematic approach.

Performing Back Physical Examination

78

Kawthar Al Ameri and Shammah Al Memari

Learning Objectives
- How to perform a back examination on a patient?

1. Introduce yourself.
2. Wash your hands and maintain privacy.
3. Explain what you are going to do.
4. Expose the body parts to be examined appropriately and take permission to examine the patient.
5. Inspect:
   (a) Gait (walking without shoes), check tip toe walking (S1), and heel walking (L5).
   (b) Posture looks at the patients from the back looking for signs of scoliosis (thoracolumbar) and sides for signs of kyphosis (thoracic) and lordosis (cervical and lumbar).
   (c) Check shoulder and pelvic levels (should be symmetrical).
   (d) Skin (erythema, swelling, scars, hair, fat pads "lipoma").
   (e) Muscle wasting.

K. Al Ameri
Ambulatory Healthcare Services, Abu Dhabi, United Arab Emirates

S. Al Memari (✉)
Abu Dhabi, United Arab Emirates

© The Author(s), under exclusive license to Springer Nature Singapore Pte Ltd. 2024
S. Lari et al. (eds.), *Family Medicine OSCE: First Aid to Objective Structured Clinical Examination*, https://doi.org/10.1007/978-981-99-5530-5_78

6. Palpate:
   (a) Temperature bilaterally.
   (b) Tenderness (using your thumb): over spinous process, paraspinal muscles, paravertebral area, sacroiliac joint, and anterior and posterior iliac spines.
   (c) Masses or muscle spasms.
7. Percuss: lightly on the back for any tenderness using a fist.
8. Check the range of motion:
   (a) Flexion: bending forward (if limited indicates disc pathology).
   (b) Extension: bending backward (if limited indicates spinal stenosis, spondylolisthesis, or usually facet pain).
   (c) Lateral rotation: bending to both sides (if limited indicates muscular pathology).
   (d) Rotation: fix the hip and ask the patient to turn left and right (if limited indicates muscular pathology).
9. Special tests:
   (a) **Straight leg raising test (SLR)**: (positive if shooting sciatica pain between 30 and 70°: pain radiates below the knee that is sometimes associated with numbness and paresthesia, indicating herniated disc).
   (b) **Bragard test** [used to confirm a positive straight leg raising (SLR) test]: passively lower the leg an inch from the level at which the patient felt pain with an SLR test and dorsiflex the foot (positive if shooting sciatica pain reoccurs also indicates herniated disc).
   (c) **Contralateral leg raising test**: elevating the other leg causes back pain on the involved side.
   (d) **Bowstring sign or tibial stretch sign:** passively bend the patient's knee and press at the popliteal fossa (positive if sciatica pain is elicited and indicates herniated disc).
   (e) **Figure four or FABER test**: Flexion, abduction, and external rotation at the sacroiliac joint [positive if pain is produced at the **sacroiliac (SI)** joint and indicates SI joint dysfunction or sacroiliitis while pain in the **groin** indicates iliopsoas strain, iliopsoas bursitis, or intra-articular hip disorder (osteoarthritis or labral tear)]. While pain in the **posterior hip** indicates posterior hip impingement.
   (f) **Femoral stretch sign**: The patient is placed in a prone position, and with the knee flexed, the hip is raised into extension [positive if anterior thigh pain elicited and indicates involvement of L2–L3 (or L4) nerve root].
10. Neurological examination:
    (a) Sensation of the foot: medial side (L4), dorsum (L5), and lateral side(S1).
    (b) Power: dorsiflexion (L4–L5) and plantar flexion (Sl) of the foot.
    (c) Reflexes: knee jerk (L3–L4), ankle jerk (Sl–S2), and ankle clonus: sudden passive ankle dorsiflexion that results in repetitive uncontrolled ankle twitches (indicates upper motor neuron lesion).
11. End your exam with
    (a) A quick examination of the neck and hip
    (b) An abdominal palpitation to exclude abdominal aortic aneurysm
    (c) A digital rectal exam to check for anal sphincter tone
12. Give feedback and thank the patient.
13. Ensure a systematic approach.

Performing Shoulder Physical Examination

79

Eiman Al Murar and Shammah Al Memari

Learning Objectives
- How to conduct a comprehensive and systematic shoulder examination?

1. Introduce yourself.
2. Wash your hands.
3. Explain why and what you are going to do and take permission to examine the patient.
4. Expose the body parts to be examined appropriately and take permission to examine the patient (neck, shoulders, arms, and back).
5. Inspect (any swelling, posture, muscle wasting, asymmetry):
    (a) Anteriorly: sternoclavicular joint, clavicle, acromioclavicular joint, and deltoid.
    (b) Laterally: swelling of the joint.
    (c) From the above: swelling, clavicle deformity, and supraclavicular fossa.
    (d) From behind: scapular winging (ask the patient to push up against the wall, scapula becomes prominent).
6. Palpate:
    (a) Anteriorly: sterno-clavicular joint, clavicle, acromioclavicular (AC) joint, and coracoid process.
    (b) Laterally: bicipital tendon, upper humeral shaft, and gleno-humeral joint.

E. Al Murar
Ambulatory Healthcare Services, Abu Dhabi, United Arab Emirates

S. Al Memari (✉)
Abu Dhabi, United Arab Emirates

   (c) Posteriorly: supraspinatus, spine of scapula, and infraspinatus.

   (d) Armpit: palpate the head of the humerus.

7. Check the range of motion (active then passive): flexion, extension, abduction, adduction, and internal and external rotation (apply scratch test).

8. Check muscle strength or power:

   (a) Speed's test: provide downward resistance against a flexed shoulder at 90° with a supinated arm (test biceps).

   (b) Resist internal rotation (test subscapularis).

   (c) Resist external rotation (test infraspinatus and teres minor).

   (d) Resist abduction (test supraspinatus and deltoid).

   (e) Empty can test: Position the patient with shoulders elevated at 90° in scapular plane and full internal rotation, with thumbs facing downward. Apply a downward force just proximal to the patient's wrist while the patient resists (test supraspinatus).

9. Special tests:

   (a) Impingement tests: refer to Table 79.1 for details.

   (b) Joint instability testing: refer to Table 79.2 for details.

   (c) Labrum grind test: Performed with abducted shoulder at 120° and flexed elbow at 90°. The humeral head is compressed into the glenoid while internally and externally rotating the humerus (pain or clunk indicates labrum injury).

10. Check one joint above (neck for cervical spine) and one joint below (elbow). A quick neck exam includes checking for the range of motion and Spurling's test.

11. Give feedback and thank the patient.

12. Ensure a systematic approach.

Table 79.1 Impingement tests

Test	How performed	Diagnosis suggested by positive results
Crossover test	Extreme active adduction of the arm across the front of the chest	Tendon impingement at acromioclavicular joint
Neer's test	Passive forced forward flexion of the pronated arm	Rotator cuff tendon impingement
Hawkins–Kennedy test	Passive shoulder forward flexion and elbow flexion at 90° followed by medial rotation of the shoulder. Examiner grasps the patient's elbow with one hand and their wrist with the other. Examiner passively internally rotates and horizontally adducts the shoulder	Supraspinatus tendon impingement

Table 79.2 Shoulder instability tests

Test	How preformed
Anterior instability	Perform with shoulder and elbow at 90°, and apply an anterior force to the posterior shoulder, pushing the humeral head anteriorly. A stable joint will not move
Posterior instability	Perform with shoulder and elbow at 90°, and apply a posterior force to the anterior shoulder, pushing the humeral head posteriorly. A stable joint will not move
Inferior instability (sulcus sign)	Performed with arms hanging at the side. Downward pull of the arm causes a sulcus to form between the acromion and the humeral head if the patient has inferior instability

Performing Elbow Physical Examination

80

Eiman Al Murar and Shammah Al Memari

Learning Objectives
- How to conduct a comprehensive and systematic elbow examination?

---

1. Introduce yourself.
2. Wash your hands.
3. Explain why and what you are going to do and take permission to examine the patient.
4. Expose the body parts to be examined appropriately and take permission to examine the patient (neck, shoulders, arms, and back).
5. Inspect (while the elbow is flexed at 90° and extended):
   (a) Skin changes (erythema, rash, scars over the medial condyles for ulnar nerve injury, psoriatic plaques), swellings (adaptive hypertrophy in the dominant elbow of throwers, joint effusion, rheumatoid nodules, tophi, olecranon bursitis), bone deformity, and muscle wasting.
   (b) Carrying angle: The angle formed by the upper and lower arm in anatomical position (normally 5–10° in males, 10–15° in females and may increase in athletes). An abnormal angle is indicative of elbow instability or malunion.

E. Al Murar
Ambulatory Healthcare Services, Abu Dhabi, United Arab Emirates

S. Al Memari (✉)
Abu Dhabi, United Arab Emirates

© The Author(s), under exclusive license to Springer Nature Singapore Pte Ltd. 2024
S. Lari et al. (eds.), *Family Medicine OSCE: First Aid to Objective Structured Clinical Examination*, https://doi.org/10.1007/978-981-99-5530-5_80

305

6. Palpate (while the elbow is flexed at 90° and extended):
    (a) Temperature, swellings, or masses.
    (b) Tenderness: anterior aspect of joint, olecranon process, lateral epicondyle, medial epicondyle, and the ulnar nerve behind it.
7. Check the range of motion:
    (a) Active: flexion, extension, pronation (palm down), and supination (palm up).
    (b) Passive: same movements (check for crepitus).
8. Check muscle strength and power:
    (a) Resisted elbow extension (test triceps strength).
    (b) Resisted elbow flexion (test biceps strength).
9. Special tests:
    (a) Stretch tests: refer to Table 80.1 for details.
    (b) Elbow instability: refer to Table 80.2 for details.
10. Reflexes: biceps (C5), brachioradialis (C6), and triceps (C7,8).
11. Check one joint above (shoulder) and one joint below(wrist). State that it can be referred to as pain from the cervical spine. A quick neck exam includes checking for the range of motion and Spurling's test.
12. Give feedback and thank the patient.
13. Ensure a systematic approach (do not forget to check and examine the joint bilaterally).

Table 80.1 Elbow's special tests

Test	How performed	Interpretation of pain elicited by the test
Tennis elbow test	Actively flex elbow, then pronate and extend the wrist while the examiner resists at the hand	Pain indicates lateral epidcondylitis
Golfer elbow test	Actively flex the elbow, then supinate and flex the wrist	Pain indicated Medical epicondylitis

Table 80.2 Elbow's instability tests[a]

Test	How performed	Interpretation of pain elicited by the test
Valgus displacement or stress test	– Perform with externally rotated shoulder and elbow flexed at 20–30°. – Place your first palm over the medial elbow and the second above the lateral wrist. – Create an abduction or varus stress at the distal forearm.	Pain or laxity indicates medial collateral ligament (MCL) injury
Varus displacement or stress test	– Perform with externally rotated shoulder and elbow flexed at 20–30°. – Place your first palm over the medial elbow and the second above the lateral wrist. Create an adduction or varus stress at the distal forearm.	Pain or laxity indicates lateral collateral ligament injury
Milking maneuver	– Bend the affected elbow at 90° along with supination and thumb extension. – Move the opposite arm under the involved elbow for the patient to grasp the thumb of the affected limb with the opposite hand. Instruct the patient to pull laterally on the thumb creating valgus stress.	Pain indicates medial collateral ligament injury

[a]Remember that the medial collateral ligament is injured much more commonly than the lateral

Performing Wrist and Hand Physical Examination

81

Khuloud Al Hammadi, Dana Al Marzooqi, and Shammah Al Memari

> **Learning Objectives**
> - How to conduct a comprehensive and systematic wrist examination?
> - How to conduct a comprehensive and systematic hand examination?

Refer to Table 81.1 for details in most common causes of hand and wrist conditions

1. Introduce yourself.
2. Wash your hands.
3. Take permission to examine the patient and explain what you are going to do.
4. Expose examined body parts appropriately (hands up to elbows).
5. Inspect (bilaterally):
   (a) Skin (rash, erythema, palmar pallor).
   (b) Nails (nail pitting in psoriasis, nail bed pallor).
   (c) Dorsal surface for bone deformity, nodes, joint effusion, and drop wrist sign: refer to Table 81.2 for details.
   (d) Inspect the **palmar** surface of the hand for **muscle wasting** (thenar muscles in carpal tunnel syndrome, and hypothenar muscles in ulnar tunnel syndrome). Look for **Dupuytren's contracture** (fixed flexion contracture of the hand) and any swelling (mass or ganglion cyst). If any swelling is found, comment on the location, size, color, consistency (soft or hard), mobile, or fixed, any tenderness or fluctuation, relation to surrounding tis-

K. Al Hammadi · D. Al Marzooqi
Sheikh Khalifa Medical City, Abu Dhabi, United Arab Emirates

S. Al Memari (✉)
Abu Dhabi, United Arab Emirates

© The Author(s), under exclusive license to Springer Nature Singapore Pte Ltd. 2024
S. Lari et al. (eds.), *Family Medicine OSCE: First Aid to Objective Structured Clinical Examination*, https://doi.org/10.1007/978-981-99-5530-5_81

309

Table 81.1 Common diseases of the hand and wrist and their examination findings

Disease	Examination findings
Median nerve entrapment	Wasting of the thenar muscles, loss of sensation over the lateral 3.5 fingers, weak thumb abductors and wrist flexors, as well as positive Phalen's, Tinel's, and Flick tests
Ulnar nerve injury	Claw hand, hypothenar wasting, loss of sensation over the medial 1.5 fingers, weak small finger's abductors and interossei, as well as positive Formant's
Radial nerve injury	Drop wrist because of loss of wrist extensors and thumb abductors
De Quervain's tenosynovitis	Tenderness over the abductor pollicis longus and extensor pollicis brevis tendons, as well as a positive Finkelstein test

Table 81.2 Abnormalities to observe during wrist inspection

General observation	Description
Bone deformity	• Ulnar or radial deviation • Prominent ulnar styloid • Swan neck deformity (proximal interphalangeal joint hyperextension and distal interphalangeal joint hyperflexion) • Boutonniere deformity (proximal interphalangeal joint hyperflexion and distal interphalangeal joint hyperextension) • Z thumb deformity (metacarpophalangeal joint hyperflexion and interphalangeal joint hyperextension) • Mallet (inability to actively extend distal interphalangeal joint) or jersey (inability to actively flex distal interphalangeal joint) fingers • Claw hand (evident on resting the hand on a hard surface in case of ulnar nerve injury; also, called Tabletop test)
Nodes	Heberden (distal Interphalangeal joint) or Bouchard (proximal interphalangeal joint)
Joints for any effusion	Look for loss of spaces between the knuckles when the patient puts his hand into a fist
Drop wrist	Evident on hand stretching in case of radial nerve injury

sue (subcutaneous or intratendon or intrasheath by checking whether it appears or disappears with flexing and extending the wrist). Scars: at the wrist for carpal tunnel release.

(e) Elbow for skin: Psoriatic plaque, eczematous rash, or rheumatoid nodules. Scars at the medial epicondyles for ulnar nerve release surgeries.

6. Palpate:
   (a) Temperature (increase in rheumatoid arthritis).
   (b) Any sweating (in autonomic nerve dysfunction).
   (c) Pulses (radial and ulnar).
   (d) Capillary refill.
   (e) Any tenderness over the following: Metacarpophalangeal and interphalangeal joints, carpal bones, ulnar and radial styloid processes (to check for Colles' fracture), and snuff box (to check for scaphoid fracture). Abductor pollicis longus and extensor pollicis brevis tendons (for De Quervain's tenosynovitis).

Table 81.3 Range of motion of wrist, fingers, and thumb

Test	Range of motion
Wrist	• Flexion and extension (dorsiflexion and palmer flexion) • Pronation and supination • Lateral flexion (ulnar and radial deviation)
Fingers	• Flexion at MPJ and extension of IPJ (first and second lumbricals muscle supplied by median nerve while third and fourth by ulnar nerve) • Adduction and abduction (interossei muscles supplied by ulnar nerve) • Ask the patient to hold a paper between the third and fourth fingers against your resistance (interossei muscles)
Thumb	• On passive assessment look for clasp sign (flexor longus muscle – median nerve) • Extension (stick your thumb out to the side) • Flexion (involves bending the thumb at one or more joints, resulting in a decrease in the angle between the thumb and its adjacent structures) • Abduction (point your thumb up to the ceiling to test abductors supplied by the median nerve) • Adduction (returning the finger toward the other hand fingers) • Opposition (oppose the tip of your thumb to the tip of your little finger) • Functionality: – Power grip (patient squeezes examiner's fingers) – Pincer grip (try to break the pinch between his thumb and first finger to test opponens pollicis muscle supplied by the median nerve) – Buttoning and unbuttoning shirt – Holding pen and writing name

(f) Sensation: Check for sensation on the lateral 3.5 fingers for median nerve innervation. Check for the medial 1.5 fingers for ulnar nerve innervation and snuff box for radial nerve innervation.

7. Check the range of motion (active, passive, and resisted for power): refer to Table 81.3 for details.

8. Special tests: refer to Table 81.4 for details and try to mention a brief description of what you are doing as you perform them.

9. Check one joint above (elbow).

10. State that it can be referred to as pain from the cervical spine. A quick neck exam includes checking for the range of motion and Spurling's test.

11. Give feedback of your findings and cover the patient.

12. Thank the patient.

13. Maintain a systematic approach (do not forget to check and examine the joint bilaterally).

Table 81.4 Special wrist tests

Condition	Test	How performed
Carpal tunnel Syndrome (to check for median nerve)	Phalen's test	Ask the patient to flex his or her wrist maximally for 1 min, positive if numbness develops over the lateral 3.5 fingers
	Tinel's test	Tap on the volar side of the wrist over the median nerve, positive if numbness develops over the lateral 3.5 fingers
	Flick test	Command: "shake your hand," positive if the test relieves the numbness (has the highest sensitivity and specificity)
Ulnar tunnel syndrome (to check for ulnar nerve)	Froment's sign test	Ask the patient to hold a paper between his thumb and index finger against your resistance (test for adductor pollicis muscle, positive if notable to maintain pinch or flexes the thumb to compensate)
De Quervain's tenosynovitis (tenosynovitis of the sheath that surrounds both abductor pollicis longus and extensor pollicis brevis)	Finkelstein's test	Command the patient to the thumb, make a fist, and deviate the wrist ulnarly, positive test results in pain along the sheath of abductor pollicis "adduct longus"
Testing the ligament and tendon injury (in trauma cases)	Digital collateral ligament test	Apply varus and valgus stress to the injured fingers (laxity indicates tear)
	Digital DIP extensor and flexor tendons' test	Stabilize the PIP joint and ask the patient to flex and extend the DIP joint Classify the defects as follows: – Inability to extend the finger indicates extensor tendon rupture (mallet finger) – Inability to flex the finger indicates flexor tendon rupture (jersey finger)
	Ulnar collateral ligament of the thumb's test	Apply extension stress to the thumb (laxity or weakness indicates skier's thumb)

Performing Hip Physical Examination

82

Dana Al Marzooqi
and Shammah Al Memari

Learning Objectives
- How to perform a comprehensive, well-structured, and systematic hip exam?

1. Introduce yourself.
2. Wash your hands.
3. Explain why and what you are going to do and take permission to examine the patient.
4. Expose the body parts to be examined appropriately and take permission to examine the patient (ideally the back and lower extremities).
5. Inspect:
   (a) Observe from the front side for the posture (symmetry of legs and pelvis, any pelvic tilting), muscle wasting, and rotational deformity. From the side look for scars, lumbar lordosis, and from behind look for scoliosis, gluteal muscle wasting, and scars.
   (b) Assess gait (observe from front and back) noting any limp such as antalgic gait (a limp adopted in an effort to avoid pain by shortening the stance phase of the gait on the injured side) or Trendelenburg gait (a limp in compensation occurs by leaning the torso toward the involved side during stance phase on the affected extremity).

D. Al Marzooqi
Abu Dhabi, United Arab Emirates

S. Al Memari (✉)
Abu Dhabi, United Arab Emirates

© The Author(s), under exclusive license to Springer Nature Singapore Pte Ltd. 2024
S. Lari et al. (eds.), *Family Medicine OSCE: First Aid to Objective Structured Clinical Examination*, https://doi.org/10.1007/978-981-99-5530-5_82

6. Palpate (look at the face of the patient in case of tenderness):
   (a) Temperature.
   (b) Joint effusion.
   (c) Tenderness: anterior joint line (osteoarthritis, fracture, or a vascular necrosis), anterior superior iliac supine (ASIS) for sartorius attachment, anterior inferior iliac supine (AIIS) for rectus femoris attachment, greater trochanter (bursitis), iliotibial band, posterior superior iliac supine (PSIS), sacroiliac joint, gluteus muscle, ischial tuberosity (hamstring attachment), and hamstring muscle.
7. Check the range of motion (active and passive) and power (resisted range of motion)
   (a) Abduction and adduction.
   (b) Internal rotation: flex the knee to $90°$ in sitting position and move the foot away from the midline.
   (c) External rotation: flex the knee to $90°$ in sitting position and move the foot toward the midline.
   (d) Flexion (up to $90°$ if the knee extended and up to $120°$ if the knee flexed).
   (e) Extension (lift the leg off the table while in a prone position).
8. Check muscle strength and power:
   (a) Resist extension (for gluteus maximus and hamstrings)
   (b) Resist flexion (for iliopsoas, rectus femoris, and sartorius)
   (c) Resist abduction (for gluteus maximus, medius, and minimus)
   (d) Resist adduction (for adductors longus, brevis, magnus, and gracilis)
9. Evaluate sensation:
   (a) Meralgia paresthetica: Numbness in the lateral thigh distally. Is common in pregnancy (innervated by lateral femoral cutaneous nerve).
   (b) Medial aspect of the thigh and knee (obturator nerve).
10. Special tests:
    (a) Leg length measurement: from the ASIS until the medial malleolus (look for discrepancy).
    (b) Log roll test: Gently rolling thigh internally and externally (pain indicates fracture, infection, or synovitis). Most sensitive test for hip pathology.
    (c) Trendelenburg's test: ask the patient to stand on the affected leg, then ask him to lift the other leg off the ground, and if the pelvis drops toward the contralateral side, the test is considered positive.
    (d) Hop test: ask the patient to hop on each leg in turn (positive if pain is reproduced in the groin, indicating femoral neck stress fracture).
    (e) FABER or Patrick test: performed by crossing the ankle over the front of contralateral knee and then forcing the knee of the involved extremity down on the table to make a figure 4 (pain indicates SI joint pathology).

    (f) Ober's test: Ask the patient to lie on the side with the upper knee flexed at 90°. Measure the distance of the flexed knee from the table. Inability to bring the knee down to the table suggests iliotibial band tightness.

11. Check one joint above and one joint below: Knee and back (lumbosacral spine). A quick back exam includes checking for the range of motion and straight leg raise test.

12. Cover the patient and give feedback.

13. Thank the patient.

14. Ensure a systematic approach.

Performing Knee Physical Examination

83

Kawthar Al Ameri and Shammah Al Memari

Learning Objectives
- How to perform a structured knee exam?

---

1. Introduce yourself.
2. Wash your hands and maintain privacy.
3. Explain what you are going to do and take permission to examine the patient.
4. Expose the body parts to be examined (mid-thigh down to the foot).
5. Inspect:
   (a) Both knees for symmetry, shape, and size of patella.
   (b) Skin (erythema, swelling, scars, deformity, bruising).
   (c) Quadriceps muscle wasting measures the quads bulk with measuring tape 20 cm above the tibial tuberosity.
   (d) Gait.
6. Palpate:
   (a) Temperature bilaterally and all sides.
   (b) Tenderness: Position the knee in slight flexion and check for tenderness over multiple anatomical positions. Refer to Table 83.1 for details.

K. Al Ameri
Ambulatory Healthcare Services, Abu Dhabi, United Arab Emirates

S. Al Memari (✉)
Abu Dhabi, United Arab Emirates

S. Lari et al. (eds.), *Family Medicine OSCE: First Aid to Objective Structured Clinical Examination*, https://doi.org/10.1007/978-981-99-5530-5_83

Table 83.1 Tender points in knee examination: location and associated diseases

Location of the tenderness	Associated disease
Tibial tubercle	Osgood Schlatter disease
Patellar tendon	Tendinitis
Patellar plate	Pre-patellar bursitis
Medial knee joint line	Meniscal injury
Medical collateral ligament insertion point	Pes-anserine bursitis
Lateral collateral ligament and iliotibial band insertion point	Iliotibial band syndrome

7. Effusion (check while the patient is supine with extended knee):
   (a) Fluctuation test (ice cube test): tap over the patella by one finger(positive if patella moves up, indicating large effusion).
   (b) Patellar tap or ballottement sign: Squeeze the suprapatellar pouch with the index finger and the thumb starting 15 cm above the knee to the level of the upper border of the patella. Using the tips of the fingers of the free hand and push the patella with force downward (positive if patellar ballottement indicates moderate effusion).
   (c) Milking or bulge sign, cross-fluctuation sign, or fluid displacement test: repeatedly milk the effusion up into the suprapatellar area by moving the hand in an upward motion along the medial patellar margin, then press behind the patellar lateral margin (positive if swelling reappears, indicating minor effusion).
8. Check the range of motion (flexion and extension): normal range of motion is 130–140° in flexion and 0° in extension.
   (a) Passive (look for limitations and crepitus)
   (b) Active
   (c) Against resistance (for power)
9. Special tests:
   (a) Medial collateral ligament (MCL): valgus stress test: with the knee flexed at 30° (to isolate the collateral ligament), push medially against the lateral surface of the knee with one hand and pull laterally at the ankle with the other hand (pain indicates MCL tear).
   (b) Lateral collateral ligament (LCL): varus stress test: with the knee flexed at 30°, push laterally against the medial surface of the knee with one hand and pull medially at the ankle with the other hand (pain indicates LCL tear).
   (c) Anterior cruciate ligament (ACL): Perform **a Lachman test** (considered the most definitive test) by flexing the knee at 20° and applying anterior directed force on the tibia while stabilizing the thigh. Also, perform **the anterior drawer test** by flexing the knee at 90°, placing the examiner's thumbs on the medial and lateral joint lines, and placing the fingers on the hamstring insertions. Pull tibia forward (positive if tibia slides forward, indicating ACL tear).
   (d) Posterior cruciate ligament (PCL): Perform posterior drawer test by positioning the patient and examiner's hand as in the anterior drawer test. Push

the tibia backward (positive if the tibia slides backward, indicating PCL tear).

(e) Menisci: perform the McMurray test by starting with a flexed knee and while extending it and apply: **varus stress** and internal rotation (pain or click indicates lateral meniscal tear) and **valgus stress** and external rotation (pain or click indicates medial meniscal tear).

(f) Patellae: **Patellar apprehension test** is performed while the patient is lying supine with extended knees, pushing the patella medially and laterally (subluxation indicates patellar dislocation). **The patella grind test** is performed while the patient is lying supine with extended knees, and pushes the patella posteriorly into the trochlear groove of the femur. Grind back and forth (pain indicates patellofemoral syndrome).

(g) Popliteal fossa (while the patient is in a prone position): **Inspect** for any mass, swelling (baker cyst), or erythema and **palpate** for tenderness, popliteal pulsation, and any mass or swelling (measure the circumference bilaterally).

10. Check one joint above the "hip" and one joint below the "ankle." State that it can be referred to as pain from the lumbosacral spine. A quick back exam includes checking for the range of motion and the straight leg rise test.

11. Give feedback and thank the patient.

12. Ensure a systematic approach (do not forget to examine the joint bilaterally).

Performing Ankle Physical Examination

84

Eiman Al Murar and Shammah Al Memari

Learning Objectives
- How to perform a comprehensive, well-structured, and systematic ankle exam?

1. Introduce yourself.
2. Wash your hands.
3. Explain why and what you are going to do and take permission to examine the patient.
4. Expose the ankles and feet up to the knees and maintain privacy.
5. Inspect:
   (a) The foot: from front, back, lateral, medial, and plantar aspects (while the patient is lying). Look for any scars (at the big toe or tendon Achilles), deformity (hallux valgus, Charcot joint), foot shape, and arch when standing, any flat feet, muscle wasting, swelling, corns, or calluses.
   (b) The gait: ask the patient to stand on toes, heal, and outer and inner border of the foot.
   (c) Footwear: look for abnormal foot patterns.

E. Al Murar
Ambulatory Healthcare Services, Abu Dhabi, United Arab Emirates

S. Al Memari (✉)
Abu Dhabi, United Arab Emirates

© The Author(s), under exclusive license to Springer Nature Singapore Pte Ltd. 2024
S. Lari et al. (eds.), *Family Medicine OSCE: First Aid to Objective Structured Clinical Examination*, https://doi.org/10.1007/978-981-99-5530-5_84

Table 84.1 Ankle examination: areas of palpation and associated anatomical structures

Area of palpation	Anatomical structure
The medial side of the ankle	The medial malleolus, posterior tibiotalar, tibiocalcaneal, tibionavicular, deltoid, and calcaneonavicular ligaments
The lateral side of the ankle	The lateral malleolus, anterior talofibular ligament (ATFL), peroneal longus tendon, calcaneofibular ligament (CFL), and posterior talofibular ligament (PTFL)
The posterior side of the ankle	Achilles tendon (tendonitis), calcaneus, and tibialis posterior tendon
Foot	Base of the fifth metatarsal bone, mid-foot bones (especially the navicular bone)

6. Palpate:
   (a) Temperature.
   (b) Tenderness at the lower leg or different position of the ankle. Refer to Table 84.1 for details.
   (c) Squeeze the forefoot, and check capillary refill and sensation over the dorsum of the foot.
   (d) Pulses (dorsalis pedis, posterior tibialis).
7. Check the range of motion:
   (a) Active: dorsiflexion, plantar flexion, eversion, and inversion
   (b) Passive (check for crepitations)
8. Check muscle strength or power:
   (a) Resist eversion (peroneal longus and brevis) – L4
   (b) Resist dorsiflexion (tibialis anterior) – L4,5
   (c) Resist inversion (tibialis anterior and posterior) – L5 or S1
   (d) Resist plantar flexion (gastrocnemius, peroneal longus, tibialis posterior) – S1, 2
9. Special tests:
   (a) Tinel's test for tarsal tunnel syndrome: tap repeatedly on the tibial nerve behind the medial malleolus to reproduce pain and paresthesia along the course of the nerve.
   (b) Squeeze test: while the patient is sitting, squeeze the proximal tibia and fibula together (distal discomfort indicates tibiofibular ligament injury, aka syndesmosis sprain).
   (c) Anterior drawer test: stabilize the lower leg with one hand while cupping the heel with the other, then pulling forward on the calcaneus or talus complex (positive if lax or slides forward, indicating ATFL ligament tear).
   (d) Talar tilt test: Stabilize the lower leg with one hand while cupping the heel with the other, then invert the ankle joint. Laxity when compared to the opposite uninvolved side suggests CFL ligament tear, while pain suggests CFL ligament injury.
   (e) Thompson test: while the patient is prone, squeeze at the base of the calf muscle anticipating an ankle plantar flexion (lack of the plantar flexion indicates Achilles tendon rupture).

10. Check the ankle reflex (S1,S2).
11. Check one joint above (knee) and one joint below(foot). State that it can be referred to as pain from the lumbosacral spine. A quick back exam includes checking for the range of motion and straight leg rise test.
12. Give feedback and thank the patient.
13. Ensure a systematic approach (do not forget to examine the joint bilaterally).

Performing Physical Examination for a Patient Diagnosed with Diabetes Mellitus

85

Shaima Lari and Shammah Al Memari

> **Learning Objectives**
> - How to perform a comprehensive, well-structured, and systematic diabetic patient exam?

1. Introduce yourself, acknowledge (annual exam looking for organ damage and proper control of diabetes mellitus), and wash your hands.
2. Explain what you are going to do and take permission to examine the patient.
3. Expose the body parts to be examined appropriately.
4. Inspect: comment on obesity, underweight, moon-face, acromegalic facies, dehydration, gait, and footwear.
5. Measure:
   (a) Biometrics (weight, height, body mass index) and vitals (blood pressure, pulse rate).
   (b) Capillary blood glucose.
6. Examine eyes:
   (a) Xanthelasma, arcus senilis, cataract, and rubeosis iridis (neovascularization of the iris)
   (b) Visual acuity (check roughly with finger count or hand waving and mention that it should be checked with Snellen's chart)

S. Lari
Sheikh Shakhbout Medical City, Abu Dhabi, United Arab Emirates

S. Al Memari (✉)
Abu Dhabi, United Arab Emirates

  (c) Visual field with confrontation
  (d) Pupillary reaction
  (e) Red reflex
  (f) III, IV, VI cranial nerves
  (g) Fundoscopy
7. Examine ears: otitis externa and fungal infections.
8. Examine oral cavity: hygiene, caries, and aphthous ulcers.
9. Examine neck: carotid pulse and bruit, thyroid gland palpation, acanthosis nigricans, and skin tags.
10. Examine heart sounds, air entry at lungs, and abdomen (look for lipodystrophy at injection sites, listen for renal bruit).
11. Examine the feet to check for signs of neuropathy:
  (a) Inspect for edema, skin thinning, pigmentation, corns, callosities, tinea pedis, hair loss, ulcers, nail changes, amputation, Charcot's deformity, necrobiosis lipodica diabeticorum, granuloma annulary, nail changes (onychomycosis, paronychia, ingrown nails), and trimming technique.
  (b) Palpate: pulses, temperature, and dorsal and plantar flexion power.
  (c) Check sensation at 10 points by monofilament (10 g).
  (d) Check vibration sense (128 Hertz tuning fork).
  (e) Check proprioception in the big toe.
  (f) Check ankle reflex (S1, S2) and knee reflex (L3, L4).
12. Give feedback and thank the patient.
13. Ensure a systematic approach.

Performing a Physical Examination on a Patient Diagnosed with Hypertension

86

Shaima Lari and Shammah Al Memari

Learning Objectives
- How to perform a comprehensive, well-structured, and systematic exam on a hypertensive patient?

---

1. Introduce yourself.
2. Wash your hands.
3. Explain what you are going to do and take permission for examining the patient.
4. Expose the body parts to be examined appropriately and take permission to examine the patient.
5. Inspect: obesity, malar rash, moon-face, acromegalic facies, exophthalmos, marfanoid features, and hemiplegic gait.
6. Measure:
    (a) Weight, height, and body mass index (BMI).
    (b) Blood pressure: both arms, sitting then standing upright.
    (c) Pulse rate.
    (d) Capillary blood glucose.
7. Examine eyes:
    (a) Xanthelasma, arcus senilis, cataract, and rubeosis iridis
    (b) Visual acuity with Snellen's chart

S. Lari
Sheikh Shakhbout Medical City, Abu Dhabi, United Arab Emirates

S. Al Memari (✉)
Abu Dhabi, United Arab Emirates

© The Author(s), under exclusive license to Springer Nature Singapore Pte Ltd. 2024
S. Lari et al. (eds.), *Family Medicine OSCE: First Aid to Objective Structured Clinical Examination*, https://doi.org/10.1007/978-981-99-5530-5_86

    (c) Visual field with confrontation

    (d) Pupillary reaction

    (e) Fundoscopy

8. Examine hands: comment on clubbing, nicotine staining, sweating, water hammer or collapsing pulse (aortic regurgitation).

9. Examine oral cavity: comment on hygiene, caries, high arch palate, and cyanotic tongue.

10. Examine neck: check carotid pulse and bruit, palpate the thyroid gland, observe any signs of acanthosis nigricans, skin tags, or distended vessels.

11. Examine chest: inspect for pectus excavatum, palpate for any heave or thrill, auscultate heart sounds, and air entry at lungs and basal crackles.

12. Examine abdomen: palpate for aortic pulsation, radio-femoral delay, and auscultate for renal bruit.

13. Examine central nervous system (CNS): comment on cranial nerves, power, tone, sensations, reflexes (if you ran out of time explain: to complete I would do a CNS exam to rule out neuropathic end-organ damage).

14. Give feedback and thank the patient.

15. Ensure a systematic approach.

Performing a Physical Examination on a Patient Presenting with Dizziness

87

Shammah Al Memari

Learning Objectives
- How to perform a comprehensive, well-structured, and systematic exam on a patient presenting with dizziness?

1. Introduce yourself.
2. Wash your hands.
3. Explain why and what you are going to do and ensure a systematic approach.
4. Expose the body parts to be examined appropriately and take permission to examine the patient.
5. Gait: Observe for any imbalance, check Romberg's test. (Ask the patient to stand with his feet together. Then ask the patient to close his/her eyes. Remain close to the patient in case he/she begins to sway or fall. Positive for cerebellar lesion if the patient is unable to maintain this position even with his/her eyes open.)
6. Vital signs:
   (a) Comment on heart rate, respiratory rate, and blood pressure.
   (b) Check the blood pressure both lying, sitting, and standing (any postural hypotension with decrease in systolic blood pressure by 20 mmHg and diastolic blood pressure by 10 mmHg within 3 min of standing compared with blood pressure from the sitting or supine position).

S. Al Memari (✉)
Abu Dhabi, United Arab Emirates

© The Author(s), under exclusive license to Springer Nature Singapore Pte Ltd. 2024
S. Lari et al. (eds.), *Family Medicine OSCE: First Aid to Objective Structured Clinical Examination*, https://doi.org/10.1007/978-981-99-5530-5_87

329

7. Eye: if any nystagmus comments on:
   (a) Type of movement: pendular (smooth movement) or jerky
   (b) Direction of movement: horizontal, vertical, rotatory, or mixed, fixed, or changing
8. ENT:
   (a) Ear canal inspection: any discharge, foreign body, and tympanic membrane infection or perforation.
   (b) Hearing: grossly by whispering or rubbing fingers, precise by Rinne and Weber tests.
9. Cardiac: listen to carotids and feel pulse for arrhythmias.
10. Neurological:
    (a) Check gross power and sensation, deep tendon reflexes, and cranial nerves.
    (b) Cerebellar signs: gait (cerebellar ataxia), finger-nose test, dysdiadochokinesia (rapid alternating movements), and heel-shin test (moving the heel over the opposite leg).
11. Dix–Hallpike maneuver: seat the patient at the edge of the examination table, then assist him or her to lie down suddenly with the head hanging 45 degrees backward and turned 45 degrees to one side (once to right, once to left, and once in the middle) while keeping the eyes open.
    Check for the development of vertigo or nystagmus. Interpret as follows:
    (a) Severe vertigo or nystagmus of fixed direction with characteristic onset after 3–10 seconds, and that lessen with repetition indicating peripheral cause of vertigo.
    (b) Mild vertigo or nystagmus of variable direction with the immediate onset and continuous presence with repetition, indicating the central cause of vertigo.
    (c) Can be followed by Epley's maneuver as a therapeutic option for BPPV to remove debris from the semicircular canals and deposit it in the utricle where hair cells are not stimulated.
12. Give feedback, thank the patient, and ensure a systematic approach.

Part VIII

Counseling: Adult Health

Breaking Bad News to a Patient Newly Diagnosed with Diabetes

88

Kawthar Al Ameri, Noora Al Blooshi, and Shammah Al Memari

Learning Objectives
- How to take a focused history addressing the risk factors from a patient newly diagnosed with diabetes?
- How to effectively use the SPIKES model in breaking bad news to a patient newly diagnosed with diabetes?
- How to implement good communication skills in counseling a patient newly diagnosed with diabetes?

Focus areas on Risk include factors to develop diabetes mellitus, the complication of diabetes mellitus and how to prevent them, and how to diagnose and manage diabetes.

K. Al Ameri
Ambulatory Healthcare Services, Abu Dhabi, United Arab Emirates

N. Al Blooshi
Ambulatory Healthcare Services, Abu Dhabi, United Arab Emirates

S. Al Memari (✉)
Abu Dhabi, United Arab Emirates

© The Author(s), under exclusive license to Springer Nature Singapore Pte Ltd. 2024
S. Lari et al. (eds.), *Family Medicine OSCE: First Aid to Objective Structured Clinical Examination*, https://doi.org/10.1007/978-981-99-5530-5_88

1. Introduce yourself.
2. Establish good rapport: "How are you today?"
3. Setting:
   (a) Close the door, ensure no interruptions (call the nurse and ask her not to allow any interruptions and put your phone on silent), and ensure proper setting (tissue around with some water).
   (b) Ask if any family members are with the patient: "Are you here alone?"
4. Perception: Check using open-ended questions: "Mr. X, how can we help you today?" "Do you know why you are here?" "Do you know what tests you had last time and why were they done?" "Do you have any idea what the results might be?" "Some people like to have someone (family or friend) with them when they receive their results!"
5. Invite the patient to share in the discussion:
   (a) "Before we review the results, tell me, Mr. X, are you the sort of person who likes to know details or not?"
   (b) "Mr. X, I am afraid I have bad news."
   (c) "Mr. X, your blood glucose levels are high. I am sorry to tell you that this means that you are diabetic." Pause ... Hand in the patient some tissue paper.
   (d) Encourage expression of feelings: "I am sorry I had to give you such bad news. I wish things were different. It must be difficult to hear; how do you feel about it?" "I understand that it can be difficult to take the news."
   (e) "It is okay. Take your time. I am here for you."
   (f) "Would you like to have some rest in the treatment room before we proceed?"
   (g) Remember to facilitate verbal and nonverbal cues.
   (h) Remember to listen attentively and ask several times about the extent of understanding.
6. Knowledge check and sharing:
   (a) How much of the patient already knows? "Can you tell me what you know about diabetes?"
   (b) "It is not easy to hear that you are diabetic, but we will work with you to improve your health and well-being, and prevent diabetes complications."
   (c) "As you know diabetes is common worldwide. Many are diagnosed with it and are doing well, and so would you."
   (d) "Simply, there are two main types of diabetes, yours is type II, where your body is not responding to the insulin that is produced by the pancreas."
   (e) "Insulin is needed to make use of the glucose, the basic fuel that we get from food, for energy)."
   (f) "When glucose is in excess and is not utilized by the body, it accumulates and harms the eyes, heart, kidneys, nerves, and vessels."
   (g) "To decrease the glucose to normal, patients need to adjust their diet, start to exercise, take an oral tablet, and/or take insulin injections."

7. Empathy expression: "Tell me, Mr. X, how do you feel now?"
   (a) Acknowledge your limitations in breaking bad news.
   (b) Reinforce support provision and give clinic phone number.
   (c) Ask about feelings and emotional acceptance.
8. Summarize briefly what has been discussed and the upcoming plan: "What you can do is":
   (a) Start eating healthy food. I will refer you to a dietician to help you with that.
   (b) Exercise using the right shoes for 30 minutes 5 times a week.
   (c) Take your medications regularly.
   (d) Come back for your appointments: every 3 months with an annual checkup.
   (e) From our side, we will help you with regular labs [HbA1C, lipids, kidney functions, and electrocardiogram (ECG)], foot exam, education about foot care, and referral to an ophthalmologist for retinal screening annually. Referral to the dentist for screening and follow-up every 6 months. Vaccinations (influenza, hepatitis B, pneumococcal virus).
   (f) Direct associations and support groups.
   (g) Answer any queries and address concerns clearly.
9. Arrange:
   (a) Give hope but not a false one: "I know it's difficult to handle this, we are always available to support you and answer your questions."
   (b) Safety netting: "Diabetics are at risk of decreased blood glucose level. You need to be aware of the symptoms to be able to help yourself with half a cup of juice. the symptoms of hypoglycemia are sweating, shivering, dizziness, palpitation, and syncope."
   (c) Give a follow-up appointment soon and arrange the referrals as mentioned above.
   (d) Give away reading material and support groups contact if available!
   (e) Ensure patient's safety: "Do you think you can drive back home, or would you like me to arrange for you an appropriate transportation?"
   (f) Housekeeping: ensure you take a break after breaking bad news to regain emotional stability.
10. Communication skills: ensure an organized approach, mixed questioning style (open and close-ended questions), active listening, clear language, and reflection on the patient's ideas, concerns and expectations (ICE).

Breaking Bad News of Human Immunodeficiency Virus (HIV) Infection to a Newly Diagnosed Patient

89

Kawthar Al Ameri, Sakina Al Bloushi, Sumiya Taheri, and Shammah Al Memari

---

Learning Objectives
- How to take a focused history addressing the risk factors from patients newly diagnosed with HIV infection?
- How to effectively use the SPIKES model in breaking bad news to patients newly diagnosed with HIV infection?
- How to implement good communication skills in counseling patients newly diagnosed with HIV infection?

Focus areas include risk factors to develop HIV infection, sexual history, past medical history, and management of HIV patients.

K. Al Ameri
Ambulatory Healthcare Services, Abu Dhabi, United Arab Emirates

S. Al Bloushi · S. Taheri
Ambulatory Healthcare Services, Abu Dhabi, United Arab Emirates

S. Al Memari (✉)
Abu Dhabi, United Arab Emirates

© The Author(s), under exclusive license to Springer Nature Singapore Pte Ltd. 2024
S. Lari et al. (eds.), *Family Medicine OSCE: First Aid to Objective Structured Clinical Examination*, https://doi.org/10.1007/978-981-99-5530-5_89

1. Introduce yourself.
2. Establish good rapport: "How are you today?"
3. Setting:
   (a) Close the door, ensure no interruptions (call the nurse and ask her not to allow any interruptions and put your phone on silent), and ensure proper setting (tissue around with some water).
   (b) Ask if any family members are with the patient: "Are you here alone?"
4. Perception: Check using open-ended questions: "Mr. X, how can we help you today?" "Do you know why you are here?" "Do you know what tests you had last time and why were they done?" "Do you have any idea what the results might be?" "Some people like to have someone (family or friend) with them if they receive their results. Are you that type or you are happy to be alone?"
5. Invite the patient to share in the discussion:
   (a) "Since this is the first time I see you, I would like to ask you a few questions about your health." Any chronic medical and psychiatric conditions? Any current medications that may affect treatment options? Any history of sexually transmitted infections? Any known co-infections, such as tuberculosis (TB), hepatitis B, or hepatitis C infection? Rule out the risk factors (multiple sexual partners, tattoos, blood transfusion, previous surgeries).
   (b) Enquire about occupation, marital status, flu-like symptoms, or lymph node enlargement.
   (c) "Before we review the results, tell me, Mr. X, are you the sort of person who likes to know details or not?"
   (d) "After I reviewed your lab results, Mr. X, I am afraid I have bad news for you."
   (e) "Mr. X, I am sorry to tell you that your results have come back positive for human immunodeficiency virus (HIV)." Pause and hand the patient some tissue papers.
   (f) Encourage expression of feelings: "This must be very hard for you. I can see how difficult it can be to handle this."
   (g) "Would you like to have some rest in the treatment room before we proceed?"
   (h) Remember to facilitate verbal and nonverbal cues.
   (i) Listen attentively and ask several times about the extent of understanding.
6. Knowledge check and sharing:
   (a) Check how much the patient already knows: "Can you tell me what you know about human immunodeficiency virus (HIV) infection?"
   (b) "Human immunodeficiency virus (HIV) is a viral infection that attacks your immune system."
   (c) "It gets transmitted by body secretions (blood or sexual intercourse)."
   (d) "Having positive antibodies means that you carry the virus and may infect others."
   (e) "The infection has three main stages, and symptoms usually start with flu-like illness."

    (f) "Fortunately, treatments have been developed to slow the progression of the disease and they are available locally. Although it is not curative, it is important to know that the earlier you start on the medications, the later you develop the complications. We will work together with our consultants in infectious diseases on that together in order to help you."

    (g) "Moreover, I would encourage you to share the diagnosis with your family and medical attendants. I know many consider it as a social stigma, but we can collaborate with social workers and psychologists to sit with your family and help them understand and create a supportive environment for you."

    (h) "Remember to protect yourself from other infections and others from your infection:

    (i) Avoid sharing injections or shaving tools.

    (j) Do not donate blood.

    (k) Practice safe sex (use condoms). If lubricants are needed, use water-based gels such as K-Y gel rather than oil-based ones such as Vaseline as the latter may cause the condom to slip and therefore decreases its efficacy.

    (l) Screen your family for human immunodeficiency virus (HIV) infection so that they can start early treatment if they do."

7. Empathy expression: Explore emotions and show empathy, saying, "I can see how difficult it is for you, there are many people out there with similar diagnoses and they are doing well. I am sure you can deal with it too."

8. Summarize: "We have discussed multiple things Mr. X so please allow me to wrap up the important messages. As I told you, human immunodeficiency virus (HIV) is a viral disease that affects your immune system. There is treatment but no cure. You need to take precautions and screen your family. Does that make it clearer? Now, how about outlining a customized plan?" "Let us start with":

    (a) Lab tests: as detailed in Table 89.1.

    (b) Referral to the infectious diseases consultant who will review your results and decide the best treatment. You will be started on antiviral therapy (ART) to prevent your disease progression and transmission of HIV to others, along with regular follow-ups to monitor response, side effects, and complications.

    (c) Answer any queries and address concerns clearly: "Would you like to ask me anything? Do you feel better?"

Table 89.1 Lab investigations indicated for a newly diagnosed HIV patient

Test category	Details
Baseline and HIV activity status	Complete blood count, kidney function tests, liver function tests, CD4 count, and HIV viral load
Assessment for diabetes and hyperlipidemia	Fasting blood glucose and lipids
Screening for other STIs	Syphilis, hepatitis B, hepatitis C, gonorrhea, and chlamydia
Testing for concurrent or latent infections	TB, toxoplasma, and cytomegalovirus

9. Arrange:
    (a) Give hope but not false ones: "I know it's difficult to handle this, but we are always available to support you and answer your questions (if you have any please write them on a piece of paper so that we discuss them during the next visit)."
    (b) Arrange to follow up soon, mentioning: "Let us schedule a follow-up visit in a few days, at your comfort, to continue the treatment. How about that?" "Next visit, we will review the results and consider necessary vaccines: **For all patients:** hepatitis B vaccine, hepatitis A vaccine, influenza vaccine, pneumococcal vaccine, meningococcal vaccine, and Td or TdaP. **Patients with a CD4 count greater than or equal to 200 cells/mm^3:** MMR and Varicella (if CD4).
    (c) Safety netting: "If you develop any fever, rash, lung infection, decreased appetite, or unexpected weight loss, please come back immediately."
    (d) Give away reading material and support groups contact if available. If not explain: "I apologize, I do not have reading material for you, but you can book an appointment any time for any worries or questions you have."
    (e) Ensure patient's safety: "Do you think you can drive back home, or would you like me to arrange for you appropriate transportation?"
10. Communication skills: ensure organized approach, mixed questioning style (open and close-ended questions), active listening, clear language, and reflection on the patient's ideas, concerns and expectations (ICE).

Assessing and Counseling a Patient with Hepatitis C Virus (HCV) Infection

Kawthar Al Ameri, Sumiya Taheri, and Shammah Al Memari

Learning Objectives
- How to take a focused history addressing the risk factors from patients with HCV infection?
- How to effectively use the 5 As model to counsel a patients diagnosed with HCV infection?
- How to implement good communication skills in counseling patients with HCV infection?

Focus areas include Risk factors to develop hepatitis C infection, management of hepatitis C infection, and the complication of hepatitis C and prognosis.

K. Al Ameri
Ambulatory Healthcare Services, Abu Dhabi, United Arab Emirates

S. Taheri
Ambulatory Healthcare Services, Abu Dhabi, United Arab Emirates

S. Al Memari (✉)
Abu Dhabi, United Arab Emirates

© The Author(s), under exclusive license to Springer Nature Singapore Pte Ltd. 2024
S. Lari et al. (eds.), *Family Medicine OSCE: First Aid to Objective Structured Clinical Examination*, https://doi.org/10.1007/978-981-99-5530-5_90

1. Introduce yourself and establish a good rapport.
2. Ask:
   (a) Ideas, concerns, and expectations (ICE).
   (b) Since when? How? Any treatment? check patient understanding of the disease? "Just so that we are on the same page, can you tell me what you know about HCV?"
   (c) Any complaints: weight loss, jaundice, loss of appetite, fever, fatigue, dark urine, clay-colored stool, abdominal pain, nausea, and vomiting.
   (d) Past medical and social history (smoking, sexual activity, illicit drug use).
   (e) Ask about the risk factors: illicit injection use, exposure to needle sticks in a healthcare setting, history of transfusions or organs, unregulated tattooing, long-term hemodialysis, HIV-positive status, sexual activity with HCV or HIV-infected persons, and maternal HCV infection during pregnancy/birth.
3. Advise:
   (a) "Being your doctor, I think it's very important for you to understand that HCV infects the liver primarily."
   (b) "It is usually transmitted through sharing contaminated needles, shavers, toothbrushes, or having multiple sexual partners (small risk if solitary heterosexual partner). It can less likely be transmitted through surgeries/ blood transfusions since blood from donors is tested nowadays and devices are adequately disinfected. HCV doesn't spread by sneezing coughing, hugging, eating utensils, or through food and water."
   (c) "Initially only a few symptoms appear including flu-like illness, yellowish discoloration of the eyes and skin, fatigue, or joint pain."
   (d) "Depending on how strong the body's defense mechanism is, the HCV can either be cleared or continue, causing long-lasting inflammation beyond the first 6 months, a condition called chronic infection. Unfortunately, HCV is the most common viral cause of chronic hepatitis where 70–80% of infected individuals develop chronic infection."
   (e) "It is essential that you know that, at later stages of the infection, especially if not properly managed, a chronic infection for 20–30 years can lead to liver cell damage. This can cause liver cirrhosis in 15–30% of patients or even progress to hepatocellular cancer (HCC)."
   (f) "The good news is that we have treatment that slows down the damage and there are medications as well to help decrease the infectiousness and progression of the disease and they are locally available. We will work together with our experienced liver doctor (hepatologist) to ensure the best care for your health."
4. Assess: Patient understanding and clarify any ICE.
5. Assist: "Let us share a plan that is suitable for helping you. You can resume your normal daily life activities with no restrictions. However, you must make a few adjustments to protect yourself from other infections:
   (a) Ensure a daily balanced diet with lots of water and stop or limit your alcohol to once a day.
   (b) Avoid strenuous exercises, increased workload, or stress.

    (c) Do not take medications without doctors' advice (some may damage the liver), including herbs.

    (d) Practice safe sex: use male condoms.

    (e) Get hepatitis A and B vaccines to prevent co-infection."

6. Educate the patient about the expected evaluation and follow-up:

    (a) Lab tests reflect your liver function and to rule out other sexually transmitted diseases.

    (b) Ultrasound to check how well your liver has been coping.

    (c) To assess for liver fibrosis or cirrhosis to arrange for further monitoring and management.

    (d) Assessment of viral and patient factors that help in choosing the optimal antiviral selection (viral genotype, liver fibrosis stage, history of prior antiviral treatment, renal function, and concurrent medication use).

    (e) Tests for human immunodeficiency virus and hepatitis B virus are given the common modes of transmission and the association of these co-infections with more rapid disease progression.

    (f) Referral to a hepatologist to start on antiviral medications that are the cornerstone of treatment (cure defined as undetectable RNA level 12 weeks following the completion of therapy).

    (g) If liver damage occurs, we can start you on drugs: interferon/antivirals (such as lamivudine). These can cure up to 80% of people with hepatitis C.

    (h) Protect your loved ones.

    (i) Maintain good hygiene: Do not share toothbrushes, shavers, or needles. Wipe up blood spills with household bleach. Cover cuts and wounds with firm dressings.

    (j) Do not donate blood.

    (k) I encourage you to discuss the issue with your spouse. You can also bring him or her to the clinic so that we help you with that and prepare him or her psychologically. This is very important and will ensure that you have a supportive environment and that your spouse is tested.

7. Arrange:

8. Positive reinforcement: "Many others did it before you, you can definitely do it, we are always available to support you."

9. Follow up soon.

10. Refer to:

    (a) Dependence unit to treat alcohol dependence and intravenous (IV) drug abuse if any.

    (b) Hepatologist for lab investigations, imagining, liver biopsy if indicated, and initiation of antiviral medications.

11. Safety netting: "If you develop any yellowish discoloration, itchiness, bleeding, or suffer from difficulty with sleep, please come back immediately."

12. Brief assessment of the underlying conditions and age-appropriate screening.

13. Give away reading material if available.

14. Communication skills: ensure organized approach, mixed questioning style (open and close-ended questions), active listening, clear language, and reflection on the patient's ICE.

How to Deal with an Angry Patient

91

Shaima Lari, Noora Al Blooshi,
and Shammah Al Memari

Learning Objectives
- How to effectively manage emotions and de-escalate the situation when dealing with angry patients?
- How to establish a productive dialogue, address the patient's concerns, and work toward a mutually satisfactory outcome?

Focus areas include how to handle patients with various concerns, such as those wanting to be discharged against medical advice, expressing dissatisfaction with waiting times, requesting unnecessary tests or sick leaves, concerns related to junior staff training, and addressing patients wanting to raise complaints.

1. Introduce yourself, establish a good rapport, and maintain friendly gestures.
2. What to do?
   (a) Acknowledge the person's anger and validate his or her feelings. Say, "I can see that you are upset about …."
   (b) Find out the reason for the patient's anger and let him or her express the anger, or any feelings that led to his or her anger, such as frustration, fear, or

S. Lari
Sheikh Shakhbout Medical City, Abu Dhabi, United Arab Emirates

N. Al Blooshi
Ambulatory Healthcare Services, Abu Dhabi, United Arab Emirates

S. Al Memari (✉)
Abu Dhabi, United Arab Emirates

© The Author(s), under exclusive license to Springer Nature Singapore Pte Ltd. 2024
S. Lari et al. (eds.), *Family Medicine OSCE: First Aid to Objective Structured Clinical Examination*, https://doi.org/10.1007/978-981-99-5530-5_91

345

guilt: If patient anger was related to waiting time your answer should be: "I am very sorry that you had to wait so long to be seen. We have not forgotten about you, but we are very busy today. We always make sure that each patient's problems are fully evaluated, and some problems take longer than others. If the patient expresses frustration about having seen multiple physicians, you could respond with:" I am sorry you have had to repeat your medical history so many times. This is a teaching hospital, and that means that we have medical students and residents here, but we all work together. Sometimes, being seen by more than one person can help tease out some important details. Moreover, senior physicians always supervise all of your care. We treat all patients the same here regardless of their insurance status or ability to pay. Is there any specific reason you do not wish to be discharged? Are you worried about a problem at home or work?" (Rotte and Lopez 2011).

(c) Offer to do something for him or her: "You are right to expect to be treated quickly when you come to our hospital. Here is what I can do get your X-rays done as soon as possible." "I am here to help you now and I will spend as much time with you as you need" (Rotte and Lopez 2011).

3. How to do it:
    (a) Be aware of your own safety and know your escape route.
    (b) Setting: sit at the same level as the patient while respecting his or her personal space.
    (c) Maintain two arm's distance and provide space for easy exit.
    (d) Mind nonverbal cues: speak calmly and do not raise your voice, use concise and simple language, and avoid dismissive or threatening body language.
    (e) Be responsive: Empathize as much as you can and encourage the person to speak. Ask open rather than closed questions and use verbal and nonverbal cues to show that you are listening and identify feelings or desires: "What are you hoping for?" Listen closely to what the patient is saying and restate what the patient said to improve mutual understanding (e.g., "Tell me if I got this right …").
    (f) Address violence directly: The patient should be asked relevant questions, such as, "Do you feel like hurting yourself or someone else?"

4. What NOT to do:
    (a) Nonverbal cues: glare at the person, approach the patient from behind or move suddenly, get too close or touch him or her, or block his exit route.
    (b) Verbal cues: confront, interrupt, argue, or command the patient to calm down, patronize him or her, put the blame on others or exonerate yourself: "I was not there when you had this test ordered, so I cannot say exactly what was the doctor's plan and I cannot speak for that doctor," lie to the patient or make unreasonable promises, or breach confidentiality (especially if the angry person is a relative).

5. Arrange: *"Before we finish, let us quickly review what we have decided today ..."*
   (a) Be realistic and do not break the rules or do harm: *patient demanding unnecessary sick leave "I am not able to give you more than 3 days off work. If you are still having serious symptoms after 3 days, you should come back to my office to be re-examined. Parent requesting unnecessary test or medication: "I know you only want what is best for your child. We do, too. But ordering extra tests or medications will not help him or her out at this point. I am willing and able to get your child any tests or medications he or she needs, but right now, I think it would be best to start with some basic tests. If anything, abnormal shows up, we can order additional tests, as needed"* (Rotte and Lopez 2011).
   (b) Follow up as needed.
   (c) If a patient wants to make a complaint, offer details on how to and assure them it will get acknowledged by the manager in (X) number of working days.
   (d) Housekeeping is very important—take care of your own well-being too.
   (e) If medications are prescribed, explain: "You are a vital part of your own care, and it is important that you take this medicine every day, as directed. My job is to give you my opinion on the best way to deal with your medical problem. You are in charge of your own health, so it is entirely up to you whether you want to take the advice" (Rotte and Lopez 2011).
   (f) Brief assessment of the underlying conditions and age-appropriate screening.
   (g) Give away reading material if available.
6. Communication skills: ensure organized approach, mixed questioning style (open and close-ended questions), active listening, clear language, and reflection on the patient's ICE.

Medical Error Disclosure

92

Shaima Lari, Noora Al Blooshi,
and Shammah Al Memari

Learning Objectives
- How to take a focused history when disclosing a medical error to patients?
- How to effectively use the 5 As model when disclosing medical error to patients?
- How to implement good communication skills when disclosing a medical error?

Focus areas include communication skills, hospital policy, and mitigating consequences.

1. Introduce yourself and establish a good rapport.
2. Ask:
   (a) The reason behind the visit.
   (b) Specific ideas or concerns for this visit (medication, vaccination, care related to underlying condition).
   (c) Why was the test done or the medication prescribed?
3. Medical error disclosure.

S. Lari
Sheikh Shakhbout Medical City, Abu Dhabi, United Arab Emirates

N. Al Blooshi
Ambulatory Healthcare Services, Abu Dhabi, United Arab Emirates

S. Al Memari (✉)
Abu Dhabi, United Arab Emirates

© The Author(s), under exclusive license to Springer Nature Singapore Pte Ltd. 2024
S. Lari et al. (eds.), *Family Medicine OSCE: First Aid to Objective Structured Clinical Examination*, https://doi.org/10.1007/978-981-99-5530-5_92

    (a) Give a warning statement: "I am sorry, but I have bad news for you today."

    (b) State the error clearly in simple language (wrong dose or diagnosis was given or provided).

    (c) Mention why the error occurred. Avoid making excuses or blaming others (a colleague, system, program, clerk, etc.).

    (d) Pause and wait for the patient's reaction. Encourage feelings and emotional expression. Show empathy and avoid medical jargon. "I understand your frustration."

4. Express accountability:

    (a) Apologize personally: "I am very sorry that this happened. I am sure it was a terrible experience" (Rotte and Lopez 2011).

    (b) Express responsibility: "I apologize for what happened. I feel awful that I made that mistake" (Rotte and Lopez 2011).

    (c) Remain calm and don't argue: "I take responsibility for this error. You have been my patient for several years now and I appreciate you letting me take care of you. I am glad to see that you are doing well, and I want you to know that I am going to work hard to make sure that you get better" (Rotte and Lopez 2011).

5. Assist:

    (a) Put a plan to remedy harm taken place.

    (b) Pressure that this will not happen again and state possible actions to avoid similar events: "I want to make sure that such an error does not happen to you again. I will therefore highlight this allergy on your medical record, write an incident report, and keep you updated during your close follow-up" (Rotte and Lopez 2011).

    (c) Support the patient's wishes to complain but also offer alternatives. Let the patient write the complaint and assure them it will be investigated, and he or she will get a response.

    (d) Explain that it will be addressed openly and improvement will be made to avoid this in the future.

    (e) Invite questions from the patient, "What questions do you have for me?"

6. Arrange:

    (a) Follow up if no improvement at any time.

    (b) Safety net as appropriate.

    (c) Brief assessment of the underlying conditions, age-appropriate screening, and vaccination.

    (d) Give away reading material if available.

7. Communication skills: ensure organized approach, mixed questioning style (open and close-ended questions), active listening, clear language, and reflection on the patient's ideas, concerns and expectations (ICE).

Assessing and Counseling a Patient with Heartburn or Gastroesophageal Reflux Disease

93

Sakina Al Bloushi, Kawthar Al Ameri, and Shammah Al Memari

Learning Objectives
- How to take a focused history addressing the risk factors from patients complaining of heartburn?
- How to effectively use the 5 As model to counsel patients complaining of a heartburn?
- How to implement good communication skills in counseling a patient complaining of heartburn?

Focus areas include diagnosis of heartburn and red flags of heartburn.

1. Introduce yourself and establish a good rapport.
2. Ask:
   (a) Discover the problem: nature of symptoms (heartburn, regurgitation, chronic cough, halitosis, or hoarseness of voice), the onset of symptoms, aggravating factors (bending over or lying down), and relieving factors (antacids).
   (b) Exclude red flags (pain radiating to left shoulder, shortness of breath, dysphagia, odynophagia, upper or lower GI bleeding, weight loss), and risk factors (refer to Table 93.1 for details).

S. Al Bloushi
Ambulatory Healthcare Services, Abu Dhabi, United Arab Emirates

K. Al Ameri
Ambulatory Healthcare Services, Abu Dhabi, United Arab Emirates

S. Al Memari (✉)
Abu Dhabi, United Arab Emirates

© The Author(s), under exclusive license to Springer Nature Singapore Pte Ltd. 2024
S. Lari et al. (eds.), *Family Medicine OSCE: First Aid to Objective Structured Clinical Examination*, https://doi.org/10.1007/978-981-99-5530-5_93

Table 93.1 Risk factors of heartburn or GERD

Risk factor	Examples
Exaggerated physiological state	Older age, pregnancy
Past medical history	Obesity, diabetes mellitus (gastroparesis), hiatal hernia
Medications	Nonsteroidal anti-inflammatory drugs (NSAIDs) use
Social habits	Diet (caffeinated or carbonated foods or drinks, peppermint or mint, chocolate, citrus, high-fat food, milk, onions, garlic, spicy foods, tomato juice), smoking, alcohol use
Family history	Gastroesophageal reflux disease or heartburn

    (c) The treatment used so far (antacids, proton pump inhibitors, surgeries).

    (d) Patient's ideas, concerns and expectations (ICE) about the condition.

3. Advise:

    (a) "Heartburn is not a standalone condition; rather, it manifests as a symptom marked by a burning discomfort in the chest, frequently accompanied by an acidic taste in the mouth. This sensation, often referred to as indigestion or dyspepsia, is commonly linked to the intake of food and beverages."

    (b) "It typically arises from the reflux of stomach acid contents back into the esophagus, and occasionally into the throat. Peptic ulcers can also be a contributing factor. The reflux happens due to incomplete closure of the muscular ring valve at the junction of the esophagus and stomach, and it may be linked to a hiatus hernia."

    (c) "Things that aggravate the problem include particular food (as onion, pies, pastries, fries), certain drinks (as wine, coffee), chewing gum, stress, pregnancy, old age, certain drugs (as aspirin), obesity."

4. Assess: knowledge about red flags and precautions to take: "If you have any of the following, go immediately to the emergency department":

    (a) Severe chest pain.

    (b) Vomiting blood.

    (c) Dark, tarry stool.

    (d) Difficulty swallowing.

    (e) Palpitation with abdominal pain.

5. Assist:

    (a) Ways to prevent heartburn: have small frequent meals, make new lifestyle modifications, make a plan to lose some weight and avoid excessive physical activity such as running, avoid foods that upset you, tight-fitting clothes, and bedtime eating or snacks, stay upright for greater than or equal to 3 h after a meal and elevate the head of your bed (use three pillows or incline the bed to 45°), avoid nonsteroidal anti-inflammatory (NSAIDs) drugs, and quit smoking.

   (b) What complications to avoid: esophageal ulcer, hemorrhage or perforation, Barrett's esophagus (a change in the lining of the esophagus that can increase the risk of cancer), esophageal stricture (a narrowing of the esophagus due to scarring), bronchospasm (irritation and spasm of the airways due to acid), chronic cough or hoarseness of voice, or dental problems.

6. Arrange:
   (a) Follow up if no improvement at any time.
   (b) Other management options include pharmacological (proton pump inhibitors or antacids).
   (c) Safety net as appropriate.
   (d) Brief assessment of the underlying conditions, age-appropriate screening, and vaccination.
   (e) Give away reading material if available.

7. Communication skills: ensure organized approach, mixed questioning style (open and close-ended questions), active listening, clear language, and reflection on the patient's ICE.

Assessing and Counseling a Patient with Epilepsy

94

Dhuha Al Ameri and Shammah Al Memari

Learning Objectives
- How to take a focused history addressing the risk factors from patients complaining of epilepsy?
- How to effectively use the 5 As model to counsel patients complaining of epilepsy?
- How to implement good communication skills in counseling patients complaining of epilepsy?

Focus areas include History and knowledge of epilepsy and lifestyle changes of epileptics.

1. Introduce yourself and establish a good rapport.
2. Ask:
   (a) Patient's ideas, concerns and expectations (ICE) (newly diagnosed epileptic and does not know how to cope, epileptic noncompliant due to medication side effects, pre-employment counseling, epileptic who wants to drive, pre-marital counseling).
   (b) Other medical problems.

D. Al Ameri
Ambulatory Healthcare Services, Abu Dhabi, United Arab Emirates

S. Al Memari (✉)
Abu Dhabi, United Arab Emirates

© The Author(s), under exclusive license to Springer Nature Singapore Pte
Ltd. 2024
S. Lari et al. (eds.), *Family Medicine OSCE: First Aid to Objective Structured
Clinical Examination*, https://doi.org/10.1007/978-981-99-5530-5_94

355

(c) Medications and compliance.
(d) Social history: age, marital status, smoking, alcohol, driving, and occupation.
3. Advise:
   (a) Knowledge about epilepsy: "It is a common disorder (1 in every 100 people) that runs in families, in which a person is prone to have recurring seizures. A minor fault, in the complex electrical circuits in the CNS for an unknown reason, results in brief brain dysfunction. The various symptoms depend on what part of the brain is affected. Seizures can range from generalized seizures to partial ones". *"As your doctor, I think it's very important for you to know that most patients with epilepsy can achieve complete seizure control and lead a normal life (marry, have normal sexual life, and have children)."*
   (b) Medications: emphasize compliance ("Take your medication regularly. If you suddenly stop them, this could precipitate a severe fit.") and explain side effects ("If you get a fever, rash, mouth ulcers, bruising, or bleeding, please contact your physician.").
   (c) Avoid precipitating factors (fatigue, physical exhaustion, stress, sleep deprivation, hunger, and flashing devices such as television and cinema screens).
   (d) Driving: Inform the driving licensing authority: "You will not be able to drive till you are fit-free for a certain period of time depending on the type of license and vehicle."
   (e) Occupation: "People with epilepsy can hold down most jobs except that they should not operate heavy machinery because the medications commonly cause drowsiness."
   (f) Home environment: avoid potentially dangerous sites or activities when alone (kitchen, bathtub) and do not lock the bathroom doors.
   (g) Sports: avoid swimming, cycling, or rock climbing when alone, avoid boxing, but you can enjoy playing football.
   (h) "Wear an epileptic card or bracelet with details of your fits, medications, and your physician and hospital number."
   (i) Female patients: Antiepileptics may reduce the efficacy of oral contraceptive pills. You will need dual contraceptive methods [Mirena intrauterine device (IUD) or injectable are more suitable). If you wish to get pregnant, discuss this with your doctor first. You will need prenatal folic acid supplements to prevent backbone (and spinal cord) anomalies (neural tube defects) and prophylactic vitamin K to prevent neonatal bleeding.
4. Assess:
   (a) Re-explore ICE.
   (b) Level of understanding.
   (c) Knowledge about the red flags and precautions to take.
5. Assist: "Let us share a plan that is suitable for helping you."
   (a) "Ensure compliance and regular follow-up."
   (b) "Ensure a safe environment during attacks."
   (c) Inform a responsible person at work or school: "When in seizure, do not restrain, try to stop the fit, or force anything into the mouth, just roll the seizing patient to one side and keep her or him in a safe environment."

(d) "Have rectal valium at home in case of intractable seizures (status epileptics)."

6. Arrange:
   (a) Follow up and monitor drug levels.
   (b) A first-time seizure should be seen within 4 weeks by a specialist, the risk of recurrent seizure is high within 3–6 months of the first seizure.
   (c) If new onset seizure (carbamazepine, oxcarbazepine, phenytoin for focal seizure, lamotrigine, levetiracetam, topiramate, valproate for focal or generalized seizure).
   (d) Invite the patient to bring close relatives, friends, or colleagues to be educated about dealing with him or her in case he or she develops a fit. Say, "When it lasts more than 5 min with no consciousness between attacks, this is called status epileptic. You will need a suppository to stop it and then you must be taken immediately to the emergency."
   (e) Emergency therapy like IV lorazepam or 10 mg IM midazolam or rectal diazepam is used in case of recurrent or prolonged seizures lasting ≥5 min or tonic–clonic seizures lasting ≥2 min.
   (f) Anticipate complications, safety netting, and red flags.
   (g) Brief assessment of the underlying conditions and age-appropriate screening.
   (h) Give away reading material if available.

7. Communication skills: ensure organized approach, mixed questioning style (open and close-ended questions), active listening, clear language, and reflection on the patient's ICE.

Assessing and Counseling a Patient with Obesity

95

Shaima Lari and Shammah Al Memari

Learning Objectives
- How to take a focused history addressing the risk factors from a patient presenting with obesity?
- How to effectively use the 5 As model to counsel a patient presenting with obesity?
- How to implement good communication skills in counseling a patient presenting with obesity?

Focus areas include causes and complications, motivational interviewing techniques, and pharmacological and nonpharmacological options for obesity management.

1. Introduce yourself and establish a good rapport: "The decision to reduce weight is probably the best one that you take in your life, and we are here to support and help you." "Would it be OK to talk about your weight today?"
2. Ask:
   (a) Current weight, height, and body mass index?
   (b) How long has the patient been obese?

S. Lari
Sheikh Shakhbout Medical City, Abu Dhabi, United Arab Emirates

S. Al Memari (✉)
Abu Dhabi, United Arab Emirates

© The Author(s), under exclusive license to Springer Nature Singapore Pte Ltd. 2024
S. Lari et al. (eds.), *Family Medicine OSCE: First Aid to Objective Structured Clinical Examination*, https://doi.org/10.1007/978-981-99-5530-5_95

   (c) What about during your childhood: obesity, dysmorphic features, short stature, and stunted growth?
   (d) Medical history: diabetes mellitus, hypertension, coronary artery disease, hyperlipidemia, smoking, obstructive sleep apnea, knee osteoarthritis, gastroesophageal reflux disease, and cancers.
   (e) Regular use of any medications, including steroids, oral contraceptive pills, antidepressants, antipsychotics, and antiepileptics.
   (f) Rule out organic causes: hypothyroidism (constipation, fatigue, cold intolerance) or polycystic ovarian syndrome (irregular menses, hirsutism, acne).
   (g) Previous trials to reduce weight (medical or surgical, reasons for failure).
   (h) Social history: self-image or feeling and impact of obesity in social life.
   (i) Explore ideas, concerns and expectations (ICE).
3. Advise: "I can see that you're eating or lifestyle habits are putting you at risk for multiple diseases" (you can relate to specific diseases such as diabetes or hypertension if the patient has a family history). ("It is up to you to decide to make a lifestyle change, I am here to support you") if the patient agrees or shows interest. "Obesity is a behavioral, sociocultural problem and occurs when you have an unbalance between your intake and energy use." Explain to the patient the 5Rs:
   (a) Relevance: List the personal and health advantages of losing weight. Establish a connection between obesity and any existing medical conditions: "Losing weight will help improve your sugar control, knee pain, etc. Moreover, weight loss will give you a nice body shape, and this will boost your self-esteem."
   (b) Risks: "Do you know how the increase in weight can affect your life?" Explain how obesity can affect the patient by mentioning the following: "Obesity is scientifically linked to several health risks, including diabetes mellitus, hypertension, ischemic heart disease, infertility, and various cancers. Furthermore, it can adversely affect mood and social interactions, as supported by studies."
   (c) Rewards: "I am confident that achieving your target weight and losing excess weight will bring about numerous rewards, significantly influencing your overall well-being."
   (d) Roadblocks: "*Set a date and share it with family and friends. Do you think of anyone who can stand between you and this achievement? Are you worried about the reaction of a friend or family to your decision? How about you ask family members to help you and list down roadblocks that you might face and ways to avoid them?*"
   (e) Repetition: "Remember it's all about your health, you can do it."
4. Assess: Ask the patient:
   (a) "*Do you know about the different methods that are available to help you?*"
   (b) "*On a scale of 0 to 10, how confident are you that you can lose weight?*"
   (c) "*On the same scale, how motivated you are to lose weight?*"
   (d) Stage on behavioral change cycle according to motivation and willingness to lose weight (pre-contemplation, contemplation, preparation, action, maintenance).

Table 95.1 Managing a patient with obesity

Management options		Details
Lifestyle modification	Diet	• "Be sensible with your plan. Do not crash diet but set a goal over 6–12 months" • "Avoid fast food, dense carbohydrates, and fried food. Avoid spicy food, peanuts, chocolates, and ice cream. Go for natural food and eat rather than drink your calories" • "Have grilled or boiled meat and egg 3 times per week" • "Increase fruit and vegetable intake (boiled and fresh)" • "Do not eat too fast. Chew food adequately" • "Do not eat in front of the television, or while driving" • "Eat on small plates and do not eat leftovers." • "Eat 5–6 times a day, 3 meals with small healthy snacks" • Explain to the patient the idea of the healthy plate (1/2 of the plate should consist of vegetables or fruits, 1/4 of it whole grains and 1/4 protein) • Keep a diary to record the type of food you eat and your total calories
	Exercise	• "Choose a sport that you like (tennis, swimming, golf, or cycling) and do it regularly" • "A good start can be a brisk walk for 20–30 min per day at least 5 times per week" • "Choose to be active during your whole day: Walk at every opportunity. Take the stairs instead of lifts"
	Other modifications	• Avoid shopping when feeling hungry • Always shop with a previously prepared list or let someone else shop for you • Weight yourself weekly
Medications (used as an adjacent to lifestyle intervention; consider stopping the medication if there is no more than 5% weight loss in 3 months; consider initiation of treatment in cases with a BMI of 30 or BMI of 27 with comorbidities; for FDA-approved option)	Orlistat	• Side effects include flatulence, oily stool, and severe liver disease (rare; therefore, monitor the liver functions)
	Lorcaserin	• Avoid use in psychiatric conditions. • Side effects: Headache, nausea, dry mouth, and dizziness
	Naltrexone/bupropion	• Mean weight loss 3% of total body weight. contraindicated on siezure disorders and uncontrolled hypertention
	Phentermine (P)/topiramate (T)	• Mean weight loss 8.5%. • contraindicated in psychiatric conditions or in uncontrolled hypertension
	Liraglutide	• 3.0 mg per day injectable, Mean weight loss 4.8% of total body weight
	Semaglutide	• 2.4 mg injectable on a weekly basis. Mean weight loss 11 to 13% body weight.
	Tirzepatide	15 mg max weekly. Mean weight loss 15–21% of total body weight. injectable

(continued)

Table 95.1 (continued)

Management options		Details
Surgeries*	Gastric band	Adjustable band around the stomach creating a smaller pouch, limiting food intake.
	Intragastric balloon	Surgical removal of a portion of the stomach, reducing size and limiting food intake. irreversible. Non-surgical procedure involving a balloon in the stomach to promote fullness and restrict food intake.
	Sleeve gastrectomy	Surgical removal of a portion of the stomach, reducing size and limiting food intake. irreversible
	Roux-en-Y gastric bypass	Surgical procedure creating a small stomach pouch and rerouting the digestive tract, reducing calorie absorption. Success rate in reducing weight is higher.
	Single-anastomosis duodenoileal bypass with sleeve gastrectomy (SADI-S)	Combined procedure inducing weight loss through sleeve gastrectomy and rerouting of the digestive tract.

*(if body mass index is more than or equal to 40, or index more than or equal to 35 with obesity-related comorbidities or index of 30–34.9 with either difficult-tocontrol diabetes mellitus type 2 or metabolic syndrome)

5. Assist: refer to Table 95.1 for details.
6. Arrange:
   (a) Positive reinforcement: *"Many others did it before you, you can definitely do it, we are always available to support you. We will work together even after losing weight to help you in maintaining your weight for the first 2 years. This will help in stabilizing your weight onward."*
   (b) Examination: short stature, moon-face, body mass index, hirsutism, striae, and waist–hip ratio (truncal obesity).
   (c) Labs to investigate the secondary causes of obesity and obesity-related complications: thyroid-stimulating hormone, insulin-like growth factor, cortisol, and cardiovascular risk factors: fasting glucose, lipids, liver enzymes, consider growth hormone in select patients with a pituitary disease or brain surgery, and consider referral for genetic testing with a strong suspicion of monogenetic obesity (prepubertal onset of obesity, dysmorphic features, developmental problems, severe hyperphagia, and /or family history of significant weight difference among first-degree relatives).
   (d) Follow up in 2 weeks: "I expect you to lose 1–2 kg by then. Please come any time in between that you feel you are out of track."
   (e) Referral to a dietician, bariatric medicine or surgery clinic, and stress management sessions.
   (f) Teach coping strategies (how to cope with life stressors).
   (g) Brief assessment of the underlying conditions and perform age-appropriate screening.
   (h) Give away reading material if available.
7. Communication skills: ensure organized approach, mixed questioning style (open and close-ended questions), active listening, clear language, and reflection on the patient's ICE.

Smoking Cessation Counseling

96

Shaima Lari and Shammah Al Memari

Learning Objectives
- How to take a focused history addressing the risk factors from patients presenting for smoking cessation counseling?
- How to effectively use the 5 As model to counsel patients presenting for smoking cessation counseling?
- How to implement good communication skills in counseling patients presenting for smoking cessation counseling?

Focus areas include smoking cessation benefits and pharmacological options for smoking cessation.

1. Introduce yourself and establish a good rapport.
2. Ask:
   (a) "At what age did you start smoking?"
   (b) Types, amount, and frequency of use:
       Smoking shisha approximately accounts for 39–40 cigarettes. Smoking pipe almost accounts for 7–10 cigarettes per inhalation (there are mild, moderate, and heavy types depending on the amount of pure nicotine that it contains).

S. Lari
Sheikh Shakhbout Medical City, Abu Dhabi, United Arab Emirates

S. Al Memari (✉)
Abu Dhabi, United Arab Emirates

© The Author(s), under exclusive license to Springer Nature Singapore Pte Ltd. 2024
S. Lari et al. (eds.), *Family Medicine OSCE: First Aid to Objective Structured Clinical Examination*, https://doi.org/10.1007/978-981-99-5530-5_96

(c) "Have you ever felt you should cut down on your smoking?"
(d) "Have people annoyed you by criticizing your smoking?"
(e) "Have you ever felt bad or guilty about your smoking?"
(f) First smoking session of the day [eye opener (occurs within 15 min of waking up and indicates severe addiction)].
(g) Previous attempts to quit (number, length, methods used, perceived reason for failure).
(h) Past medical history: diabetes, hypertension, coronary artery disease, and asthma.
(i) Alcohol or drugs use.

3. Advise: "Being your doctor, I think it is very important for you to quit smoking."Discuss the 5Rs with the patient:
(a) Relevance: Link smoking to current medical conditions. Briefly list the advantages of quitting: refer to Table 96.1 for details.
(b) Risks: "Do you know how smoking can affect your life?" If no, explain.
(c) Rewards: "I am sure that you will gain many rewards from quitting. It will have a significant impact on your general well-being."
(d) Roadblocks: "Set a date and share it with family and friends. Do you think of anyone who can stand between you and this achievement? Are you worried about the reaction of a friend or family to your decision?"
(e) Repetition: "Remember it's all about your health, you can do it."

4. Assess:
(a) "On a scale of 0–10, how confident are you that you can quit?"
(b) "On the same scale, how motivated you are to quit smoking?"
(c) Stage on behavioral change cycle according to motivation and willingness to quit (pre-contemplation, contemplation, preparation, action, maintenance).

5. Assist: "Let us share a plan that is suitable to help you quit smoking."
(a) Set a quit date.
(b) Address psychosocial fears, and family and friend support.

Table 96.1 Advantages of quitting smoking

Time after quiting	Health benefits
20 min	BP, pulse, and peripheral temperature normalize
8 h	Carbon monoxide levels in the blood normalize
2 days	Improved ability to smell and taste
3 days	Breathing gets easier as bronchial tubes relax and lung capacity increases
1 month	Mucous in the lung loosens and lung functions and circulation improve
2 months	Blood flows more easily to the arms and legs and lung function increases up to 30%
3 months	Lungs become healthier, you breathe easier, and you get fewer colds
1 year	Risk of sudden death from heart attack is lowered by 50%
5 years	50% reduction in lung cancer death rate for the average smoker
10 years	Risk of sudden heart attack and stroke equalizes to that of nonsmokers and the risk of cancer drops significantly

(c) Avoid smoking cues: coffee, stress, etc.
(d) The patient can keep cigarettes box away to take time to reach them.
(e) He or she may stay away from a smoking environment to decrease his need and the feeling of urge to go back to that habit.
(f) A gradual reduction in the amount of smoke (progressive restriction).
(g) Use alternatives: gum, hand activity, and get involved in sports.
(h) Pharmacological methods: refer to Table 96.2 for details.
(i) Educate the patient about the side effects of smoking cessation, including weight gain, headache, anxiety, nausea, and craving for more tobacco (as nicotine creates a chemical dependency).

6. Arrange:
(a) Positive reinforcement: "Many others did it before you, you can definitely do it, we are always available to support you."
(b) Follow up soon.
(c) Referral to smoking cessation clinic.
(d) Anticipate withdrawal and weight gain.
(e) Brief assessment of the underlying conditions and age-appropriate screening.
(f) Give away reading materials if available.

7. Communication skills: ensure organized approach, mixed questioning style (open and close-ended questions), active listening, clear language, and reflection on the patient's ICE.

Table 96.2 Pharmacological options for aiding smoking cessation

Medication	Initiation	Dosage	Side effects
Nicotine replacement therapy (patches, gum, inhaler, spray, or lozenges)			Gastrointestinal distress; mouth, throat, or skin irritation (American Academy of Family Physicians, 2012)
Bupropion (effectiveness increases if combined with nicotine replacement therapy)	Begin therapy 1–2 weeks before the quit date and continue until 12 weeks to 6 months after the quit date	150 milligrams (mg) in the morning for 3 days, then increased to 150 milligrams (mg) twice daily	• Insomnia and dry mouth • Contraindicated in patients with seizure or eating disorders and in those who have used a monoamine oxidase inhibitor in the past 14 days. May increase suicidality in patients with depression (American Academy of Family Physicians, 2012)
Varenicline (Chantix) (it is expensive and should not be combined with nicotine replacement therapy, otherwise no other drug interactions)	Begin therapy 1 week before the quit date and continue for 12 weeks	First 3 days: 0.5 milligrams (mg) per day, the next 3 days: Milligrams twice daily, thereafter 1 mg twice daily	• Headache, nausea, insomnia, abnormal dreams, neuropsychiatric symptoms, flatulence, and increase risk of cardiovascular events in patients with cardiovascular disease (fewer side effects in comparison to bupropion) (American Academy of Family Physicians, 2012)

Immunization Counseling for a Patient Diagnosed with Diabetes Milletus

97

Dana Al Marzooqi, Buthaina Al Maskari,
and Shammah Al Memari

Learning Objectives
- How to take a focused history addressing the risk factors from diabetic patients presenting for vaccination counseling?
- How to effectively use the 5 As model to counsel diabetic patients presenting for vaccination counseling?
- How to implement good communication skills in counseling diabetics patients presenting for vaccination counseling?

Focus areas include risk factors of diabetes mellitus, vaccines, and their side effects.

---

1. Introduce yourself and establish a good rapport.
2. Ask:
   (a) Ideas, concerns and expectations (ICE).
   (b) History (onset of diabetes mellitus, treatment, control, other chronic diseases, screening).
   (c) Risk factors: health worker, surgery, contact, travel, asplenia, intravenous drug use, homosexual, chronic liver, renal, or heart disease.
3. Advise: "As your doctor, I think it is very important for you to get proper information about the needed vaccines for patients with diabetes. This is because diabetes decreases immunity and therefore you need to be protected."

S. Al Memari (✉) · D. Al Marzooqi · B. Al Maskari
Abu Dhabi, United Arab Emirates

© The Author(s), under exclusive license to Springer Nature Singapore Pte
Ltd. 2024
S. Lari et al. (eds.), *Family Medicine OSCE: First Aid to Objective Structured
Clinical Examination*, https://doi.org/10.1007/978-981-99-5530-5_97

4. Assess:
   (a) "Have you taken any vaccines as an adult so far?"
   (b) "Have you ever had a severe allergic reaction to vaccines taken before?"
5. Assist: "Let us share a plan that is suitable for you ...."
   (a) Protection against seasonal flu annually: By intramuscular injection of inactivated influenza vaccine or influenza nasal spray. The latter is contraindicated in pregnant ladies and immunocompromised. It is relatively contraindicated if the patient has taken antiviral drugs within the previous 48 h, has had a severe allergic reaction to vaccine components or egg, or had a severe reaction to the injection previously (e.g., Guillain–Barre syndrome). Refer to Table 97.1 for details of the administration of influenza vaccine if patient has a history of egg allergy.
   (b) Tetanus, diphtheria, and acellular pertussis (TDaP vaccine) against diphtheria, whooping cough, and tetanus (lockjaw): One dose of tetanus, diphtheria, and acellular pertussis (TDaP) for adults above 18 years of age, otherwise tetanus and diphtheria (Td) booster every 10 years. Also recommended in the third trimester of each pregnancy if high risk (outbreak of pertussis in the community).
   (c) Pneumococcal vaccination: For adults aged 19–64 years, one dose of pneumococcal conjugate vaccine (PCV15) or one dose of (PCV 20); if PCV 15 is used, it should be followed by the pneumococcal polysaccharide vaccine (PPSV23) ≥ 1 year. Adults aged ≥65 who have not received any pneumococcal vaccines should receive one dose of pneumococcal conjugate vaccine (PCV15) or one dose of (PCV 20); if PCV 15 is used, it should be followed by the pneumococcal polysaccharide vaccine (PPSV23) ≥ 1 year.
   (d) Hepatitis B vaccination: Doses depend on the type of vaccine. Usually, it is recommended to take three doses at 0, 1, and 6 months.
   (e) Hepatitis A vaccine: Two doses 6–12 months apart, in high-risk individuals, living in or traveling to endemic areas or food handlers or healthcare providers.
   (f) Recombinant zoster vaccine (Shingrix): Age 50 years or older, two dose series, 2–6 months apart.

Table 97.1 Influenza vaccination in patients with egg allergy: guidelines for administration based on reaction history

Allergic history	Recommended action for influenzas virus vaccination
No reaction to lightly cooked egg (scrambled eggs)	Administer any influenza vaccine
Reaction limited to hives	Administer any influenza vaccine and observe the patient for 30 min
Symptoms other than hives (e.g., hypotension, wheezing, perioral swelling)	The vaccine can still be administered but referral to the infectious disease department where expertise in the management of severe allergic reaction is available is preferable

(g) Human papillomavirus (HPV) vaccine: For males and females up to the age of 26 years, 2–3 doses depending on age at initial dose, and between the ages of 27–45 it is a shared clinical decision.

(h) Measles, mumps, and rubella (MMR) vaccine: One or two doses, if born at or after 1957 and have not gotten the vaccine, have no immunity to these diseases by laboratory evidence, or are an international traveler.

(i) Varicella vaccine: Two dose series, 4–8 weeks apart if born at or after 1980 and have not gotten two doses of this vaccine or have not developed natural post-infection immunity to this disease.

6. Arrange:

(a) Positive reinforcement.

(b) Anticipate complications: Observe for 15 minutes post-vaccine in order to early detect and manage anaphylaxis or vasovagal syncope. Apply cold compression at the site of the injection to decrease swelling and pain. Take paracetamol for any fever.

(c) Safety netting: "If you develop any skin rash, lips swelling, or shortness of breath, please seek medical attention immediately."

(d) Follow up: for annual diabetes examination or to follow up lab results.

(e) Brief assessment of the underlying conditions and screening for age.

(f) Give away reading material if available.

7. Communication skills: ensure organized approach, mixed questioning style (open and close-ended questions), active listening, clear language, and reflection on the patient's ICE.

Assessing and Counseling a Patient Diagnosed with Diabetes Mellitus about Foot Care

98

Shaima Lari, Noora Al Blooshi, and Shammah Al Memari

Learning Objectives
- How to take a focused history addressing the risk factors in patients diagnosed with diabetes mellitus for effective foot care?
- How to effectively use the 5 As model to counsel patients diagnosed with diabetes mellitus on preventive foot care measures?
- How to implement good communication skills in counseling patients diagnosed with diabetes mellitus to educate and prevent diabetic foot complications?

Focus areas include history of diabetes and its complications, and diabetic foot care.

1. Introduce yourself and establish a good rapport.
2. Ask:
   (a) "How long have you been diabetic? Treatment used? Level of control?"
   (b) Any previous foot injury, infections, nail problems, or accidental foreign bodies (indicates loss of sensation).

S. Lari
Sheikh Shakhbout Medical City, Abu Dhabi, United Arab Emirates

N. Al Blooshi
Ambulatory Healthcare Services, Abu Dhabi, United Arab Emirates

S. Al Memari (✉)
Abu Dhabi, United Arab Emirates

© The Author(s), under exclusive license to Springer Nature Singapore Pte Ltd. 2024
S. Lari et al. (eds.), *Family Medicine OSCE: First Aid to Objective Structured Clinical Examination*, https://doi.org/10.1007/978-981-99-5530-5_98

(c) Any end-organ damage: kidney [deranged glomerular filtration rate (eGFR) or microalbuminuria], eye, or cardiac disease (angina or myocardial infarction).

(d) Patient's ideas, concerns and expectations (ICE): medication, vaccination, and care related to an underlying condition.

(e) Brief past medical, family, and social histories along with vaccination status.

3. Advise: "Feet problems among diabetes patients are common, treating them early is very important to prevent serious complications. This is because; healing is slow in diabetics due to the decreased blood supply and less sensitive nerves."

4. Assess the current care routine, the ability of the patient to take care of the foot (limited by obesity), and the availability of family support.

5. Assist: "Most people can prevent any serious foot problem by following some simple steps. So let us share a plan that suits you ..."

(a) "Daily, make sure to wash and thoroughly dry the spaces between your toes. Avoid testing water temperature with your foot and use petroleum jelly to prevent dryness in your feet."

(b) "Opt for non-tight footwear, choose cotton socks, and refrain from walking barefoot."

(c) "Examine your feet using a mirror every night. Check for any issues like wounds, corns, calluses, moist skin between toes (indicative of fungal infection), ingrown toenails, or cracked heels. If you find a wound, wash it with tap water, cover it with clean gauze, and consult your doctor within a maximum of 2 days."

(d) "Regularly trim your toenails into a square shape. Seek assistance if reaching them is challenging."

(e) "Ensure proper blood circulation in your feet. Elevate your feet while sitting, wiggle your toes, and move your ankles up and down for 5 minutes, two or three times a day. Avoid crossing your legs for extended periods, and refrain from smoking."

(f) "Maintain excellent control of your diabetes mellitus through regular visits to your doctor."

6. Arrange: follow up:

(a) Every 3–6 months labs to check control level and screen for cardiovascular risk factors (hypertension or hyperlipidemia).

(b) Annual foot exam and retinal screening, with referral to a foot care specialist in case of a history of foot ulceration or amputation, neuropathic foot deformities, or peripheral vascular disease.

7. Provide a brief assessment of the underlying conditions and age-appropriate screening.

8. Give away reading materials if available.

9. Communication skills: ensure organized approach, mixed questioning style (open and close-ended questions), active listening, clear language, and reflection on the patient's ICE.

Assessing and Counseling a Patient with a Recent Episode of Myocardial Infarction (MI)

99

Reem Al Mansoori, Kawthar Al Ameri, and Shammah Al Memari

Learning Objectives
- How to take a focused history addressing the risk factors from patients presenting with a recent episode of myocardial infarction?
- How to effectively use the 5 As model to counsel patients presenting with a recent episode of myocardial infarction?
- How to implement good communication skills in counseling patients presenting with a recent episode of myocardial infarction?

Focus areas include post-MI advice and prevention of complications.

---

1. Introduce yourself and establish a good rapport, and explore the patient's ideas, concerns and expectations (ICE).

R. Al Mansoori
Ambulatory health services, Abu Dhabi, United Arab Emirates

K. Al Ameri
Ambulatory Healthcare Services, Abu Dhabi, United Arab Emirates

S. Al Memari (✉)
Abu Dhabi, United Arab Emirates

© The Author(s), under exclusive license to Springer Nature Singapore Pte Ltd. 2024
S. Lari et al. (eds.), *Family Medicine OSCE: First Aid to Objective Structured Clinical Examination*, https://doi.org/10.1007/978-981-99-5530-5_99

373

2. Ask and discuss:
    (a) "Are you aware of what happened to you?" If not, explain: "You had chest pain because your heart was short of oxygen due to a narrowing of the coronary arteries by a fat-like deposit."
    (b) "Now that you are out of the hospital, do you feel any residual symptoms?" Fever, fatigue, lightheadedness, breathlessness, tingling sensation in the left side of the chest, and palpitation (as an indication of an ectopic beat).
    (c) "It must have been difficult to pass through. Can you describe your mood?" Look for anxiety (excess worries, irritability) or depression (loss of interest, poor concentration, lack of energy, appetite, sleep, feeling of guilt) (use Patient Health Questionneire-9).
    (d) "Have you been able to go back to your normal life?"
    (e) "What medications have you been put on? Have you been able to take them regularly?"
    (f) Evaluate the patient's lifestyle and coronary risk: "So tell me about your routine. Do you exercise?"
3. Advise: "As your doctor, I think it's very important for you to prevent a recurrence. You will need to minimize your risk factors":
    (a) Reduce your weight.
    (b) Diet: "To prevent further fat deposits in the coronary arteries by reducing fat, sugar and salt and increasing fluid and fiber intake."
    (c) Exercise: "To improve your heart pumping capability, blood circulation in the body, and prevent a second event." Explore: What are the exercises suitable for him or her? For example, walking and jogging. Advise: "Start slowly and gradually 3 times per week, 10–30 min. Warm up before exercising."
    (d) Avoid stress.
    (e) Stop smoking.
    (f) Take your medications: emphasize compliance with aspirin, angiotensin-converting enzyme inhibitor, and beta-blockers. Avoid using anti-inflammatory drugs for 7–10 days after the acute myocardial infarction.
4. Assess:
    (a) Patient understanding ICE.
    (b) Stage on behavioral change cycle according to motivation and willingness to undergo lifestyle modification (pre-contemplation, contemplation, preparation, action, maintenance).
5. Assist:
    (a) Returning to different life activities: refer to Table 99.1 for details; post-myocardial infarction evaluation).
    (b) Examination: vitals, body mass index, and cardiovascular system examination (any signs of heart failure).
    (c) Investigations: electrocardiogram (post-myocardial infarction baseline), cardiovascular risk assessment [hemoglobin A1c, lipid profile, heart failure markers; B-type natriuretic peptide (BNP)], and echocardiography (measuring the ejection fraction).

Table 99.1 Guidelines for returning to activities following myocardial infarction

Activity	Recommendation
Driving	After 3 weeks (only short distances and avoiding heavy traffic)
Sexual activity	After 1 week post-discharge
Air traveling	After 2 weeks exceptions prior that only if symptom-free, having nitroglycerin as needed, having a travel companion, and avoiding exertion
Occupation	• After 4–12 weeks if an exercise test is done and permits • Check how strenuous is his or her work to decide if further assessment by occupational medicine specialist is required

Table 99.2 Required referrals for patients with a recent myocardial infarction

Referral to	Recommendation
Smoking cessation clinic	To quit smoking
Dietician	Mediterranean diet
Psychologist	Relaxation therapy and stress management techniques
Cardiologist	If a patient is a good candidate for revascularization
Electrophysiologist	If ejection fraction is low: To insert implantable defibrillator
Health educator	CPR training for the family

6. Arrange:
   (a) Positive reinforcement: "Many others did it before you, you can definitely do it, we are always available to support you."
   (b) Prescribe any medications required.
   (c) Referral as detailed in Table 99.2.
   (d) Brief assessment of the underlying conditions and screening for age.
   (e) Follow up in 2 weeks or earlier if any red flags [recurrence of chest pain, rupture of papillary muscles (dizziness), congestive heart failure (lower limb edema), or Dressler syndrome (fever, shortness of breath, pericarditis)]. Use TIMI score to identify 2-week risk of death or need for revascularization.
   (f) Safety netting: "If you develop any chest pain or shortness of breath, take nitroglycerin spray and come to the emergency."
   (g) Give away reading material if available.
7. Communication skills: ensure organized approach, mixed questioning style (open and close-ended questions), active listening, clear language, and reflection on the patient's ICE.

Assessing and Advising a Patient for a Safe Travel

100

Shaima Lari and Shammah Al Memari

Learning Objectives
- How to take a focused history to identify the risk factors and provide appropriate travel advice to patients?
- How to effectively use the 5. As model to counsel and provide appropriate travel advice to patients?
- How to implement good communication skills in counseling and provide appropriate travel advice to patients?

Focus areas include history taking with risk factor identifications and prevention of travel-related illnesses.

1. Introduce yourself and establish a good rapport.
2. Ask:
   (a) "First allow me to ask about your travel if you do not mind." When, where why, and duration of stay and type of activity.
   (b) "Do you have any idea about the travel precautions?"
   (c) Patient's ideas, concerns and expectations (ICE): "Do you have any specific concerns or worries?" "Have you traveled earlier and had a problem with jet lag or motion sickness?" Examples include pre-visa vaccinations, taking care of an underlying condition, or its medications. Tailor accordingly.

S. Lari
Sheikh Shakhbout Medical City, Abu Dhabi, United Arab Emirates

S. Al Memari (✉)
Abu Dhabi, United Arab Emirates

© The Author(s), under exclusive license to Springer Nature Singapore Pte Ltd. 2024
S. Lari et al. (eds.), *Family Medicine OSCE: First Aid to Objective Structured Clinical Examination*, https://doi.org/10.1007/978-981-99-5530-5_100

377

(d) Past medical history: recent myocardial infarction (fit to fly after 2 weeks, surgery, or stroke (fit to fly after 2 weeks). Epilepsy or psychiatric disorders. Current pregnancy and last menstrual period (contraindication for some vaccines or medications; only fit to fly if less than 32 weeks of pregnancy).

(e) Drugs (anticoagulants) and allergies (latex, egg, or aspirin).

(f) Vaccination status.

3. Advise, assess, and assist: check the endemic diseases at the destination on CDC yellow pages and refer to Table 100.1 for details.

4. Arrange:

(a) Refill meds print a prescription or a simple report of the underlying conditions (to be taken with him or her in case he or she ran out of them or had difficulty passing through the airport).

(b) Follow up PRN.

(c) Safety netting: if there are any red flags, seek immediate medical advice.

(d) Brief assessment of the underlying conditions and screening for age.

(e) Give away reading material if available.

5. Communication skills: ensure organized approach, mixed questioning style (open and close-ended questions), active listening, clear language, and reflection on the patient's ICE.

Table 100.1 Details of advise, assessment, and assistance of a traveling patient

Element	Details
General advice	(a) "Avoid swimming in lakes or rivers" (b) "Use safe transportation" (c) "If you get sick, seek tertiary or university hospitals as they usually follow updated practice" (d) "Avoid casual sex or sex with a pregnant partner, especially in the zika-endemic area. Use a condom and safe sex practice. Do not inject drugs, and do not share needles or any devices that can break the skin. That includes needles for tattoos, piercings, and acupuncture. If you receive medical or dental care, make sure the equipment is disinfected or sanitized" (Center for Disease Control and Prevention, travelers health)
Chronic disease management	(a) "Take enough stock of your medications and carry them in your handbag rather than in the luggage. Do not change the containers but keep them in your own package. Take a copy of your prescription with you" (b) "Wear a bracelet that mentions your condition and medications taken" (c) If diabetic on insulin explain dose adjustment: Flying east and the day is less than 6 h shorter, drop one dose. If flying west and the day is more than 6 h longer, add one dose
Immunization	(a) Routine vaccines Ensure up-to-date regular vaccines (b) Give recommended vaccines as per the Center for Disease Control's (CDC) yellow pages. Common ones are detailed on the right **Yellow fever vaccine:** – Single shot every 10 years – Only in patients 9 months to 59 years old – Contraindications: Severe egg or latex allergy, or immunocompromised patients **Japanese encephalitis vaccine:** – Two shots before travel, 28 days apart – Only in a patient more than 2 months old – Provide annual booster if more than 17 years old **Hepatitis A virus vaccine:** – Two shots, 6 months apart **Typhoid vaccine:** – Available in intermuscular and oral form – The IM form is available in one shot, booster every 2 years – The oral form is available in four doses 48 h apart; a booster is every 5 years **Rabies vaccine as pre-exposure prophylaxis:** – Primary series: Three doses on days 0, 7, 21, or 28 high-risk areas. If bitten by an animal, two booster doses are required – Also advise the patient to "avoid reptiles and wild animals' bites. If any, seek medical advice immediately" **Cholera:** – One dose of the vaccine without the need for a booster **Meningococcal vaccine:** – For patients going to Saudi Arabia for pilgrimage (Haj and Umrah) and to countries in the meningitis belt during the dry season (December to June) as per the CDC

(continued)

Table 100.1 (continued)

Element	Details	
Motion sickness	(c) Explain	"A series of unpleasant symptoms (feeling unwell, drowsy, dizzy, irritable, headache, fullness in the stomach, nausea or vomiting) that occur due to sensitive inner ear canal when in a moving vehicle"
	(d) Red flags	Fever, chills, sweating, nausea, or vomiting
	(e) Prevention	Choose a seat between the wings of the airplane, avoid reading or looking at a computer screen – Avoid drinking alcohol – Avoid eating spicy, greasy, or acidic food – Eat light meals before the trip Buscopan – 20 mg tablet 30 min prior to departure – Repeat every 6 h if long flight Benadryl or ginger chewing gum
Deep vein thrombosis (DVT)	(a) Red flags	Swelling, redness, and pain in one or both legs
	(b) Prevention	In long air flights, take lots of fluids on board, minimize alcohol, have light meals, and perform calf exercises
Jet lag	(a) Explain	"Your body has an internal clock that regulates your temperature, BP and hormones. When you cross more than 5 time zones in 1 day, especially when you travel eastward, your clock can get out of order leading to sleeping problems (mostly in the first 2 days)"
	(b) Prevention	To lower your chances of getting jet lag, try to: – Get enough rest and avoid changing sleep patterns before your flight – During your flight: Drink lots of nonalcoholic drinks like water and only have short naps if needed – On arrival: Try to change your daily routine to the new time schedule as soon as possible. Some people find it helpful to take melatonin at bedtime as they arrive. However, if you have epilepsy or taking medication to stop blood clotting, you should not take melatonin

Traveler's diarrhea	(a) Explain	Seek medical attention if symptoms don't improve after 48 h
	(b) Prevention	"Watch what you eat":
		– "Avoid eating from open buffets, street-sellers, and undercooked and reheated food"
		– "Avoid drinking tap water or ice cubes that are made from it"
		– "Avoid unpasteurized dairy products, ice cream, cold sauces, or toppings"
		– "Practice hand hygiene and alcohol-based hand sanitizer to reduce the risk of infection"
		Bismuth
		– Dose: 262 mg, 4 times a day, for the duration of the trip
		– 60% effective
		– Contraindications include patients with aspirin allergy or patients on doxycycline for malaria prophylaxis
		– Side effects include black stool, black tongue, and tinnitus
	(c) Red flags	Dehydration (dry skin, dizziness, decrease urine output, increase heartbeat)
	(d) Treatment	Fluid replacement	Most important treatment
		Antimotility agents	– Can be combined with antibiotics except if there is blood in stool
			– Loperamide (imodium: Take two tablets of the 2 mg doses with the first loose motion, then take one tablet with each bout of diarrhea without exceeding four tables in 24 h) or phynoxylate

(continued)

Table 100.1 (continued)

Element	Details	
Mosquito-borne infections (malaria, yellow or dengue fevers, Japanese encephalitis)	(a) General prevention:	– Apply repellent with N, N-diethyl-meta-toluamide (DEET) at concentrations of more than 30–50%, either alone or in combination with permethrin cream. Alternatively, consider using natural alternatives such as lemon or eucalyptus repellents. – Avoid sleeping outdoors – Use bed nets that are sprayed with DEETs – Wear light-colored clothes that are long sleeves (daytime to prevent yellow or dengue fevers and night-time to prevent malaria) – Use air conditioning as the transmission of malaria occurs mostly between 25 and 30 °C
	(b) Malaria and chemoprophylaxis	Atovaquone and proguanil (Malarone) – Most expensive – Dose: 250 and 100 (mg) tablets daily. Take 1–2 days prior, during, and 1 week after travel – Side effects: Uncommon – Contraindications: Breastfeeding or pregnancy
		Mefloquine – Dose: 250-mg tablet weekly. Take 1–2 weeks prior, during, and 4 weeks after leaving the malaria-endemic area – Side effects: Nightmares and depression – Contraindications: Psychiatry, epileptic, or cardiac patients
		Chloroquine – Dose: 500 (mg) tablets weekly. Take 1–2 weeks prior, during, and 4 weeks after travel – Safe in pregnancy and for long travelers – Contraindications: Psoriasis
		Doxycycline – Has a low cost – Dose: 100 (mg) tablets daily. Take 1–2 days prior, during, and 4 weeks after the malaria-endemic area – Side effects include stomach upset, and flare-ups of vaginal yeast – Contraindications: Pregnancy or young children
		Primaquine – Dose: 56 mg tablet. Take 1–2 days prior, during, and 1 week after leaving the malaria-endemic area – Contraindicated in G6PD

Assessing and Counseling a Patient Over the Telephone

101

Eman Al Hayayi, Noora Al Blooshi, and Shammah Al Memari

> **Learning Objectives**
> - How to conduct a medical consultation over the phone?
> - How to effectively use the 5 As model to counsel the patient over the phone?
> - How to safely triage and manage cases over the phone?

1. Prerequisites:
   (a) Make sure you go through the patient's file before the tele-consultation starts to familiarize yourself with the patient's history, medical history, and recent consultation.
   (b) Have a notepad or paper to write your notes on during the consultation.
2. Ask: "Hello, this is Dr. X, the Family medicine resident on-call, may I know whom I am talking to?" (Make sure you take the caller's name and contact number to be able to call him or her back if the call disconnects.)
   (a) Clarify patient identity: name, age, address, electronic medical record number, primary doctor healthcare center, and relation of the caller.
   (b) Clarify the problem: complaint (e.g., vomiting), nature (bilious, bloody, with or without food content, projectile), duration, aggravating and relieving factors, and any associated symptoms [fever, irritability, jaundice, skin rash, cough, runny nose, abdominal pain or distension or obvious mass, diarrhea

E. Al Hayayi
Etihad Airways Medical Center, Abu Dhabi, United Arab Emirates

N. Al Blooshi
Ambulatory Healthcare Services, Abu Dhabi, United Arab Emirates

S. Al Memari (✉)
Abu Dhabi, United Arab Emirates

(bloody, jelly, pale), constipation, dysuria, decreased oral intake, weight loss, history of trauma or toxin ingestion or allergy].

(c) Clarify if the case is emergency or not: in case of infants and children; with nonresponding fever, stiff neck, bloody vomitus or bloody diarrhea, skin rash, nontolerance to oral feeds, anuria for hours, or toxic ingestion.

(d) Clarify management took and duration.

(e) Explore the patient's ideas, concerns, and expectations (ICE).

3. Advise: *"Mrs. X, from the information that you have told me so far, it seems like your child does not have any alarming features and that he or she has simple gastroenteritis. In such cases, the treatment is supportive, and the most important thing is to avoid dehydration, so:*

(a) 'Increase fluid intake, you may use oral rehydration solution if available.'

(b) 'Offer healthy food to him or her.'"

4. Assess: answer any questions and check the caller's level of understanding.

5. Assist and arrange:

(a) Safety netting: *"As of now, the illness is probably not serious, especially since your child is still interested in playing, eating, and drinking. However, if he or she deteriorates, becomes drowsy or irritable, develops a stiff neck, skin rash, nonresponsive fever, bloody vomitus, or diarrhea, refuses oral feeds, or does not pass urine for hours, please take your child immediately to the emergency department for full assessment."*

(b) Ask the caller to repeat what he or she understood and allow the caller to end the call first.

(c) Follow up in the morning in the clinic for further assessment and treatment as needed.

6. Communication skills: ensure organized approach, mixed questioning style (open and close-ended questions), active listening, clear language, and reflection on the patient's ICE.

Assessing and Counseling a Patient or their Family Regarding a "Do Not Resuscitate" Order

102

Sakina Al Bloushi, Noora Al Blooshi, and Shammah Al Memari

> **Learning Objectives**
> - How to effectively use the 5 As model to counsel patients/relatives on a "Do Not Resuscitate" order?
> - How to implement good communication skills to counsel patients/relatives on a "Do Not Resuscitate" order?

1. Introduce yourself and establish a good rapport.
2. Ask:
   (a) About the ideas, concerns, and expectations (ICE).
   (b) About the patient's mental status.
   (c) State that it is the patient's right to make this decision.
3. If discussing with a relative, explore and explain:
   (a) Whether he or she has ever discussed life-sustaining treatment with the patient before, and if yes what are the patient's preferences.
   (b) Whether he or she discussed it with other family members.
   (c) Any possible hidden agendas, for example, financial issues, and other stressors such as pressure from the spouse or other siblings.
   (d) State that he or she would always want to be involved in a decision about his or her own life (e.g., put yourself in that situation).
   (e) State that the patient may welcome the discussion of her illness and "Do Not Resuscitate" order.

S. Al Bloushi · N. Al Blooshi
Ambulatory Healthcare Services, Abu Dhabi, United Arab Emirates

S. Al Memari (✉)
Abu Dhabi, United Arab Emirates

© The Author(s), under exclusive license to Springer Nature Singapore Pte Ltd. 2024
S. Lari et al. (eds.), *Family Medicine OSCE: First Aid to Objective Structured Clinical Examination*, https://doi.org/10.1007/978-981-99-5530-5_102

   (f) Refuse to write the "Do Not Resuscitate" order without the patient's consent. Consider the patient's mental status, whether it supports consenting or not.

   (g) Arrange a meeting with the patient and the family and reassure them that it will be handled in a sensitive way.

4. Discuss advanced directives '' living well''; this allows the patient to consent or refuse medical treatment while he or she is too ill to communicate their decisions. Through this, the patient can:

   (a) Name a person who will speak on behalf of the patient in the event of life-threatening situations.

   (b) Make specific requests regarding future treatment (treated at home or hospital).

   (c) Do not resuscitate in case of deterioration.

   (d) Specify the type of treatment in a specific situation.

5. Communication skills: organized approach, mixed questioning styles (open and close-ended questions), active listening, clear language, and reflection on the parent's ICE.

Eman Al Hayayi, Noora Al Blooshi,
and Shammah Al Memari

Learning Objectives
- How to evaluate patients undergoing a cardiac procedure?
- How to explain in nonmedical terms an angiography using the 5 As model?
- How to educate patients about the management options and potential complications?

---

1. Introduce yourself: "Good afternoon Mr. or Mrs. X."
2. Establish good rapport: "How are you today?"
3. Ask:
   (a) Explore the reason for the visit: Why did he or she visit the clinic today?
   (b) Explore the nature of symptoms: chest pain, shortness of breath with exertion, orthopnea (suggestive of acute coronary syndrome, or pulmonary embolism), weakness in the extremities and slurred speech (suggestive of stroke), pain in lower extremities especially while walking (suggestive of peripheral vascular disease), history of tumors, renal disease, or any plans for an organ transplant.
   (c) Ask about the nature of angiography planned (elective or emergency).
   (d) Exclude red flags (bleeding disorder, kidney and liver disease, pregnancy).

E. Al Hayayi
Etihad Airways Medical Center, Abu Dhabi, United Arab Emirates

N. Al Blooshi
Ambulatory Healthcare Services, Abu Dhabi, United Arab Emirates

S. Al Memari (✉)
Abu Dhabi, United Arab Emirates

© The Author(s), under exclusive license to Springer Nature Singapore Pte Ltd. 2024
S. Lari et al. (eds.), *Family Medicine OSCE: First Aid to Objective Structured Clinical Examination*, https://doi.org/10.1007/978-981-99-5530-5_103

Table 103.1 Procedural risk factors in angiography

Risk factors	Examples
Older age	
Past medical history	Coronary artery disease (history of angina, heart attack), stroke, diabetes mellitus, hypertension, dyslipidemia, obesity, arterial aneurysm, kidney disease, cerebral vascular malformation, chronic liver disease, and tumors
High-risk medications	Warfarin and diabetes medications (insulin, metformin)
Allergies to contrast agents	
Social habits	Smoking and alcohol use
Family history	Of heart disease (coronary artery disease) or stroke

(e) Inquire about the risk factors: refer to Table 103.1.

(f) Explore the patient's ideas, concerns, and expectations (ICE) about the condition and the procedure.

4. Advise:

(a) "Angiography is a procedure that an interventional cardiologist or an interventional radiologist will do to visualize your blood vessels and detect a suspected disease. With angiography, we can detect a narrowing or a disease in the vessels of the various organs in the body such as the brain, neck, heart, chest, kidney, liver, arms, or legs."

(b) "During the procedure, the doctor will insert a small tube called a catheter into your vessels through a small incision, most of the time in the groin area. The doctor then will inject a contrast material through this tube, which can be visualized through an imaging study. The doctor will take serial pictures of your vessels and may treat diseased vessels by inserting a stent or a balloon to widen them if he found them narrow."

(c) "This procedure may be scheduled as an elective procedure; however, it could be an emergency in case of heart attacks."

(d) "During the procedure, you will be minimally sedated to reduce your anxiety. A numbing medication will be given at the catheter insertion site. The procedure will last from 30 min to 2 h."

(e) "After the procedure, you will be observed for a few hours and allowed to go home on the same day."

(f) "You are allowed to drink and eat immediately after the procedure."

(g) "You will not be able to drive, and you should arrange for a drive back home after the procedure."

5. Assess knowledge about red flags and precautions to take after the procedure: "If you have any of the following, go immediately to the nearest emergency department":

(a) Chest pain after the procedure.

(b) Severe pain, coldness, or bluish discoloration in the leg that held the catheter.

(c) Fever over (38 °C).

(d) Redness, bleeding, or discharge at the catheter insertion site.

6. Assist:
   (a) Stop the following medications prior to the procedure: warfarin and dipyridamole (72 h before the procedure and 48 h after the procedure), and clopidogrel (5 days prior to the procedure).
   (b) Adjust diabetic medications as follows: continue long-acting insulin, reduce detemir or NPH insulin dosage to half, and stop metformin 48 h before and after the procedure. Ask your doctors further if any changes are required to keep your sugar levels controlled.
   (c) You should continue taking blood pressure-lowering medications and maintain your blood pressure readings before the procedure.
7. Communication skills: organized approach, mixed questioning styles (open and close-ended questions), active listening, clear language, and reflection on the parent's ICE.

Preprocedural Evaluation and Counseling of a Patient Undergoing Upper Endoscopy (Esophagogastroduodenoscopy - EGD)

104

Eman Al Hayayi, Buthaina Al Maskari, and Shammah Al Memari

> **Learning Objectives**
> - How to evaluate patients undergoing an upper endoscopy procedure?
> - How to explain in nonmedical terms an upper endoscopy using the 5 As model?
> - How to educate patients about the management options and potential complications?

1. Introduce yourself and establish a good rapport.
2. Ask:
   (a) Discover the reason for attendance and any symptoms: heartburn, difficulty swallowing, the sensation of food sticking in the throat, abdominal pain, black stool, or weight loss.
   (b) Inquire about any family history of gastrointestinal cancer.
   (c) Ask about the past medical history of *Helicobacter pylori* infection, lung disease, heart disease (heart valve replacement), or diabetes.
   (d) Briefly explore drug history, allergies, blood thinners, and the need for antibiotics before a dental or surgical procedure.
   (e) Inquire about previous surgical history: previous endoscopy and findings.
   (f) Last menstrual period.

E. Al Hayayi
Etihad Airways Medical Center, Abu Dhabi, United Arab Emirates

B. Al Maskari
Ambulatory Healthcare Services, Abu Dhabi, United Arab Emirates

S. Al Memari (✉)
Abu Dhabi, United Arab Emirates

© The Author(s), under exclusive license to Springer Nature Singapore Pte Ltd. 2024
S. Lari et al. (eds.), *Family Medicine OSCE: First Aid to Objective Structured Clinical Examination*, https://doi.org/10.1007/978-981-99-5530-5_104

   (g) Background knowledge about upper endoscopy.

   (h) Patient's ideas, concerns, and expectations (ICE).

3. Advise:

   (a) Explain the procedure: "An esophagogastroduodenoscopy (EGD) is a simple outpatient procedure where we check the upper part of your digestive system, including the esophagus, stomach, and the first part of your small intestine (the duodenum). A gastroenterologist, a doctor who specializes in digestive health, usually performs this examination. It helps us understand and address any concerns related to your digestive well-being."

   (b) Before the upper endoscopy, you will be instructed to sign a consent form, which will provide you with information about upper endoscopy and possible complications.

   (c) In order to have a successful upper endoscopy, your doctor will provide you with instructions to follow prior to the procedure, but generally, you must not eat or drink anything for 6–8 h before your test.

   (d) Make sure someone accompanies you as you will not be able to drive after the procedure because of the sedation.

   (e) On the day of the procedure, you will be asked to lie on the examination table wearing a hospital gown. You will be attached to a monitor to monitor your blood pressure, heart rate, and breathing, with an intravenous line inserted into your veins, through which a sedating medication will be given that will make you feel relaxed and drowsy and will diminish gagging. Moreover, your throat may be sprayed with a local anesthetic, or you will be asked to gargle a solution that will help to numb the area.

   (f) During the procedure: a slender and flexible tube known as an endoscope, equipped with a light and a tiny camera on its tip, will be gently passed through your mouth and into the back of your throat. You'll be asked to swallow as the scope moves down into your esophagus, stomach, and duodenum. The doctor can either look directly through the scope or view images displayed on a TV monitor.

      The endoscope has an open passage that allows instruments to be passed for tasks such as taking tissue samples, treating bleeding, or removing polyps. Typically lasting around 15–20 minutes, the procedure duration may vary based on findings and necessary interventions. It's essential for you to try to stay relaxed and take deep, slow breaths through your nose.

      During the endoscopy, you might experience some discomfort, such as a sore throat and bloating or cramping in your stomach. This is normal, and it occurs as air is gently blown into your digestive tract to facilitate the movement of the endoscope.

   (g) After the procedure, you will be transferred to a recovery room for monitoring until the effects of the medication wear off. This step is crucial to ensure that you can cough and swallow normally before resuming eating. If everything goes smoothly, you will be allowed to go home. A family member or someone else can drive you. It's important to avoid alcohol, driving, and operating machinery for the next 24 hours.

If a biopsy or polyps were removed, and you are on blood thinners, the doctor will provide guidance on when it is safe to resume taking medications. You may experience a sore throat, bloating, or cramping, which are normal side effects and should subside within 24 hours.

4. Assess the level of understanding and preparedness, risk of bleeding versus the risk of thromboembolism if a patient is on an anticoagulant. The decision on whether it will be a high-risk or a low-risk procedure will be based on history.

5. Assist with discussing what complications to expect: "An EGD is a common and safe procedure. Complications are rare, but they can occur. These risks include aspiration, bleeding, perforation, infection, and allergic reaction to the medication given for the procedure and complications from preexisting diseases if any."

6. Arrange:
   (a) Referral to a gastroenterologist.
   (b) Liaise with a cardiologist or internal medicine specialist regarding anticoagulant management preoperatively.
   (c) Give educational material.
   (d) Discuss the possible red flags: "If you have any of the following symptoms after an upper endoscopy, go immediately to the emergency department if you experience fever, not able to eat or drink, having blood in your stool, severe or persistent abdominal pain, nausea or vomiting (blood), swallowing difficulties, feeling dizzy, fainting, or having shortness of breath."

7. Communication skills: organized approach, mixed questioning styles (open and close-ended questions), active listening, clear language, and reflection on the patient's ICE.

Preprocedural Evaluation and Counseling of a Patient Undergoing Lower Endoscopy (Colonoscopy)

105

Sakina Al Bloushi, Sumiya Taheri, and Shammah Al Memari

> **Learning Objectives**
> - How to evaluate patients undergoing a colonoscopy procedure?
> - How to explain in nonmedical terms a colonoscopy using the 5 As model?
> - How to educate patients about the management options and potential complications?

1. Introduce yourself and establish a good rapport.
2. Ask:
   (a) Discover the reason for attendance and any symptoms such as abdominal pain, bleeding per rectum, weight loss, or change in bowel habits.
   (b) Enquire if it is a regular screening test or diagnostic.
   (c) Is there a family history of colon cancer, and if yes, at what age?
   (d) Inquire about past medical history: lung disease, heart disease (heart valve replacement), or diabetes.
   (e) Explore drug history (blood thinners, need to take antibiotics before a dental or surgical procedure).
   (f) Previous surgical history: previous colonoscopy and its findings.
   (g) Last menstrual period.
   (h) Knowledge about colonoscopy.
   (i) Patient's ideas, concerns, and expectations (ICE).

S. Al Bloushi · S. Taheri · S. Al Memari (✉)
Ambulatory Healthcare Services, Abu Dhabi, United Arab Emirates

© The Author(s), under exclusive license to Springer Nature Singapore Pte Ltd. 2024
S. Lari et al. (eds.), *Family Medicine OSCE: First Aid to Objective Structured Clinical Examination*, https://doi.org/10.1007/978-981-99-5530-5_105

3. Advise:
   (a) Explain the procedure: "A colonoscopy is an outpatient procedure in which the inside of the colon is examined. It is used to assess symptoms, such as bleeding per rectum, abdominal pain, or changes in bowel habits. Colonoscopies are also performed if there is iron-deficiency anemia, personal history of polyps or colon cancer, and as a screening method for colon and rectal cancer in people without any complaints."
   (b) Before the colonoscopy, you will be instructed to sign a consent form, which will provide you with information about colonoscopy and possible complications.
   (c) To have a successful colonoscopy, your doctor will provide you with instructions to follow prior to the procedure. This is very important to have clear images of your entire colon and prevent failure of colonoscopy and the need to repeat the procedure.
   (d) You might receive instructions for dietary and fluid restrictions leading up to the procedure, and you may be prescribed laxatives to use in the days before. To summarize, you can consume clear liquids, such as water, clear soups (beef, chicken, or vegetable), and coffee or tea (without milk) until several hours before your procedure. However, it's advised to avoid red liquids. Additionally, your doctor may recommend abstaining from high-fiber foods, including seeds and nuts, for the week preceding the procedure.

   To ensure a clean colon, you will need to take a potent laxative to empty your bowels. The preparation may involve taking the entire dose the night before the test, or it may be divided into two doses, with the second taken 4–6 hours before the colonoscopy.
   (e) Make sure someone accompanies you as you will not be able to drive after the procedure because of sedation.
   (f) On the day of the procedure, you will be requested to lie on your left side on the examination table, donning a hospital gown. You'll be connected to a monitor to track your blood pressure, heart rate, and breathing. An intravenous line will be inserted into your veins to administer medication that induces a relaxed and drowsy state.
   (g) The procedure, usually performed by an experienced surgeon or gastroenterologist, typically lasts between 30 to 60 minutes. A specialized instrument called a scope, which is a long, flexible tube approximately 1/2 inch in diameter and equipped with a camera and light at its end, is used by the doctor to visualize the lining of your colon. This scope is gently inserted through the anus. As the doctor advances the scope, air is blown into your colon to enhance visibility, and this may cause mild cramping during the procedure.
   (h) During the colonoscopy, if the doctor sees something that looks abnormal, small amounts of the tissue can be removed for further workup; this is called a biopsy (any abnormal growths, or polyps, can be identified and removed).
   (i) At the end of the procedure, the scope is slowly withdrawn while the lining of your bowel is carefully examined.

   (j) After colonoscopy: You will be taken to a recovery room for observation; if no problems occurred, you will be discharged home.

   (k) You may experience some abdominal cramping that should be resolved quickly, and a family member or anyone else can drive you home.

   (l) Avoid alcohol, driving, and operating machinery for 24 h following the procedure. You can return to your diet after the procedure.

   (m) You may notice rectal bleeding if a biopsy is taken or a polyp is removed for 1–2 days.

   (n) If you are on blood thinners and the doctor did a biopsy or polyps were removed, the doctor will tell you when it is safe to resume taking your medications.

4. Assess the level of understanding and preparedness; risk of bleeding versus the risk of thromboembolism if a patient is on an anticoagulant. The decision on whether it will be a high-risk or a low-risk procedure will be based on history.

5. Assist with discussing what complications to expect: Colonoscopy is a safe procedure, and complications are rare but can occur; this includes bleeding, perforation, sedative medication's side effects, missing some abnormalities, and thought as normal.

6. Arrange:

   (a) Referral to a gastroenterologist.

   (b) Liaise with a cardiologist or internal medicine specialist about when to stop anticoagulants prior to the procedure.

   (c) Give educational material.

   (d) Discuss the possible red flags: "If you have any of the following after a colonoscopy, go immediately to the emergency department: a large amount of rectal bleeding, high or persistent fever, or severe abdominal pain within the next 2 weeks."

7. Communication skills: organized approach, mixed questioning styles (open and close-ended questions), active listening, clear language, and reflection on the patient's ICE.

Part IX

Counseling: Pediatrics and Adolescents Health

Counseling Regarding the Health Maintenance in an Adolescent

106

Dana Al Marzooqi, Buthaina Al Maskari, and Shammah Al Memari

> **Learning Objectives**
> - How to identify and address common health issues related to pediatric and adolescents through comprehensive history-taking?
> - How to provide age-appropriate advice to adolescents on topics such as nutrition, exercise, sexual health, substance use, mental health, screening, and preventive measures using the 5 As model?
> - How to implement good communication skills in counseling and provide appropriate advice for adolescent patients?

1. Introduce yourself.
2. Establish a good rapport.
3. Ensure privacy (consider meeting privately with the adolescent for sensitive topics).
4. Ask:
   (a) Ideas, concerns, and expectations (ICE) [e.g., obesity, depression, partner with sexually transmitted infections (STIs), or unwanted pregnancy].

Adolescents are defined as patients who are 10–19 years old according to the WHO.

D. Al Marzooqi
Sheikh Khalifa Medical City, Abu Dhabi, United Arab Emirates

B. Al Maskari
Ambulatory Healthcare Services, Abu Dhabi, United Arab Emirates

S. Al Memari (✉)
Abu Dhabi, United Arab Emirates

© The Author(s), under exclusive license to Springer Nature Singapore Pte Ltd. 2024
S. Lari et al. (eds.), *Family Medicine OSCE: First Aid to Objective Structured Clinical Examination*, https://doi.org/10.1007/978-981-99-5530-5_106

(b) Medical, surgical, medications, allergies, immunizations, family, and social histories (explore relations and role of parents).

(c) Explore important factors (use the mnemonic "HEADSS"): **H**ome and external environment, **E**ducation and employment, **A**ctivities and hobbies, **D**rugs, **S**ubstance, alcohol abuse and/or smoking, **S**exual activities, **S**uicidal thoughts, or plans.

5. Advise and assess: Review the file before seeing the patient. Start with routine general medical screening and then move on to more sensitive topics, like sexual health and illicit drug use (to gain trust).

(a) Explain: "As your doctor, I think it is very important for you to share with me some medical and personal information that will help me understand what kind of health advice you might need. I'm here to educate you and give you information. I am hoping you will make good decisions. If you ever make a mistake, I hope you will trust me enough to help take care of you. By law, I must keep anything you tell me confidential unless I am concerned about your safety or someone else's safety, then I am afraid, the law sometimes requires me to notify others."

(b) Healthy diet: "At times we get confused about what we should or should not eat. Briefly, we have to follow some general rules." Refer to Table 106.1 for details.

(c) Depression screening for patients 12–18 years: Use 9-item Patient Health Questionnaire for Adolescents or use the two screening questions (mood and interest in the last 2 weeks). If positive, offer selective serotonin reuptake inhibiter, psychotherapy, or both.

(d) "Young adults like yourself love to experience new things. Have you ever tried any?" (Refer to Table 106.2 for details.)

(e) Blood pressure checks: from 18 years (at every visit) to screen for hypertension.

(f) Weight, height, and body mass index screen yearly If the abnormal screen for obesity and eating disorders: offer behavioral-based intervention to achieve better overall health and decrease any peer pressure.

(g) Hyperlipidemia if indicated, and tuberculosis if at risk.

Table 106.1 General healthy nutritional rules for adolescents

Nutritional group	Recommendation
Protein-rich foods	Five ounces per day, including meat, poultry, fish, beans, eggs, etc.
Caffeinated beverages: such as tea, coffee, and chocolate	Limit to 2–4 portions per day
Takeaway food	Limit to once per week (high in salt and fat)
Fruits	1–2 cups per day and vegetables: 2–3 cups per day
Water	8–10 glasses per day
Dairy products	3–4 cups per day, examples include milk, yogurt, cheese, etc.
Regular exercise	For example, 30 min of brisk walking each day

Table 106.2 Guidance and recommendations for adolescents regarding specific risky behaviors

Risky behavior	Advice and recommendations
Driving or cycling	Advice to use seat belts and bicycle helmets
Smoking or alcohol	Offer motivational interview and smoking cessation
Sexual activity	– Defined as being sexually involved with anyone (guys, girls, or both) – Advise participation in school, faith, or community-based sex education programs – Screen females for chlamydia and gonorrhea, discuss contraception, and offer pap smear and HIV screen annually
Violence	– Sensitively ask about the history of abuse, low commitment to school, involvement in gangs, and fear of assault: "We do have to ask some very personal or painful questions about what might have happened to you. I know it will be hard to answer some of these questions, but we are asking them so that we can take care of you to the best of our abilities" (Rotte and Lopez 2011) – If at risk: connect families with school-based programs and arrange psychologists' referrals

(h) Physical, sexual, and emotional abuse as well as learning or school problems.

(i) Intravenous drugs and substance abuse (CRAFFT questionnaire: Car, Relax, Alone, Forget, Family or Friends, Trouble).

(j) Ask about high-risk sexual behavior and screen for sexually transmitted infections accordingly.

6. Assist: "Let us share a plan that is suitable to help you …"

(a) Education about lifestyle modification, injury prevention, and safe sex.

(b) Immunization: influenza, HPV, and varicella.

7. Arrange:

(a) Offer age-appropriate immunizations, including one dose of Tdap, one dose of meningococcal disease (MenACWY), HPV vaccine two doses, and influenza vaccine annually.

(b) Positive reinforcement: "Many others did it before you, you can definitely do it, we are always available to support you."

(c) Referral for dental screening every 6 months.

(d) Follow-up, safety netting, and red flags (suicidality if depressed).

(e) Give away reading material.

8. Communication skills: ensure organized approach, mixed questioning style (open and closed-ended questions), active listening, clear language, and reflection on the patient's ICE.

Assessment and Counseling for a Child's Well-Child Visit

107

Dana Al Marzooqi, Buthaina Al Maskari, and Shammah Al Memari

> **Learning Objectives**
> - How to evaluate children according to their age groups and expected develop milestone stages?
> - How to provide age-related advice, in relation to sleeping, feeding, driving, indoor safety, oral health, reading, and discipline, using the 5 As model?
> - How to implement good communication skills in counseling and provide appropriate advice for adolescents?

Focus areas include age-appropriate advice on sleep, diet, oral health, discipline, and safety.

1. Introduce yourself and establish a good rapport.
2. Ask:
   (a) Mother's reason for the visit.
   (b) Child's health state, growth, and development.
   (c) Birth history, prior screenings, immunizations, medical, surgical, and family and social histories.

D. Al Marzooqi
Sheikh Khalifa Medical City, Abu Dhabi, United Arab Emirates

B. Al Maskari
Ambulatory Healthcare Services, Abu Dhabi, United Arab Emirates

S. Al Memari (✉)
Abu Dhabi, United Arab Emirates

© The Author(s), under exclusive license to Springer Nature Singapore Pte Ltd. 2024
S. Lari et al. (eds.), *Family Medicine OSCE: First Aid to Objective Structured Clinical Examination*, https://doi.org/10.1007/978-981-99-5530-5_107

405

(d) Explore feeding, oral health, sleeping, reading, car seat use, and safety measures.

(e) Check parents' ideas, concerns, and expectations (ICE).

3. Advise: tailor it according to the child's age: refer to Table 107.1 for details.

4. Assess: answer any questions and check your level of understanding.

Table 107.1 General advice and guidance on infant care for parents

Item	Advice and recommendations
Sleeping	(a) Always put the baby to sleep on his or her back (b) Avoid loose bedding and soft toys in the crib (c) Avoid overdressing or overheating (d) By 6 months, your baby should sleep in his or her own bed in a separate room and must be lying on his or her back or side (e) By 12 months, your child should have a regular sleeping schedule and sleep through the night and nap once during the day
Feeding	(a) Breastfeed – Feed on demand not per schedule – Exclusively at least in the first 6 months – Vitamin D supplementation if exclusively breastfed – Refer to the breastfeeding counseling page for more details (b) When weaning: – Introducing solid food before the age of 4 months is not advisable. Before considering the introduction of food, assess the baby's head stability and ability to swallow – Introduce one food item at a time to detect any allergy – Start with iron-fortified cereals and pureed meat at 6 months – Add vegetables and fruits after the introduction of cereals and pureed meats – Establish a routine with three meals and two healthy snacks – Do not give fresh cow's milk or honey until 1 year of age – Do not add salt or sugar until 2 years of age – If your child wishes to have juice, then dilute it at a rate of 1/10 – Teach him or her to drink in a cup for 6 months and avoid giving tea, coffee, or soft drinks – Allow eating using his or her own fingers by 9 months and self-feed using a spoon by 9–12 months (c) Never share a spoon with the child to avoid risks of dental caries
Car seats	(a) Refer to Chap. 111 for the use of car seat
Oral health	(a) Refer to Chap. 108 for pediatric oral health
Indoor safety	(a) Maintain a smoke-free environment (b) Never leave the baby alone on high surfaces (c) Keep a safety plug on all electric sockets at home (d) Keep all detergents and medicines on the upper shelves (e) Use stair gates, safety cabinet, lock fridge door, and put barriers around heaters and stoves (f) Avoid leaving the child unattended in potentially dangerous areas such as the bathroom, kitchen, or swimming pool (g) Do not drink hot drinks while the baby is on your lap

Table 107.1 (continued)

Item	Advice and recommendations
Reading	(a) This allows IQ development and attainment of social skills and encourages teaching the child to love books (b) Start reading to your child from around 4–6 months. Use books with pictures and share stories
Discipline	(a) Start the time-out method at around 12 months of age for about 5 min followed by lots of hugging and cuddling (b) Praise good behavior and redirect the child if showed bad behavior gently (c) Share rules across all caregivers and be consistent (d) Get down to the child's eye level when talking to him or her (e) Limit screen time to 1 h or less and avoid using electronic devices to distract or calm down the child

5. Assist: "Let us share a plan that is suitable for helping you."
   (a) Coping with breastfeeding
   (b) Appropriate use of car seat
   (c) Child discipline
6. Arrange:
   (a) Positive reinforcement and reassurance: "Many others did it before, you can definitely do it and we are always available to support you."
   (b) Follow up soon and encourage the child's presence.
   (c) Give away reading material if available.
7. Communication skills: ensure organized approach, mixed questioning style (open and close-ended questions), active listening, clear language, and reflection on the patient's ICE.

Assessment and Counseling for a Child's Oral Health

108

Sakina Al Bloushi, Kawthar Al Ameri,
and Shammah Al Memari

> **Learning Objectives**
> - How to evaluate infants brought for teething and oral health?
> - How to provide age-related advice, in relation to child's oral health, using the 5 As model?
> - How to implement good communication skills in counseling parents and provide appropriate advice in child's oral health?

1. Introduce yourself and establish a good rapport.
2. Ask:
   (a) Parent's reason for the visit.
   (b) Child's health status, growth, and development.
   (c) Explore feeding, oral health, sleeping behavior, and any dental visits.
   (d) Check the mother's ideas, concerns, and expectations (ICE).
3. Advise: "I am glad that you are here today, it is important to understand how to maintain good mouth hygiene for your child." Then counsel about the details in Table 108.1.
4. Assess: Answer any questions and check your level of understanding.
5. Assist: "Let's share a plan that is suitable to help you ….."

S. Al Bloushi · K. Al Ameri
Ambulatory Healthcare Services, Abu Dhabi, United Arab Emirates

S. Al Memari (✉)
Abu Dhabi, United Arab Emirates

© The Author(s), under exclusive license to Springer Nature Singapore Pte Ltd. 2024
S. Lari et al. (eds.), *Family Medicine OSCE: First Aid to Objective Structured Clinical Examination*, https://doi.org/10.1007/978-981-99-5530-5_108

409

Table 108.1 General advise and recommendation for child's oral health

Item	Advice and recommendations
Teething	(a) Starts from 6 months to 3 years (may have tender gums when teeth erupt)
	(b) Wipe your baby's face often with a cloth to remove the drool and prevent the development of rashes
	(c) Give your baby something to chew on as a rubber teething. Make sure it is big enough to avoid the risk of swallowing and breakage into small pieces. If it contains liquid inside, it may leak, so it is better to avoid using them
	(d) A wet washcloth placed in the freezer for 30 min makes a handy teething aid but ensure washing it after each use
	(e) Teething does not cause fever, so if your child develops any, then please return
Feeding habits	(a) Your child should not fall asleep on bottles containing anything other than water
	(b) You should wean her or him from bottles at 12–14 months of age
	(c) Avoid giving juice to drink from bottles. Fruit juice should be in a cup with meals or at snack time
Thumb and finger sucking	(a) It is perfectly normal for infants and many stop sucking by age 2
	(b) Prolonged thumb sucking can create crooked teeth or bite problems. If the habit continues beyond age 3, your child will need a professional evaluation
Dental visits	(a) Ongoing dentist visits begin around the age of 1 year or after the eruption of the first tooth
	(b) The earlier the dental visit, the better the chance of preventing dental problems like caries. It also makes your child comfortable with his or her dentist, help builds a rapport, and establishes the good habit of regular dental check-ups
Cleaning	(a) Clean your baby's teeth as soon as they erupt with a clean cloth
	(b) Use toothpaste when your child can spit it out, usually around the age of 3. Choose one with fluoride and use only a pea-sized amount or less in younger kids. Do not let your child swallow the toothpaste or eat it out of the tube because an overdose of fluoride can be harmful
	(c) You can also get toddlers interested in the routine by letting them watch and imitate you as you brush and floss
	(d) Include sweetened items as part of meals rather than as separate snacks and rinse the mouth with water immediately after consumption of sweetened items
	(e) Clean teeth with an age-appropriate toothbrush for 2 min twice a day (studies showed no benefits of self-flossing in caries reduction) and no benefit of electrical brush over mechanical brushing in preschool age
	(f) Tooth whitening and bleaching are not recommended before 8 years of age
	(g) Check your baby's teeth, healthy teeth should be all one color; if you see spots or stains on the teeth, take your baby to the dentist
Fluoride supplementation	(a) Children should take fluoride supplement if they are drinking (less than 0.6 ppm F) water. Check the total dietary intake of fluoride and the age prior given any supplements

6. Arrange:
   (a) Positive reinforcement and reassurance: "Many others did it before you with their children. You can do it and we are always available to support you."
   (b) Follow up soon and encourage the child's presence.
   (c) Prescribe 1.1% NaF-containing toothpaste and educate about fluorosis related to excess consumption of fluoride leading to hypo mineralization of dental enamel.
   (d) Give away reading materials if available.
7. Communication skills: ensure organized approach, mixed questioning style (open and close-ended questions), active listening, clear language and reflection on the parent's ICE.

Assessment and Counseling for a Child with Fever

109

Shaima Lari, Sumiya Taheri,
and Shammah Al Memari

Learning Objectives
- How to take a focused history from parents with a child with fever?
- How to effectively use the 5 As model to counsel parents on managing their child's fever?
- How to implement good communication skills when advising parents on managing their child's fever?

Focus areas include Differential diagnoses of fever include upper or lower respiratory tract infection, gastroenteritis, otitis media, viral illness, and urinary tract infection.

---

1. Introduce yourself and establish a good rapport.
2. Ask:
   (a) Onset, duration, readings if any, associated symptoms (runny nose, cough, rash, nausea or vomiting, diarrhea, earache, or headache), and relieving factors (paracetamol or ibuprofen). If any medications are given, ask about the dose, frequency, and last given dose.

S. Lari
Sheikh Shakhbout Medical City, Abu Dhabi, United Arab Emirates

S. Taheri
Ambulatory Healthcare Services, Abu Dhabi, United Arab Emirates

S. Al Memari (✉)
Abu Dhabi, United Arab Emirates

© The Author(s), under exclusive license to Springer Nature Singapore Pte Ltd. 2024
S. Lari et al. (eds.), *Family Medicine OSCE: First Aid to Objective Structured Clinical Examination*, https://doi.org/10.1007/978-981-99-5530-5_109

(b) History of recent travel or contact with sick individuals.
(c) Vaccination status and recent ones.
(d) Parent's ideas, concerns and expectations (ICE) (medication, vaccination, care related to underlying condition). Correct any myths (teething does not cause fever).
(e) Past medical, family, and social history.
(f) Growth, development, and vaccine history.

3. Advise:
(a) "I understand your worries, fever is a very common source of mothers' anxiety."
(b) "Fever is a very good sign of your child's body being strong enough to fight germs and does not cause brain damage, but we must be very careful it doesn't persist or increase. This is because it can lead to dehydration so give your child lots of fluids. It can also lead to febrile convulsions."
(c) "Fever does not mean the child has a serious illness. It is normal for them to have at least 5–6 episodes of fever in a year."
(d) "There is no evidence that reducing fever reduces the morbidity or mortality from a febrile illness and response to treatment does not differentiate a viral cause from bacterial cause."
(e) "Potential benefits of treating fever with antipyretics include improvement of discomfort and decrease in insensible water loss, which may decrease the risk of dehydration. Antipyretic agents also have analgesic effects, which may enhance their overall effect. Potential downsides of treating fever include delayed identification of an underlying illness and drug toxicity; it is uncertain whether treating fever increases the risk for or complications of certain types of infections."

4. Assess:
(a) "A clinically significant fever in children younger than 3 years is a rectal temperature of at least 38 °C (100.4 °F). Axillary, tympanic, and temporal artery measurements have been shown to be unreliable."
(b) Exclude red flags (febrile convulsions, urinary symptoms, recent travel, neck stiffness, altered mental status, nonconsolable crying, rash).
(c) Perform a thorough physical examination.
(d) Reassurance when a serious illness is excluded (child interested in playing, eating, and drinking well, no skin changes, good and fast response to antipyretics).
(e) Identify if fever without apparent source ("acute febrile illness with no obvious source of fever after a thorough history and physical exam") or fever of unknown origin ("core body temperature ≥38.1 °C measured at least once daily for ≥14 consecutive days and diagnosis inapparent after careful history, physical exam, and relatively simple, noninvasive tests").
(f) Reassurance and clear addressing of the mother's concern: "For now I think you can take good care of your child with a few tips, and we will follow him or her closely."

(g) Fever in young children (less than 2 years of age): Evaluation of febrile infants younger than 29 days should include complete blood count with differentials, lumbar puncture, blood culture, chest radiography, urinalysis, and urine culture. Stool testing should be performed if diarrhea is present. Moreover, evaluation of febrile young infants (more than 28 days but less than 3 months) should include urinalysis and urine culture and complete blood count with differentials. Nevertheless, urinalysis and urine culture are recommended as part of the evaluation for all febrile infants 24 months of age or younger with unexplained fever.

5. Assist: "Let's share a plan together to help you."
   (a) "Encourage fluid intake, dress lightly, cotton, single layer and avoid covering your child with multiple or thick blankets."
   (b) "Measure body temperature and if higher than 38° for 3 consecutive days go back to your doctor."
   (c) "Give your child a warm bath. Cold towels are irritating, so try to avoid them."
   (d) "Do not use alcohol or vinegar for bathing a child with fever, it is dangerous!"
   (e) "Do not use aspirin."
   (f) "Use Adol (paracetamol) or Ibuprofen for lowering body temperature, use weight to determine the proper dose or call your doctor for help, give doses regularly every 6–8 h at least in the first 24 h of onset."
   (g) "To prevent overdosing of antipyretics, store them out of reach of children."

6. Arrange:
   (a) Admission and investigation for all neonates (younger than 28 days).
   (b) Follow up in 2 days or earlier if no improvement.
   (c) Brief assessment of underlying conditions, age-appropriate screening, and vaccination.
   (d) Give away reading materials if available.
   (e) Safety netting: "If he or she developed a rash, neck stiffness, altered mental status or nonconsolable cry, please come back to the clinic."

7. Communication skills: ensure organized approach, mixed questioning style (open and closed-ended questions), active listening, clear language, and reflection on the parent's ICE.

Assessment and Counseling for a Child with Febrile Convulsions

110

Eiman Al Murar, Sumiya Taheri,
and Shammah Al Memari

Learning Objectives
- How to conduct a focused history-taking session from parents with children experiencing febrile convulsions?
- How to effectively use the 5 As model to counsel parents on febrile convulsions?
- How to implement good communication skills when advising parents about febrile convulsions?

Focus areas include red flags of febrile convulsions and safety netting, management of fits at home, and criteria for home discharge and referral to secondary care.

1. Introduce yourself.
2. Establish a good rapport.
3. Ask:
   (a) Explore mother's ideas, concerns, and expectations (ICE).
   (b) Details of the incident: onset, type (focal, generalized tonic clonic seizure), duration (more or less than 15 min), mother's actions, and any doctor's visit or management if done.

E. Al Murar · S. Taheri
Ambulatory Healthcare Services, Abu Dhabi, United Arab Emirates

S. Al Memari (✉)
Abu Dhabi, United Arab Emirates

(c) Identify if simple (generalized tonic–clonic activity with no focal component, duration <15 min, occurs no more than once in 24 h, no previous neurological problems), or complex seizure (duration >15 min, focal component, recurrence within 24 h).

(d) Any preceding fever or symptoms of febrile infections (upper respiratory tract infections or urinary tract infections) or provoking factors (exposure to flickering lights, lack of sleep, or food).

(e) Red flags: altered mental status, rash, abnormal gait, or behavior.

(f) Perinatal, past medical and family history.

(g) Growth, development, and vaccination history.

4. Advise:

(a) "Febrile seizures occur in 2–5% of children between the ages of 6 months and 5 years. It occurs because their brain cannot handle high body temperatures, leading to disturbance in its activity that results in abnormal movements, or fits. It is totally benign and neither affects the growth or development of your child, nor his or her academic performance or intelligence."

(b) "If your child is getting a seizure for the first time, then he or she needs to be assessed by a doctor to exclude any other related conditions. Usually, no tests or imaging is needed."

(c) "In children with first febrile seizure, one-third may have recurrence, and 10% may experience greater than or equal to three febrile seizures."

(d) "Children with febrile seizures are five times more likely to develop subsequent unprovoked seizures compared with children with no febrile seizures."

(e) "The risk of epilepsy ranges from 2.4% in children with simple febrile seizures to 6–8% in children with complex seizures."

5. Assess: mother's knowledge about the condition and answer any questions.

6. Assist: "So let us share a plan that is suitable for helping you and your child to prevent or control further attacks":

(a) **Treat the fever**: whenever the child has it: bath or apply sponge tips using tap water, (avoiding vinegar or alcohol), put on light clothes, and give antipyretics.

(b) **Treat the cause of the fever**: Identify the cause of fever and treat it appropriately. Advise the mother to anticipate fever with some vaccines [common after measles, mumps, and rubella (MMR) vaccine] and start giving antipyretic regularly for at least 24 h after them.

(c) **Treat the fit**: refer to Table 110.1 for advice regarding the first aid of fits.

7. Decide discharge disposition:

(a) Discharge to home is usually appropriate if and only if all the following are met: the child had a simple febrile seizure with return to normal neurological state, focus found and appropriate treatment initiated (serious bacterial infection is excluded), caregiver educated about febrile seizures and advised what to do if seizures recur, and appropriate follow-up of the underlying cause of fever arranged.

(b) Otherwise transfer to the emergency department.

Table 110.1 First aid of fits

Item	Advice details
Initial care	(a) Do not panic (b) Note the time (c) Protect your child's airway (d) If a child has anything in his or her mouth, clear it with a finger to prevent choking. Don't try to force anything into your child's mouth (e) Place the child on the side or abdomen to help drain secretions and avoid choking (f) Don't try to restrain your child or stop seizure movements (g) Ensure that the child is safe from surroundings (h) Loosen all clothes
If the fit continues for more than 5 min	(a) Administer per rectal diazepam (b) Call for an ambulance

8. Arrange:
   (a) Positive reinforcement: "We are always available to support you."
   (b) Treat the cause of the fever.
   (c) Prescribe: adequate dose of antipyretics (e.g., paracetamol) and consider giving rectal diazepam for possible future attacks.
   (d) Consider pediatric neurology referral for: complex febrile seizure, multiple febrile seizure recurrences, or febrile status epilepticus.
9. Give away reading materials if available.
10. Communication skills: ensure organized approach, mixed questioning style (open and close-ended questions), active listening, clear language, and reflection on the patient's ICE.

Counseling Parents on the Use of Car Seats

111

Abeer Al Naqbi and Shammah Al Memari

Learning Objectives
- How to take a brief history including current or past use of car seats and give age-appropriate advice?
- How to effectively use the 5 As model to counsel parents on car seat use?
- How to implement good communication skills in advising parents on car seat use?

Focus areas include appropriate advice according to age and safety requirements.

1. Introduce yourself and establish a good rapport.
2. Ask:
   (a) Where does the child sit in the car and if parents are using a car seat.
   (b) Age of the child weight and height.
   (c) Past medical history and any special needs as the need for different restraints.
3. Advise:
   (a) "As your doctor, I think it is very important for you to understand that children car seats have to be used because car accidents cause significant injuries and deaths in children."

A. Al Naqbi
Ambulatory Healthcare Services, Abu Dhabi, United Arab Emirates

S. Al Memari (✉)
Abu Dhabi, United Arab Emirates

© The Author(s), under exclusive license to Springer Nature Singapore Pte Ltd. 2024
S. Lari et al. (eds.), *Family Medicine OSCE: First Aid to Objective Structured Clinical Examination*, https://doi.org/10.1007/978-981-99-5530-5_111

(b) "Your body protected your child when he or she was in your womb, but it is no longer sufficient. It can cause more harm than benefits in case of an accident."

(c) "Every child needs to use a car seat until he or she fits correctly in the lap and shoulder straps of the automobile safety belt."

4. Assess:
   (a) Level of understanding and answer any questions.
   (b) Motivation and willingness to use the car seat.
   (c) Previous attempts at use or failures.

5. Assist: Let us share a plan that is suitable for helping you. Explain to the parents the rules to choose the appropriate care seat, according to your child's weight, and age (refer to Table 111.1 for details). Additionally, clarify the general rules of car seat use:
   (a) "Install the car seat correctly as instructed by the manufacturer and place the chair rear-facing until your child is more than 1 year of age and more than 9 kg in weight."
   (b) "Secure the seat with safety belt or by using the lower anchors and tethers for children (LATCH) restraint system."
   (c) "Harness strap (the child seat belt) should be flat and closely fitted on your child. Never put the car belt shoulder strap behind the back or under the arm of your child."
   (d) "Advance if your child exceeds the weight limit or his or her head is 1 in. or less to the top of the car seat."
   (e) Adult seat belt may be used once the child's height is more than 145 cm and when the lap belt is across the upper thighs (not the stomach) and the shoulder belt is across the center of the shoulder and chest (not on the neck/face or off the shoulder).
   (f) All children younger than 13 years of age should ride in the back seat.
   (g) Never leave your child alone in or around cars and lock your vehicle when it is not in use.
   (h) Always read the manufacturer's directions for proper and safe use

Table 111.1 Age-appropriate care seat guidelines

Seat	Features	Child's weight	Child's height
Infant or rearward seat	– Light weighted – Portable – Inexpensive	Up to 9–10 kg	Up to 66–74 cm
Convertible seat	– Can be placed both rearward and forward	9–18 kg	Up to 102 cm
Forward-facing seats		14–18 kg	127–145 cm
Booster seat	To use when he or she outgrows the above measurements		

6. Arrange:
   (a) Positive reinforcement: "Many mothers did it before you, you can definitely do it, we are always available to support you."
   (b) Follow up soon.
   (c) Anticipate complications (non-cooperative child).
   (d) Safety netting: inform about injuries resulting from wrong positions.
   (e) Brief assessment of the underlying conditions and screening for age.
   (f) Give away reading materials if available.
7. Communication skills: ensure organized approach, mixed questioning style (open and close-ended questions), active listening, clear language, and reflection on the patient's ideas, concerns, and expectations (ICE).

Counseling Parents on Toilet-Training Their Child

112

Abeer Al Naqbi and Shammah Al Memari

Learning Objectives
- How to obtain a focused history for toilet training advice in children?
- How to effectively use the 5 As model to counsel parents on toilet training?
- How to implement good communication skills in advising parents on toilet training?

Focus areas include excluding organic causes and psychological causes of urinary incontinence; and exclude and discuss red flags with parents.

1. Introduce yourself and establish a good rapport.
2. Ask:
    (a) Parent's ideas, concerns, and expectations (ICE).
    (b) "To be able to help you, I need to know some information about your child."
    (c) Age of the patient (most children begin training between 18 and 24 months; attaining complete toilet training and control for children is between 2½ and 4 years at daytime and by 8 years at night-time).
    (d) Prenatal, natal, postnatal, and child's development history.

A. Al Naqbi
Ambulatory Healthcare Services, Abu Dhabi, United Arab Emirates

S. Al Memari (✉)
Abu Dhabi, United Arab Emirates

© The Author(s), under exclusive license to Springer Nature Singapore Pte Ltd. 2024
S. Lari et al. (eds.), *Family Medicine OSCE: First Aid to Objective Structured Clinical Examination*, https://doi.org/10.1007/978-981-99-5530-5_112

425

    (e) Past medical history (diabetes mellitus) and taken medication history.

    (f) History of constipation, dysuria, abnormal movements, anal itching, and presence of any psychological problems.

    (g) If vaccinations are up to date.

    (h) Family history of enuresis or having a family member who had problems in achieving toilet training.

3. Advise: "As your doctor, I think it is very important for you to know when your child is ready to be trained and this can be assured when he or she":

    (a) "Tells you that he or she is wet."

    (b) "Helps to undress."

    (c) "Shows interest in the toilet."

    (d) "Stays dry longer hours."

    (e) "Has regular bowel movements."

    (f) "Stable posture while sitting on the toilet."

4. Assess: Parents' knowledge and level of understanding about toilet training: "To be able to help you, I need to know what you know about toilet training."

5. Assist: "Let's share a plan that is suitable for helping you ….."

    (a) "To start, know that your child would need 4 weeks or more to be trained."

    (b) "Do not start if your child is ill."

    (c) "Stop the trial if your child gets upset and retry in 1 month."

    (d) "Remove nappies and use pants."

    (e) "Explain to your child what a potty or toilet seat is."

    (f) "Put your child on it regularly in the morning, after meals, before and after going out, and anytime in between that you feel he or she needs to go."

    (g) "Allow 5 min on the seat with encouragement and praise. Do not force."

    (h) "Handle accidents calmly."

6. Arrange:

    (a) Positive reinforcement: "Many others did it before you, you can definitely do it, we are always available to support you."

    (b) Follow up soon.

    (c) Anticipate complications: "Remember, it is common for children not to achieve toilet training from the first trial. For persistent bed-wetting or stool toilet refusal or encopresis, please come back for support and advice and check for the underlying organic and psychological cause."

    (d) Highlight the red flags: Urine frequency and fever or if not maintaining dryness may be indicative of urinary infection; if not dry at daytime, by age 4 parents must seek medical advice. Encopresis might be a sign of child abuse. Referral to the occupational therapist, developmental specialist, and other subspecialties in cases of Down syndrome, autism, and cerebral palsy.

    (e) Give away reading materials if available.

7. Communication skills: ensure organized approach, mixed questioning style (open and close-ended questions), active listening, clear language, and reflection on the patient's ICE.

113

Counseling Parents of a Child with Breath-Holding Spells

Dhuha Al Ameri and Shammah Al Memari

Learning Objectives
- How to take a focused history from parents having a child with breath-holding spells?
- How to effectively use the 5 As model to counsel parents on breath-holding spells?
- How to implement good communication skills in advising parents on breath-holding spells?

Focus areas include excluding organic causes and psychological causes of breath-holding spells; and discuss the red flags with parents.

---

1. Introduce yourself and establish a good rapport.
2. Ask:
   (a) Detailed history of attacks: Onset, duration, frequency, associated symptoms (rolling up eyes, pale or blue face, drooling, tongue biting, jerky movements, stiffness, urine incontinence, postictal confusion, or sleeping). Precipitating factors like excessive crying or fever.
   (b) Any ongoing problems, drug history, and significant past or family history.

D. Al Ameri
Ambulatory Healthcare Services, Abu Dhabi, United Arab Emirates

S. Al Memari (✉)
Abu Dhabi, United Arab Emirates

© The Author(s), under exclusive license to Springer Nature Singapore Pte Ltd. 2024
S. Lari et al. (eds.), *Family Medicine OSCE: First Aid to Objective Structured Clinical Examination*, https://doi.org/10.1007/978-981-99-5530-5_113

    (c) Child growth, development, and vaccination history.

    (d) Family dynamics and relationships.

    (e) Stress or new events in the family (newborn baby or nanny, visiting adult).

3. Advise: "As your doctor, I think it's very important for you to understand the nature of this phenomenon and its reassuring course."

    (a) Understand that the problem is stressful for the family and usually they become worried and anxious.

    (b) "This phenomenon is known as breath-holding attacks. The child simply goes into a tantrum by letting out a loud cry and then holding his or her breath, so less oxygen will go to the brain."

    (c) "He or she can then become pale or blue and can go into a simple faint. It happens when your child is angry, frustrated, in pain, or afraid."

    (d) It is common in children between 6 months and 6 years (90% happens before the age of 18 months) with positive family history in 20–35% of patients with the autosomal-dominant trait.

    (e) Assure the parents that it is self-limited (takes 10–60 s and the child will start breathing again) and that it is not harmful and has a good prognosis (children usually grow out of it before school time). Epilepsy and mental deficiency are unrelated breath-holding spells.

    (f) "You may make a video record of the event to help in the diagnosis."

    (g) Iron supplementation in an anemic patient was found to reduce the frequency of attacks.

4. Assess:

    (a) Explore the ideas, concerns and expectations (ICE).

    (b) Don't forget to exclude red flags if any (syncope, loss of consciousness, convulsions, jerky movements, and history of cardiac disease).

5. Assist: "Let's share a plan that is suitable to help you in this situation."

    (a) Reassurance.

    (b) "Don't give attention or overprotection. Don't show that you are worried but ensure the safety of the surrounding environment during attacks."

    (c) "Put the child on his or her side with both knees slightly bent together and the lower arm pulled out behind them."

    (d) "You can help in decreasing the attacks by making him or her feel secure, ensure your child is getting enough rest and help in managing his or her frustration."

    (e) Investigation: complete blood count and you may consider iron level measurement.

6. Arrange:

    (a) Follow up after 2 weeks.

    (b) Anticipate complications, safety netting, and red flags.

    (c) Brief assessment of the underlying conditions and age-appropriate screening.

    (d) Give away reading materials if available.

7. Communication skills: ensure organized approach, mixed questioning style (open and close-ended questions), active listening, clear language, and reflection on patient's ICE.

Counseling Parents of a Child with Temper Tantrum

114

Dhuha Al Ameri, Kawthar Al Ameri,
and Shammah Al Memari◉

Learning Objectives
- How to take a focused history from parents having a child with temper tantrums?
- How to effectively use the 5 As model to counsel parents on temper tantrums?
- How to implement good communication skills in advising parents on temper tantrums?

Focus areas include explore medical and psychological causes of temper tantrums; and exclude and discuss the red flags with parents.

---

1. Introduce yourself and establish a good rapport.
2. Ask:
   (a) Explore parent's ideas, concerns, and expectations (ICE).
   (b) Detailed history of the behavior, onset, frequency, type and period of behavior, child's behavior in between the attacks, history of getting injured,

---

D. Al Ameri
Ambulatory Healthcare Services, Abu Dhabi, United Arab Emirates

K. Al Ameri
Ambulatory Healthcare Services, Abu Dhabi, United Arab Emirates

Faculty of Family Medicine Residency Program, Sheikh Khalifa Medical City,
Abu Dhabi, United Arab Emirates

S. Al Memari (✉)
Abu Dhabi, United Arab Emirates

© The Author(s), under exclusive license to Springer Nature Singapore Pte
Ltd. 2024
S. Lari et al. (eds.), *Family Medicine OSCE: First Aid to Objective Structured
Clinical Examination*, https://doi.org/10.1007/978-981-99-5530-5_114

429

any provoking factors for this behavior, associated symptoms (sleeping distur-bance, agitation, hyperactivity, isolation, or enuresis), and hearing or speech problems.

(c) Any ongoing problems, hospital admissions, past or family history, and drug history.

(d) Child growth, development, and vaccination history.

(e) Family dynamics and relationship.

3. Advise: "As your doctor, I think it's very important for you to understand the nature of this phenomenon and its reassuring course."

   (a) "The problem is stressing for the family, they become worried and anxious."

   (b) "This phenomenon is known as temper tantrums. It is a behavioral disorder in children in the form of emotional outbreaks resulting in kicking, scream-ing, hitting, or breath-holding spells."

   (c) "The outbreak can range from 20 to 30 s to several hours."

   (d) "It usually starts at 12–16 months of age and may persist till 3–4 years old."

   (e) "It occurs mostly when the child is tired or bored and feels angry or frus-trated like if they said no, when things don't go their way, when they cannot manage more difficult tasks, cannot express what they want to say, when mother leaves them even for a brief period of time, and sometimes there are no obvious reasons."

4. Assess:

   (a) Family history of the same problem.

   (b) Any major recent life event (divorce, death of relative, changes in school or home).

   (c) Explore relationship with siblings, child's performance and behavior at school, and any social problem (marital problems or stresses).

   (d) Identify parent's reaction toward such behavior.

5. Assist:

   (a) Reassurance: "Tantrums are relatively common and not harmful."

   (b) Help parents on how to deal with the situation and how to prevent it: refer to Table 114.1 for details.

   (c) Encourage to keep a record of the tantrums with the possible reasons.

6. Arrange:

   (a) Follow up after 2 weeks.

   (b) Anticipate complications, safety netting, red flags (attacks of cyanosis for more than 1 min, resultant post-ictal state, injuries during the attack).

   (c) Brief assessment of the underlying conditions and screening for age.

   (d) Give away reading materials if available.

7. Communication skills: ensure organized approach, mixed questioning style (open and close-ended questions), active listening, clear language, and reflection on the patient's ICE.

Table 114.1 Advice to parents of a child with temper tantrum

Time frame	Advice and recommendations
Prevention of the attacks	• Adopt a healthy lifestyle • Sleep and eat on time • Let the child have new experiences in his life • Reward him or her for any good behavior • Make some realistic and firm rules to follow • Be flexible and decide if the demands are reasonable before saying "yes" or "no" to your child and stick to your decision • Drugs have no place in the management of temper tantrums, give the child enough attention • Keep off-limits objects out of sight and out of reach to make struggles less likely to occur • Set the stage of success when kids are playing or trying to master a new task • Know your child's limits. If he or she is tired, avoid engaging him in activities
During the attack	• "By staying calm, you will help him calm down too" • "Ignore the behavior and don't give him what he or she wants. Pretend to ignore them even when you feel you cannot. When ignored, the problem will probably get worse for a few days before it starts to improve" • "If you cannot ignore, then try to distract the child by directing his or her attention to something of interest" • "Leave the area, keep him in a quiet and safe place, but do not lock him or her in a room" • "Use punishment approach, in particular 'time-out'" • Consider firm action by taking the child to a safe room or space and insist they be quiet (about 1 min per year of his age)"
After the attack	• Do not reward the child's tantrum by giving in • Express love to him or her • Make sure the child is getting enough sleep that can reduce tantrums dramatically

Breaking Bad News of Leukemia to Parents of a Newly Diagnosed Child

115

Eman Al Hayayi, Noora Al Blooshi, and Shammah Al Memari

Learning Objectives
- How to take a focused history addressing the risk factors from parents of a child with leukemia?
- How to effectively use the SPIKES model in breaking bad news to parents of a child with leukemia?
- How to implement good communication skills in counseling parents on leukemia?

Hints Ensure proper setting, give time to process the bad news, check understanding, and address all questions and concerns.

1. Introduce yourself: "Good afternoon Mr./Mrs. X."
2. Establish a good rapport: "How are you today?"
3. Setting:
   (a) Close the door, ensure no interruptions (call the nurse and ask her not to allow any interruptions and put your phone on silent mode), and proper setting (tissue box around with some water).

E. Al Hayayi
Etihad Airways Medical Center, Abu Dhabi, United Arab Emirates

N. Al Blooshi
Ambulatory Healthcare Services, Abu Dhabi, United Arab Emirates

S. Al Memari (✉)
Abu Dhabi, United Arab Emirates

© The Author(s), under exclusive license to Springer Nature Singapore Pte Ltd. 2024
S. Lari et al. (eds.), *Family Medicine OSCE: First Aid to Objective Structured Clinical Examination*, https://doi.org/10.1007/978-981-99-5530-5_115

433

(b) Ask if any family members are with the attending parent: "Are you here alone?"

4. Perception: Check perception using open-ended questions: "Mr./Mrs. X, how can I help you today?" "Do you know why you are here?" "Do you know what tests were done last time for your child and why were they done?" "Do you have any idea what the results might be?" "Some people like to have someone (family or friend) with them if they take their results. Is there someone attending the clinic with you, or you are happy to be alone?"

5. Invite the patient to share in the discussion:

    (a) "Before we review the results, Mr./Mrs. X, are you the sort of person who likes to know about all results-related details or just in brief?"

    (b) "Mr./Mrs. X, I am afraid I have bad news." Pause, hand the patient some tissue papers.

    (c) "Mr./Mrs. X, I am sorry to tell you that your child has a blood picture that suggests blood cancer (leukemia)."

    (d) Encourage feelings expression: "I am sorry I had to give you such bad news. I wish things were different. It must be difficult to hear, how do you feel about it?" "I understand that it can be difficult to take the news. Would you like to express yourself?" (Rotte& Lopez, 2011).

    (e) "It is okay. Take your time. I am here for you."

    (f) "Would you like to have some rest in the treatment room before we proceed?"

    (g) Remember to facilitate verbal and nonverbal cues.

    (h) Remember to listen attentively and ask several times about the extent of understanding.

6. Knowledge check and sharing:

    (a) Explore how much the parent already knows? "Just so that we are on the same page, can you tell me what you know about leukemia?"

    (b) "Acute lymphoblastic leukemia is the most common cancer in children, occurring equally among males and females."

    (c) "It usually occurs between 2 and 8 years of age."

    (d) "It occurs when normal cells in the bone marrow grow abnormally, leading to bone marrow infiltration resulting in bone pain and bone marrow failure (resulting in low red blood cells causing weakness and exercise intolerance, low platelets leading to bleeding and bruising, low white blood cells lead to infections and secondary hemopoiesis, leading to enlargement of lymph nodes, liver, and spleen)."

    (e) "Poor prognostic factors include increased primitive cells (blast) count, T (9:22) translocation, no remission with first-line treatment and/or recurrence."

7. Empathy expression: "Tell me Mr./Mrs. X, how do you feel now?"

    (a) Acknowledge your limitations in breaking the bad news.

    (b) Reinforce support provision and give clinic phone number.

    (c) Ask about feelings and emotional acceptance.

Table 115.1 Required investigation and interpretation of leukemia

Investigation	Findings
Complete blood count (CBC)	• Abnormal white blood cell count, low RBC or platelets • Leukocytosis also abnormal red blood cells and abnormal platelets
Blood film	• Expect blast cells
Bone marrow aspirate	• To confirm the diagnosis (expect a reduction in erythropoiesis as will be evident by more than 20% of cells in blast form), for analysis of the tumor linage (myeloid or lymphoid), and to test for genetic mutations (Philadelphia chromosome or JAK-2 mutation)
Chest X-ray	• Expect mediastinal lymphadenopathy

8. Summarize:
   (a) Brief what has been discussed.
   (b) Reassure and discuss the upcoming plan: "With advances in medicine, patients with acute lymphocytic leukemia (ALL) have the highest chances of being curable of all leukemia. Almost all children are cured, and 80% have no recurrence in 5 years' time."
   (c) Explain the nature of investigations and expected outcomes: "The hematologist taking care of your child will be ordering more investigations. Refer to Table 115.1 for details."
9. Discuss treatment options:
   (a) Supportive treatment: "The hematologist taking care of your child will arrange for treating anemia, preventing bleeding and infections."
   (b) Curative measures: "Treatment aims at destroying the abnormal clonal cells without destroying normal stem cells, so that the latter repopulate after cure; this is achieved by chemotherapy. It is given continuously while your child is admitted until the tumor cells are destroyed. It is then continued as outpatient therapy for 3 years to prevent recurrence."
   (c) "Patients need close follow-up after that for early detection of any recurrence."
10. Arrange:
    (a) Give hope but not false ones: "I know it is difficult to handle this, we are always available to support you and answer your questions."
    (b) Arrange a referral to a pediatric hematology/oncology clinic for further workup and treatment plan design.
    (c) Safety netting: "If your child develops any fever, extreme fatigue, or stops taking orally, bring him to the emergency department immediately."
    (d) Follow up soon.
    (e) Give away reading material and support groups contact if available.
    (f) Ensure parents' safety: "Do you think you can drive back home or would you like me to arrange for you appropriate transportation?"
11. Answer any queries and address concerns clearly.
12. Communication skills: organized approach, mixed questioning styles (open and close-ended questions), active listening, clear language, and reflection on the parent's ideas, concerns, and expectations (ICE).

Counseling Parents of a Child with Autism Spectrum

116

Eman Al Hayayi and Shammah Al Memari

Learning Objectives
- How to take a focused history addressing the risk factors from parents of a child with autism?
- How to effectively use the 5 As model to counsel parents on autism?
- How to implement good communication skills in counseling parents on autism?

Focus areas include explore ongoing medical and psychological conditions; ensure proper understanding of disease prognosis and address all concerns; and provide support, discuss the red flags, and appropriate referrals.

1. Introduce yourself and establish a good rapport.
2. Ask:
   (a) Parent's or caregiver's ideas, concerns, and expectations (ICE).
   (b) History of presenting illness: onset, symptoms, duration, severity, and progression.
   (c) Other ongoing medical problems (epilepsy).
   (d) Past medical history: prenatal, postnatal, birth history, vaccination, and developmental milestones.

E. Al Hayayi
Etihad Airways Medical Center, Abu Dhabi, United Arab Emirates

S. Al Memari (✉)
Abu Dhabi, United Arab Emirates

© The Author(s), under exclusive license to Springer Nature Singapore Pte Ltd. 2024
S. Lari et al. (eds.), *Family Medicine OSCE: First Aid to Objective Structured Clinical Examination*, https://doi.org/10.1007/978-981-99-5530-5_116

(e) Effect of the problem on family dynamic and quality of life.
(f) Investigations (screening tools, imaging. etc.).
(g) Treatment used so far (behavioral, speech therapy, etc.).

3. Advice: "As your doctor, I think it's very important for you to be fully informed about autism and how to manage it. Many mothers went through it, and you can do it." Refer to Table 116.1 for details.

Table 116.1 Providing education on autisms spectrum disorder (ASD) to parents or care giver

Category	Description
Definition and prevalence	• What is autism? "Autism is a group of disorders that affect the development of the brain, leading to a failure for children to develop normal methods of communicating with other people. There is a wide spectrum of severity, with some children able to function with very close to normal communication abilities, and other children not able to communicate with other people at all" • "About 1 in 68 children has been identified with autism spectrum disorder (ASD) according to estimates from CDC's Autism and Developmental Disabilities Monitoring Network. It occurs more commonly in males (4:1). It usually starts before the age of 3" • "Development of the child may seem the same as other children of his/her age, but then he either stops developing or his/her development slows down compared to other children"
Features & key characteristics	• The child performs repetitive tasks and has his own "rituals" of how he carries out the tasks • The child dislikes change • The child has impaired communication and social interaction skills • The child is emotionally detached • Often speech develops later in life, and communication often remains impaired • The child may also have learning disabilities (1/3rd), but this is not always the case
Etiology causes and risk factors	• "The cause is not known. There are many theories, and various genetic and environmental factors that play a role. There is no supporting evidence that shows any link between the 'Measles, Mumps and Rubella (MMR)' vaccination and autism" • "Parents who have a child with ASD have a 2–18% chance of having a second child who is also affected" (autism spectrum disorder)
Treatment strategies and interventions	• "There is no cure for autism. Special education and support aim to maximize the potential of each child as they grow into adults. The earlier the intervention, the better the outcome. Most children with autism are under the care of a specialist in child psychiatry. Autism is mainly treated behaviorally, aiming to reduce unhelpful behaviors and promote the use of good communication skills. Special education to help with language and communication skills. Support and education for the family are very important. There is a large role of speech and language therapy. Occupational therapy can help the child and family adapt to their difficulties. Medication is rarely used, but sometimes may be needed to help control outbursts of excitement or aggression"
Prognosis and long-term outcome	• "Autism continues for life. As the severity can vary, it is difficult to predict the outcome for each child. Even without treatment, sometimes there is improvement in the teenage years and some people with autism become more sociable. Some adults with autism manage to work and get by with just a little support. Many need more support and live at home with parents or family"

4. Assess knowledge about the red flags and precautions to take: "If your child has any of the following, go immediately to the emergency department":
   (a) Hurting others or hurting himself
   (b) Abnormal or jerky movements
5. Assist: "I know it's difficult to handle this, we are always available to support you and answer your questions. Let us share a plan that is suitable for helping you and your child. Please bring your child for full assessment and examination next visit."
6. Arrange:
   (a) Consider referral for genetic testing; testing for chromosomal microarray and fragile X testing to predict prognosis.
   (b) Arrange for a referral to child psychiatry for further management.
   (c) Arrange for a referral with the speech and occupational therapists.
   (d) Arrange for a meeting with the social worker and health educator.
   (e) Give educational material.
   (f) Arrange for a follow-up in 4 weeks.
7. Communication skills: organized approach, mixed questioning styles (open and close-ended questions), active listening, clear language, and reflection on the parent's ICE.

117

Counseling Parents on Childhood Obesity

Buthaina Al Maskari and Shammah Al Memari

Learning Objectives
- How to take a focused history addressing the risk factors from parents of a child with obesity?
- How to effectively use the 5 As model to counsel parents on childhood obesity?
- How to implement good communication skills in counseling parents on childhood obesity?

Focus areas and activity levels, medical complications related to obesity (hypertension, diabetes type 2, dyslipidemia, nonalcoholic fatty liver), and organic causes of obesity (hypothyroidism, Cushing syndrome, Polycystic ovary disease).

---

1. Introduce yourself.
2. Establish a good rapport.
3. Identify the complaint: age at onset of increased weight and define accordingly:
   (a) Overweight: body mass index (BMI) for age above the 85th percentile and lower than the 95th percentile.
   (b) Obesity: BMI for age at or above 95th percentile.
4. Explore if the child has had any periods of normal weight or weight loss.

B. Al Maskari
Ambulatory Healthcare Services, Abu Dhabi, United Arab Emirates

S. Al Memari (✉)
Abu Dhabi, United Arab Emirates

© The Author(s), under exclusive license to Springer Nature Singapore Pte Ltd. 2024
S. Lari et al. (eds.), *Family Medicine OSCE: First Aid to Objective Structured Clinical Examination*, https://doi.org/10.1007/978-981-99-5530-5_117

5. Explore symptoms related to obesity: respiratory difficulties, heartburn, sleep disturbances or apnea, and joint pain. Additionally, in adolescent females ask about acne, hirsutism, LMP, and regular or irregular periods.
6. Dietary history: breastfed or not in infancy, who feeds the child, type of food (healthy and unhealthy), and eating patterns (mealtimes and locations).
7. Activity history: duration and type of activity, in or after school sports, screen time, and barriers to physical activity.
8. Explore the patient's or parent's ideas, concerns, and expectations (ICE).
9. Explore continuous problem and obesity-related complications: polycystic ovarian syndrome, pre-diabetes, type 2 diabetes mellitus, nonalcoholic fatty liver disease, slipped capital femoral epiphysis, anxiety, depression, binge-eating disorder, dyslipidemia, hypertension, and sleep apnea.
10. Past medical, surgical, and family histories. Social history: school performance, self-esteem issues, bullying, family situation, smoking, alcohol, and illicit drug use.
11. Medication use: antidepressants like TCAs and mirtazapine, antipsychotics like olanzapine or risperidone, glucocorticoids, and antiseizure medications.
12. Examination:
    (a) Vitals (BP to rule out hypertension, weight, and height, BMI on growth chart)
    (b) Dysmorphic features.
    (c) Skin: acanthosis nigricans suggests insulin resistance, acne and hirsutism suggest PCOS, and purple striae can indicate Cushing syndrome.
    (d) Papilledema to look for pseudotumor cerebri.
    (e) Tonsillar hypertrophy in case of obstructive sleep apnea.
    (f) Goiter in case of hypothyroidism.
    (g) Wheezing in case of asthma.
    (h) Hepatomegaly to look for nonalcoholic fatty liver disease.
    (i) Abnormal gait or limp.
    (j) Pain in hip or groin to look for slipped capital femoral epiphysis.
13. Order investigation as indicated based on history and physical exam. Lab tests to rule out comorbidities include HbA1c, fasting glucose, ALT, and lipid profile. Endocrine testing could be considered based on clinical findings. Consider genetic testing of extreme early onset of obesity or clinical features suggestive of syndrome.
14. Management:
    (a) Multidisciplinary team involving primary care physician, dietician, behavioral therapist, child, and parents.
    (b) Lifestyle modification advice: decrease overall caloric intake, fast food, processed food, and sugary drinks, increase fruits and vegetables, increase physical activity (30–60 min/day of moderate exercise) and enroll child in sports, and decrease screen time to less than 2 h/day.
    (c) Orlistat is the only medication approved by the FDA for children >12 years of age with BMI ≥ 30 kg/m^2 or ≥ 27 kg/m^2 with obesity-related comorbidities.
15. Give reading educational materials if any.
16. Discuss health maintenance and screening for age.
17. Arrange for follow up and consider referral to a pediatrician or an endocrinologist on a case-by-case basis.
18. Communication skills: organized approach, mixed questioning styles (open and close-ended questions), active listening, clear language, and reflection on the patient's ICE.

Part X

Counseling: Women's Health

Breaking Bad News to a Patient Newly Diagnosed with Abnormal Mammogram Results Using Telemedicine

118

Dana Al Marzooqi, Kawthar Al Ameri,
and Shammah Al Memari

Learning Objectives
- How to take a focused history addressing the risk factors from patients with an abnormal mammogram?
- How to effectively use the SPIKES model in breaking bad news to patients with an abnormal mammogram?
- How to implement good communication skills in counseling patients with an abnormal mammogram?

Focus areas on Breaking bad news using telemedicine will require additional preparation and requirements. Physicians shall ensure a setting preparation unique to a virtual conversation, improve body language skills for effective communications through the camera, and avoid technical failures.

D. Al Marzooqi
Sheikh Khalifa Medical City, Abu Dhabi, United Arab Emirates

K. Al Ameri
Ambulatory Healthcare Services, Abu Dhabi, United Arab Emirates

S. Al Memari (✉)
Abu Dhabi, United Arab Emirates

© The Author(s), under exclusive license to Springer Nature Singapore Pte Ltd. 2024
S. Lari et al. (eds.), *Family Medicine OSCE: First Aid to Objective Structured Clinical Examination*, https://doi.org/10.1007/978-981-99-5530-5_118

1. Make sure to prepare for the tele-visit by dressing professionally and ensure the availability of a backup plan in case of technical failures by having an additional device or videoconference link. Ensure to invite significant others such as family members to the virtual conversation either from the same room or a separate location.
2. Introduce yourself.
3. Establish a good rapport: "How are you today?"
4. Setting:
    (a) Privacy: Make sure the patient is aware of the appropriate settings for their telemedicine visits. For instance, a private bedroom in a patient's home is preferable, while driving during the consultation or being in a noisy environment is not. Before the telemedicine visit begins, make sure that you have all the necessary information about the patient and the people in the room with them. If there are concerns (having a child or housekeeper in the room), ask that the people in the room be relocated.
    (b) Make a connection with the patient: Ensure the consultation room is quiet, ensure the consultation room has a good lightening that makes it easy to interpret facial expressions, look directly at the camera when speaking to the patient, avoid multitasking or charting during the conversations, and acknowledge the emotion verbally as the touch is not possible.
5. Perception: "Ms. X, how can we help you today?" "Do you know why you are having the consultation today?"
    (a) "Do you know what tests you had last time and why were they done?"
    (b) "Do you have any idea what the results might be?"
    (c) "Some people like to have someone (family or friend) with them if they take their results. Are you that type or you are happy to be alone?" If they express a preference to have someone with them, consider asking the patient to invite the person to the room or share a link with them if they are in separate locations. (Ensure the family member or significant other is in a quiet location during the virtual conversation.)
6. Invite the patient to share in the discussion:
    (a) "Before we review the results, tell me, Ms. X, are you the sort of person who likes to know the details or in brief?"
    (b) "Ms. X, I am afraid I have bad news, your results from the mammogram showed an abnormal area." Pause. (But move slightly as silence without moving may be interpreted as a frozen screen.) *"If I were in the room right now, I would offer you a tissue." "Please take a moment if you need one, I will be waiting here for you"* (Vitto 2022). You may lean forward to the camera to show empathy.
    (c) Encourage feelings expression: "I am sorry I had to give you such bad news. I have double-checked with the radiologist (imaging doctor) to make sure that they read it right for the right patient. I wish things were different. It must be difficult to hear, how do you feel about it?" (Rotte and Lopez 2011).
    (d) Clarify: "We are not yet sure what can this abnormal-looking area be and for that reason you need to have a biopsy (which is taking a sample by

needle) from your breast to see this area under the microscope and see if they have cancer."

(e) Ask the patient about her feeling when emotions cannot be understood from facial expressions and ask the patient to repeat themselves if the video is interrupted.

(f) Body language should be exaggerated compared to face-to-face and the motion is slower.

(g) Remember to listen attentively and ask several times about understanding.

7. Knowledge check and sharing:

(a) How much the patient already knows: "Just so that we are on the same page, can you tell me what you know about abnormal mammogram and what it could be?"

(b) If the patient asks about breast cancer, explain: "Breast cancer occurs when normal cells in the breast change and grow out of control." "It is common in females but may also occur in males." "It can run in families." "Breast cancer treatment depends on the stage at which it is diagnosed, and the patient preferences. When surgery is considered, women with breast cancer can choose between mastectomy (removal of the whole breast) or breast conservative therapy/lumpectomy (removal of cancer and a section of the healthy tissue around it)." "Other therapies that can be considered are ones that help the body to kill any leftover cancer cells. These include chemotherapy, radiotherapy, or hormonal therapy." "After treatment, most patients do well. You will only need to be checked with a mammogram annually to see if cancer comes back."

8. Empathy expression: reinforce support provision, give clinic phone number, and ask about feelings and emotional acceptance.

9. Summarize:

(a) Brief what has been discussed and the upcoming plan: "I have arranged for a biopsy to be done with our radiologist and we will take it from there. The biopsy is usually taken under local anesthesia and ultrasound guidance."

(b) "During the procedure, we take one or more small samples of the abnormally looking tissue from the breast. In that way, we can look at the cells under the microscope to see if they have cancer."

(c) Answer any queries and address the concerns clearly.

10. Arrange:

(a) Give hope but not false ones: "I know it's difficult to handle this, we are always available to support you and answer your questions."

(b) Safety netting: "If you develop any fever, pain, or bleeding from the nipples, please come back immediately."

(c) Follow up soon.

(d) Send through email or appropriate channels reading material and support groups contact if available.

11. Communication skills: ensure organized approach, mixed questioning style (open and close-ended questions), active listening, clear language, and reflection on the patient's ideas, concerns, and expectations (ICE).

Dana Al Marzooqi and Shammah Al Memari

Learning Objectives
- How to take a focused history addressing the risk factors from patients with an abnormal pap smear?
- How to effectively use the SPIKES model in breaking bad news to patients with an abnormal pap smear?
- How to implement good communication skills in counseling patients with an abnormal pap smear?

Hints Ensure proper setting, give time to process the bad news, check understanding, and address all questions and concerns.

1. Introduce yourself.
2. Establish a good rapport: "How are you today?"
3. Setting:
   (a) Close the door, ensure there are no interruptions (call the nurse and ask her not to allow any interruptions and put your phone on silent), and proper setting (tissue around with some water).
   (b) Ask if any family members are with the patient: "Are you here alone?"

D. Al Marzooqi
Sheikh Khalifa Medical City, Abu Dhabi, United Arab Emirates

S. Al Memari (✉)
Abu Dhabi, United Arab Emirates

4. Perception: "Mrs. X, how can we help you today?" "Do you know why you are here?" "Do you know what tests you had last time and why were they done?" "Do you have any idea what the results might be?" "Some people like to have someone (family or friend) with them when they receive their results. Are you that type or you are happy to be alone?"

5. Invite the patient to share in the discussion:
   (a) "Before we review the results, tell me, Mrs. X, are you the sort of person who likes to know the details or not?"
   (b) "Mrs. X, I am afraid I have bad news."
   (c) "Mrs. X, your results from the pap smear turned to be abnormal." Pause and hand the patient some tissue paper.
   (d) Encourage feelings expression: "I am sorry I had to give you such bad news. I have double checked with the pathologist (tissue doctor) to make sure that they read it right for the right patient. I wish things were different. It must be difficult to hear, how do you feel about it?" (Rotte and Lopez 2011).
   (e) "The good news is that having an abnormal pap smear does not mean that you have cancer. It sometimes happens due to some infection or menopause."
   (f) "Would you like to have some rest in the treatment room before we proceed?"
   (g) Remember to facilitate verbal and nonverbal cues.
   (h) Remember to listen attentively and ask several times about the extent of understanding.

6. Knowledge check and sharing:
   (a) Check how much the patient already knows: "Just so that we are on the same page, can you tell me what you know about cervical cancer?"
   (b) "Cervix is the bottom part of the neck of the uterus or womb. Cancer happens when the normal cells of the cervix change and grow out of control."
   (c) "Cervical cancer might not cause any symptoms at first. When it does cause symptoms, it can cause vaginal bleeding that occurs between periods, after intercourse, or after menopause."
   (d) "When the pap smear turns abnormal, we should follow it up with a biopsy (cone biopsy). During a biopsy, the doctor will remove a tiny piece of abnormal-looking tissue from the cervix; this diagnostic procedure can be considered a treatment in the early stage of cancer. The doctor would do that using a magnifying lens called "colposcopy" in order to see the cervix better during the procedure."
   (e) "The biopsy sometimes finds cells in the cervix that are not cancerous but are abnormal and have a high chance of turning into cancer. If you turn out to have these "pre-cancerous" cells, the treatment is to remove them to prevent them from turning into cancer, otherwise, we might choose to watch them closely over time."

    (f) "On the other hand, if the biopsy shows cervical cancer, then it should be treated with surgery to remove cancer. Different types of surgeries can involve removing the cervix, uterus, and most upper part of the vagina in a procedure called "radical hysterectomy" or removing all or part of the cervix but leaving the uterus in place. The latter option is only done in the early stages."

    (g) "Other therapies that can be considered are the ones that help the body kill any leftover cancer cells. These include chemotherapy or radiotherapy."

7. Empathy expression: reinforce support provision, give a clinic phone number, and ask about feelings and emotional acceptance.

8. Summarize:
    (a) Brief what has been discussed and an upcoming plan: "I have arranged for a biopsy to be done with our gynecologist and we will take it from there."
    (b) Answer any queries and address concerns clearly.

9. Arrange:
    (a) Give hope but not a false one: "I know it is difficult to handle this, we are always available to support you and answer your questions." "Most women whose pap smear turn to be abnormal and treated early do very well. After treatment, you will be checked every 3–6 months (depending on the abnormality) to see if those abnormal changes reoccur. Follow-up tests can include clinic exams, pap tests, and or some imaging."
    (b) Safety netting: "If you develop any bleeding from your genital tract, pain, fever, or abnormalities with sleep, please come back immediately."
    (c) Follow up soon.
    (d) Give away reading material and support groups contact if available.
    (e) Ensure patient's safety: "Do you think you can drive back home or would you like me to arrange for you appropriate transportation?"

10. Communication skills: ensure organized approach, mixed questioning style (open and closed-ended questions), active listening, clear language, and reflection on the patient's ideas, concerns and expectations (ICE).

Dana Al Marzooqi and Shammah Al Memari

> **Learning Objectives**
> - How to take a focused history addressing the risk factors from patients exposed to varicella during early pregnancy?
> - How to effectively use the SPIKES model in breaking bad news to patients exposed to varicella during early pregnancy?
> - How to implement good communication skills in counseling patients exposed to varicella during early pregnancy?

Hints Ensure proper setting, give time to process the bad news, check understanding, and address all questions and concerns.

1. Introduce yourself: "Good afternoon Mrs. X."
2. Establish a good rapport: "How are you today?"
3. Setting:
   (a) Close the door, ensure no interruptions (call the nurse and ask her not to allow any interruptions and put your phone on silent), and proper setting (tissue around with some water).
   (b) Ask if any family members are with the patient: "Are you here alone?"

D. Al Marzooqi
Sheikh Khalifa Medical City, Abu Dhabi, United Arab Emirates

S. Al Memari (✉)
Abu Dhabi, United Arab Emirates

4. Perception: "Mrs. X, how can we help you today?" "Do you know why you are here?" "Do you know what tests you had last time and why were they done?" "Do you have any idea what the results might be?" "Some people like to have someone (family or friend) with them when they take their results. Are you that type or you are happy to be alone?"
5. Invite the patient to share in the discussion:
    (a) "Since this is the first time that I see you, I would like to ask you a few questions about your current pregnancy and your general health": history (gestational age, prenatal follow-up, varicella vaccination status), any symptoms (fever, malaise, cough, sore throat, rash, headache, lymphadenopathy, arthralgia), and status of the contact: Diagnosis of chickenpox confirmed? When?
    (b) "Before we review the results, tell me, Mrs. X, are you the sort of person who likes to know the details or in brief?"
    (c) "After I reviewed your lab results, Mrs. X, I am afraid I have some bad news for you." Pause and hand the patient some tissue paper.
    (d) "Mrs. X, I am sorry to tell you that your results have come back positive for varicella infection and the chance your baby will get affected is 2% if you are in early pregnancy and the fetus may get severe damages (if acquired soon before delivery, the risk is 20%)."
    (e) Encourage feelings expression: "This must be very hard for you. I can see how difficult it can be to handle this. Would you like to express yourself?"
    (f) "Would you like to have some rest in the treatment room before we proceed?"
    (g) Remember to facilitate verbal and nonverbal cues.
    (h) Listen attentively and ask several times about the extent of understanding.
6. Knowledge check and sharing:
    (a) Check the patient's knowledge about varicella infection.
    (b) Chickenpox is a highly contagious infection that is caused by a virus called varicella zoster. It causes fever, flu-like symptoms, vomiting, diarrhea, headache, and itchy rash (red dots and pimples that appear on the face then trunk then extremities and it may or may not involve oral mucosa, ear, or anal area). It is usually prevented by the varicella vaccine.
    (c) Contagious period: 1–2 days before the rash appears and until all blisters scab.
    (d) When a nonimmune pregnant lady gets in contact with someone with chickenpox, she may, rarely, acquire the infection, within 10–21 days (incubation period).
    (e) If the mother acquires the infection, the fetal risks are: first trimester: 0.4–2%: congenital varicella syndrome [intrauterine growth restriction (IUGR), limb hypoplasia, ocular abnormalities, central nervous system (CNS) abnormalities, cardiac defects, hepatosplenomegaly, limbs scarring, and GI abnormalities]. Five days before or 2 days post-delivery: 20–40%: neonatal varicella (chickenpox and encephalitis). The condition may cause a 30% risk of neonatal mortality. Other complications: miscarriage, stillbirth, and maternal pneumonia in 10% (more in smoker mothers).

(f) Prenatal diagnosis of varicella done through the following:
Mother: clinical diagnosis and swab from skin lesion if available.
Fetus: polymerase chain reaction (PCR) testing for VZV from the amniotic fluid between 17 and 21 weeks' gestation and the fetal ultrasound 5 weeks after maternal infection to check for congenital anomalies.

7. Empathy expression: reinforce support provision, give the clinic phone number, and ask about feelings and emotional acceptance.

8. Summarize: "Mrs. X, how are you feeling? I do not want you to leave with your thoughts missed all over. So let us make the plan clear. How about that?"

(a) Can we know if the fetus is infected? Diagnosis of VZ infection in the fetus is difficult because only 27% have an IgM response. Serology for IgG can be performed after the sixth month.

(b) Management plan and options: detailed in Table 120.1.

(c) Answer any queries and address concerns clearly: "Would you like to ask me anything? Do you feel better?"

Table 120.1 Management options for ladies with exposure to a patient with varicella antenatally

IgM	IgG	Interpretation	Management
Negative	No increase	No acute infection	• Reassurance • Advise to restrict contact with patients with rash

Positive	Significant increase	Acute infection	• Counsel according to the time of exposure:
			  1. Exposure in the first trimester:
			    – Abortion
			    – Referral to fetal medicine unit (FMU) (diagnostic: cardiovascular system, antenatal and fetal anomalies scan)
			  2. Exposure in the peripartum period:
			    – Delay delivery by 10 days, if possible, to give time for maternal IgG to be carried to the fetus by the placenta, so that the infection will be less harmful
			    – After delivery, give varicella zoster immunoglobulin (VZIG) to the neonate
			  3. In all cases, advise the lady to take the VZ vaccine (first dose before discharge and second dose 6–8 weeks later)
			• Antivirals, depending on the severity:
			  1. Uncomplicated varicella infection (fever, myalgia, and rash); oral acyclovir should be started most effectively within 24 h of the rash appearing
			  2. Complicated varicella infection (varicella pneumonia in the mother) IV acyclovir is given
			  3. Note that using acyclovir may not decrease the risk of congenital varicella syndrome
			• Immunoglobulins (Varizig) for nonimmune pregnant women with a history of exposure. It should be provided within 10 days of exposure, otherwise administer IVIG as a second option and can be given a single dose (they decrease maternal infection and maternal morbidity; there is no sufficient data to support its efficacy in decreasing the risk of congenital varicella syndrome)

9. Arrange:
   (a) Give hope but not false ones: "I know it's difficult to handle this, we are always available to support you and answer your questions."
   (b) Safety netting: "If you noticed any fever, vaginal bleeding, or new symptoms, please come back."
   (c) Give a follow-up appointment soon and arrange the referrals as mentioned above.
   (d) Give away reading material and support groups contact if available.
   (e) Ensure patient's safety: "Do you think you can drive back home or would you like me to arrange for you appropriate transportation?"
10. Communication skills: ensure an organized approach, mixed questioning style (open and close-ended questions), active listening, clear language, and reflection on the patient's ideas, concerns and expectations (ICE).

Breaking Bad News to a Pregnant Patient Diagnosed with Rubella

Dana Al Marzooqi, Buthaina Al Maskari, and Shammah Al Memari

Learning Objectives
- How to take a focused history addressing the risk factors from patients exposed to rubella during early pregnancy?
- How to effectively use the SPIKES model in breaking bad news to patients exposed to rubella during early pregnancy?
- How to implement good communication skills in counseling patients exposed to rubella during early pregnancy?

Hints Ensure proper setting, give time to process the bad news, check understanding, and address all questions and concerns.

---

1. Introduce yourself.
2. Establish a good rapport: "How are you today?"
3. Setting:
   (a) Close the door, ensure there are no interruptions (call the nurse and ask her not to allow any interruptions and put your phone on silent) and proper setting (tissue around with some water).

D. Al Marzooqi
Sheikh Khalifa Medical City, Abu Dhabi, United Arab Emirates

B. Al Maskari
Ambulatory Healthcare Services, Abu Dhabi, United Arab Emirates

S. Al Memari (✉)
Abu Dhabi, United Arab Emirates

© The Author(s), under exclusive license to Springer Nature Singapore Pte Ltd. 2024
S. Lari et al. (eds.), *Family Medicine OSCE: First Aid to Objective Structured Clinical Examination*, https://doi.org/10.1007/978-981-99-5530-5_121

    (b) Ask if any family members are with the patient: "Are you here alone?"
4. Perception: "Mrs. X, how can we help you today?" "Do you know why you are here?" "Do you know what tests you had last time and why were they done?" "Do you have any idea what the results might be?" "Some people like to have someone (family or friend) with them when they take their results. Are you that type or you are happy to be alone?"
5. Invite the patient to share in the discussion:
    (a) "Since this is the first time that I see you, I would like to ask you a few questions about your current pregnancy and your general health": history [gestational age, prenatal follow-up, measles, mumps, and rubella (MMR) vaccination status]. Any symptoms (fever, malaise, cough, sore throat, rash, headache, lymphadenopathy, arthralgia). Status of the contact (diagnosis of rubella confirmed or not and when).
    (b) "Before we review the results, tell me, Mrs. X, are you the sort of person who likes to know the details or in brief?"
    (c) "After I reviewed your lab results Mrs. X, I am afraid I have some bad news for you." Pause and hand the patient some tissue paper.
    (d) "Mrs. X, I am sorry to tell you that your results have come back positive for rubella and there is an 85% chance that the fetus gets affected if you are in early pregnancy."
    (e) Encourage feelings expression: "This must be very hard for you. I can see how difficult it can be to handle this. Would you like to express yourself?"
    (f) "Would you like to have some rest in the treatment room before we proceed?"
    (g) Remember to facilitate verbal and nonverbal cues.
    (h) Listen attentively and ask several times about the extent of understanding.
6. Knowledge check and sharing:
    Check the patient's knowledge about rubella infection.
    (a) Tell the patient: "Rubella is a viral infection that causes fever, flu-like symptoms, or itchy rash (red dots that appear 3–5 days after the onset of symptoms, progressing from the face backward. All clear within 1–2 weeks) and is usually prevented by rubella vaccine."
    (b) Contagious period: 1–2 weeks before clinically apparent infection, and infectivity decreases with appearance of rash.
    (c) When a nonimmune pregnant lady gets in contact with someone with rubella, she is 20% susceptible to acquire the infection in 2–3 weeks (incubation period). "You will be referred to an obstetrician to discuss the required testing or ultrasound to detect any fetal abnormalities (congenital heart defect, cataract, microcephaly, sensorineural deafness), a condition called 'congenital rubella syndrome.'"
    (d) "Unfortunately, there is no effective treatment to prevent the development of congenital rubella syndrome once the mother is infected. However, the risk of fetal manifestations if mother infected is: 85% before 9 weeks, 52% from 9 to 12 weeks, and rarely after 16 weeks of pregnancy."
    (e) Other complications include spontaneous miscarriage, or stillbirth.

7. Empathy expression: reinforce support provision, give clinic phone number, and ask about feelings and emotional acceptance.
8. Summarize: "Mrs. X, how are you feeling? I do not want you to leave with your thoughts messed up all over. So, let us make the plan clear. How about that?"
   (a) Investigations: repeat IgG test in 2–3 weeks (incubation period) to look for significant increase in the titer, indicating recent infection.
   (b) Management plan or options: as detailed in Table 121.1.
   (c) Answer any queries and address concerns clearly: "Would you like to ask me anything? Do you feel better?"
9. Arrange:
   (a) Give hope but not false ones: "I know it's difficult to handle this, we are always available to support you and answer your questions."
   (b) Safety netting: "If you noticed any fever, vaginal bleeding, or new symptoms, please come back."
   (c) Give follow-up appointment soon and arrange referrals as mentioned above.
   (d) Give away reading materials and support groups contact if available.
   (e) Ensure patient's safety: "Do you think you can drive back home or would you like me to arrange for you appropriate transportation?"
10. Communication skills: ensure organized approach, mixed questioning style (open and closed-ended questions), active listening, clear language, and reflection on the patient's ideas, concerns and expectations (ICE).

Table 121.1 Management options for ladies with exposure to a patient with rubella antenatally

IgM	IgG	Rubella culture	Interpretation	Management
Negative	No increase		No acute infection	• Reassurance. • Advise to restrict contact with patients with rash.
Positive	Fourfold increase	Positive	Acute infection with a high risk of congenital rubella syndrome	• Counsel ladies with exposure in first trimester as follows: 1. Pregnancy termination. 2. Treatment of acute rubella infection includes supportive measures. 3. Controversial: immunoglobulin for post-exposure prophylaxis (it has not been demonstrated to prevent asymptomatic infection, viremia, or congenital rubella syndrome) (Riley, 2021). 4. Referral to fetal medicine unit (FMU) (diagnostic: Cardiovascular system, antenatal and fetal anomalies scan). 5. Postpartum MMR vaccine as soon as possible for susceptible individuals (avoid pregnancy for 28 days post vaccine) (Riley, 2021).

Counseling a Female on the Human Papillomavirus (HPV) Vaccine

122

Eiman Al Murar, Sumiya Taheri,
and Shammah Al Memari

Learning Objectives
- How to take a focused history addressing the risk factors from patients/mothers coming for HPV vaccine?
- How to effectively use the 5 As model to counsel patients/mother on HPV vaccine?
- How to implement good communication skills in counseling patients/mother on HPV vaccination?

Hints Ensure proper setting, give time to process the bad news, check understanding, and address all questions and concerns. In this setting, you may encounter adolescents accompanied by their mothers seeking counseling for HPV. It is crucial to provide clear explanations to both individuals and to comprehend their opinions effectively.

---

1. Introduce yourself and establish a good rapport.
2. Ask:
   (a) Mother's and patient's ideas, concerns and expectations (ICE): about the vaccine and cervical cancer as a condition.

E. Al Murar · S. Taheri
Ambulatory Healthcare Services, Abu Dhabi, United Arab Emirates

S. Al Memari (✉)
Abu Dhabi, United Arab Emirates

© The Author(s), under exclusive license to Springer Nature Singapore Pte Ltd. 2024
S. Lari et al. (eds.), *Family Medicine OSCE: First Aid to Objective Structured Clinical Examination*, https://doi.org/10.1007/978-981-99-5530-5_122

461

(b) Patient's age, marital status, history of sexually transmitted illness, or previous abnormal cervical smears and treatments.

(c) Family history of cervical cancer or other gynecological cancers.

(d) General health: any chronic disease, acute illness, and allergic reaction to vaccines.

3. Advise, assess knowledge, and willingness to take the vaccine.

(a) "Human papilloma virus (HPV) is a small DNA virus that has more than 200 types and can infect both males and females. Most of the types cause cutaneous infections manifesting as warts on the hands and feet, and it is transmitted by direct contact with the lesions or fomites. Around 40 types cause epithelial infections of which 12 are oncogenic, causing cervical, anogenital, and oral cancers. HPV is considered the most common sexually transmitted infection with the highest prevalence in females aged 20–25 years.

(b) Infection is usually self-limited and asymptomatic, but when present can manifest as anogenital, periungual, and plantar warts, malignancies, including cervical, vaginal, vulvar, anal, penile, and oropharyngeal cancers.

(c) The high-risk HPV genotypes 16 and 18 cause around 70% of cervical cancers, anal cancers, and a significant proportion of oropharyngeal cancer, vulvar and vaginal cancer, and penile cancer. Other genotypes 31, 33, 45, 52, and 58 cause an additional 20%. HPV types 6 and 11 cause approximately 90% of anogenital warts.

(d) Three different types of HPV vaccine have been developed against the high-risk types. Refer to Table 122.1 for details.

(e) "HPV vaccine is recommended for routine vaccination at age 11 or 12 years. (Vaccination can be started at age 9.) ACIP also recommends vaccination for everyone through age 26 years if not adequately vaccinated when younger. HPV vaccination is given as a series of either two or three doses, depending on the age at initial vaccination. Two doses of HPV vaccine are recommended for most persons starting the series before age 15. The second dose of HPV vaccine should be given 6–12 months after the first dose. Adolescents who receive two doses less than 5 months apart will require a third dose of HPV vaccine. Three doses of HPV vaccine are recommended for those who start the series at ages 15–26 years, and for immunocompromised persons. The recommended three-dose schedule is 0, 1–2, and 6 months. Three doses are recommended for immunocompromised persons (including those with HIV infection) aged 9–26 years."

Table 122.1 Types of HPV vaccines

Type	Details
Bivalent vaccine (Cervarix)	Targets HPV types 16 and 18
Quadrivalent vaccine (Gardasil)	Targets HPV types 6, 11, 16, and 18
9-valent vaccine (Gardasil 9)	Targets the same HPV types as the quadrivalent vaccine (6, 11, 16, and 18) as well as types 31, 33, 45, 52, and 58

(f) "Vaccination is not recommended for everyone older than age 26 years. Some adults ages 27–45 years might decide to get the HPV vaccine based on discussion with their clinician. HPV vaccination of people in this age range provides less benefit, for several reasons, including that more people in this age range have already been exposed to HPV".

(g) "HPV vaccination prevents new HPV infections but does not treat existing HPV infections or diseases. HPV vaccine works best when given before any exposure to HPV."

(h) "It is important to continue cervical cancer screening even after taking the full vaccine series because it does not protect against all types of HPV and HPV virus is not responsible for 100% of cervical cancer cases."

(i) "It is a safe vaccine that gives long-life immunity. Lactating mothers but not those who are pregnant at time of visit can take it. Side effects are mild, including mild fever, soreness, or redness at the injection site."

4. Assist: "Let's share a plan that is suitable for you ...."

(a) Check patient understanding.

(b) Offer written information or give away material if available.

(c) Arrange:
   Follow-up in 2 months for second dose.

(d) Anticipate complications: "You may experience headache, get redness, swelling, or pain in the site of the injection."

5. Communication skills: ensure organized approach, mixed questioning style (open and close-ended questions), active listening, clear language, and reflection on the patient's ICE.

Counseling a Female on Family Planning and Contraception

123

Sumiya Taheri and Shammah Al Memari

Learning Objectives
- How to take a focused history highlighting the indications and contraindications for contraceptives from females coming for family planning?
- How to effectively use the 5 As model to counsel females on family planning and contraception?
- How to implement good communication skills in counseling females on family planning and contraception?

Focus areas include a review of the patient's past history to assess the success or failure of prior contraceptive use, consideration of indications and contraindications. The discussion should cover various contraceptive types, addressing questions such as how to use them, duration of use, failure rates, side effects, and contraindications.

1. Introduce yourself and establish a good rapport.
2. Explore patient's ideas, concerns and expectations (ICE) + understanding of contraception.
3. Ask:
   (a) Age, parity, and current lactation?

S. Taheri
Ambulatory Healthcare Services, Abu Dhabi, United Arab Emirates

S. Al Memari (✉)
Abu Dhabi, United Arab Emirates

© The Author(s), under exclusive license to Springer Nature Singapore Pte Ltd. 2024
S. Lari et al. (eds.), *Family Medicine OSCE: First Aid to Objective Structured Clinical Examination*, https://doi.org/10.1007/978-981-99-5530-5_123

(b) Menstrual history: last menstrual period (LMP), regularity, heaviness, and duration.
(c) Previous experience: Any problem? Compliance?
(d) Personal preference, acceptability of contraception, cost, ethical considerations, does the partner agree?
(e) Any contraindication to contraception: multiple sexual partners [risk of sexually transmitted disease (STD), pelvic inflammatory disease (PID)], smoking, personal and family history of deep vein thrombosis (DVT), ischemic heart disease (IHD), liver disease, or cancers (ovarian, breast, endometrial).
(f) Other past medical problems and medications: diabetes mellitus (DM), hypertension (HTN), tuberculosis (TB), and epilepsy.
(g) Any allergies (latex, copper).
4. Advise: Explain to the patient the choices, types of contraception methods, effectiveness of each, advantages, disadvantages, and instructions for use: "The total risks of birth control are much less than the total risks of a pregnancy!"

123.1 Hormonal

1. **Combined oral contraceptive pills (COCP):** "As the name suggests, the combination pill is a combination of two female sex hormones that prevents pregnancy by changing the hormone balance in your body to stop ovulation."
   (a) There are different types: 21-day packet or biphasic pills: "Start the pill on the fifth day of bleeding and take at the same time of each day thereafter for maximum prevention." 28-day packets: monophasic, triphasic pills: (the seven extra pills are inactive, sugar pills): "Start the pill on the first day of bleeding and take at the same time of each day thereafter for maximum prevention." Combined contraceptives also come in the form of patches and vaginal rings.
   (b) Effectiveness: pregnancy rate in the first year, also called pearl index [about 0.3% with perfect use, about 9% with typical use (includes inconsistent or incorrect use)].
   (c) Advantages: reduce period's pain, flow, risk of uterine, ovarian cancer, risk of ectopic pregnancy, and increase bone density, improvement in acne, premenstrual symptoms, menorrhagia, polycystic ovary syndrome, and endometriosis.
   (d) Side effects: "If any it will wean within 3 months: nausea, spotting, mild headaches, tender breasts, dizziness, increased risk of ischemic stroke. or slight weight gain, loss."
   (e) Interactions: oral contraceptives pills' (OCP's) effectiveness decreases when used along with antibiotics, vitamin C, anti-epilepticus, or anti-TB medications: "When taking any, use another method of contraception during the course and up to 7 days after the last dose." OCPs decrease the effectiveness of hypoglycemic agents.
   (f) Missed pills: refer to Table 123.1 for details.

Table 123.1 Missed oral contraceptive pills rules

Time frame of missing the pill	Corrective action
If one pill is late (less than 24 h since pill should have been taken) or missed (24–47 h since pill should have been taken)	a. "Take late or missed pill as soon as possible. b. Continue taking the remaining pills as scheduled (even if it means taking two on the same day). c. Back-up contraceptive protection not necessary. d. Emergency contraception not usually indicated but may be considered if combined oral contraceptive (COC) missed early in cycle or COC missed in the last week of previous cycle."
If two consecutive pills missed (48 h since pill should have been taken)	a. "Take the most recent missed pill as soon as possible (discard any other missed pills). b. Continue taking the remaining pills as scheduled (even if it means taking two on the same day). c. Use back-up contraceptive protection (such as condom) or avoid sexual intercourse until hormonal pills have been taken for 7 consecutive days."
If pills missed in the first week of the cycle (days 1–7 for a 28-day pill pack)	a. "Consider emergency contraception if unprotected intercourse occurred in pill-free interval or first week of pill taking. b. If pills missed in the second week of cycle (days 8–14 in a 28-day pill pack), emergency contraception not indicated if pills in the preceding 7 days were taken consistently and correctly. Patient should use back-up contraceptive protection (such as condom) or avoid sexual intercourse until hormonal pills have been taken for 7 consecutive days."

(g) Contraindications: hypertension, pregnancy, breastfeeding, smoker, > 35 years old, history of DVT, liver or gallbladder disease, migraine with aura, and epilepsy.

(h) Address any myths: "There is no reason to take a break from the pill unless pregnancy is wanted." "You can get pregnant anytime once you stop the contraceptive pills."

2. **Vaginal NuvaRing:**
   (a) A flexible, transparent plastic ring that is self-inserted deep into the vagina after menses and left for 3 weeks. Removed in the fourth week to allow menstruation to occur.
   (b) Mechanism of action: similar to the oral contraceptive pills.
   (c) Effectiveness: 95% at 7 days from starting use of the ring.
   (d) Side effects: similar to the OCPs' side effects in addition to vaginitis.
   (e) Contraindications: as in OCPs, repeated fall after insertion and prolapse.
3. **Progesterone-only pill (28-day packet):**
   (a) "Start the pill on the first day of bleeding and take it at the same time of each day (or within 3 days) thereafter for maximum prevention."
   (b) Indications: lactating ladies, more than 40 years old, and history of estrogen-secreting tumor.

(c) Missed pills: "If more than 3 hours late for scheduled pill (more than 27 hours since last pill), take missed pill as soon as possible (even if it means taking 2 pills in 1 day) and advise the patient to abstain from intercourse or use additional contraceptive protection (condoms) for the next 2 days (48 hours). Consider emergency contraception if unprotected intercourse occurs in 2-day interval."

4. **Depo-Provera injections (medroxyprogesterone based inhibits ovulation):**
   (a) Effectiveness: 99.7%.
   (b) Intramuscular (IM) injection in the deltoid, thigh, gluteus, in the first 5 days of bleeding, or less than or equal to 21 days of giving birth. This gives immediate effectiveness that continues for 3 months. If given on other days of the cycle, then backup protection is needed for 7 days.
   (c) Advantages: good for ladies with compliance issues, less expensive than pills, no pelvic inflammatory disease (PID) risk, and decrease dysmenorrhea.
   (d) Side effects: irregular menses, amenorrhea, headaches, depression, weight gain (2–3 kg per year), decrease high-density lipoprotein (HDL), loss of bone mineral density (if used > 2 years), acne, hirsutism, and alopecia.
   (e) Contraindications: as with oral contraceptive pills' use, drug addiction, and seizure.
   (f) Correct any myths: "You could become pregnant as soon as 3–4 months after the last shot. But some women take up 1–2 years to conceive after stopping this method."

5. **Implantable contraceptive devices:**
   (a) Subcutaneous (SC) implantation of a rod containing levonorgestrel/etonogestrel (progesterol) in the skin covering the deltoid muscle, which lasts for 3 years.
   (b) Effectiveness: 99.95%.
   (c) Ovulation restarts 6 weeks after removal of the implant.
   (d) Side effects: bad scars, difficult to remove [may migrate and need to be located by magnetic resonance imaging (MRI), high-frequency ultrasound (US)].
   (e) Same mechanism of action, efficacy, and contraindications as Depo injections.

6. **Emergency contraception:**
   (a) **"Copper intrauterine device (Cu-IUD):** considered the most effective method of emergency contraception, with about 0.14% pregnancy rate."
   (b) **"Ulipristal acetate given as single 30-mg dose:** considered the most effective when taken up to 120 hours (5 days) after unprotected intercourse. May be more effective than levonorgestrel."
   (c) **"Levonorgestrel (1.5 mg) or double-dose regimens** (2 pills containing levonorgestrel 0.75 mg each taken 12 hours apart): Considered the most effective when administered within 72 hours (3 days) of intercourse. Levonorgestrel may be used in women with contraindications to daily hormonal contraceptives." Side effects: mild nausea, spotting, or bleeding. Correcting any myths prevents ovulation. Does not cause abortion. Not for regular use."

7. **Intrauterine device (IUD):**
   (a) "Small T-shaped device that is inserted and kept in the uterus to prevent implantation of any embryo. The hormonal types also prevent ovulation. A small, connected thread is left in the cervix for easy removal when desired."
   (b) Two types: copper coils (works for 10 years) and hormonal intrauterine systems (Mirena: works for 5 years).
   (c) Effectiveness: 99.2–99.9%.
   (d) Suitable candidates: women who have contraindication or intolerant to OCPs, smokers, and more than 35 years of age.
   (e) Advantages: easy office-based insertion, good for ladies with compliance issues, reversible, and decreased heavy bleeding (only Mirena).
   (f) Side effects: pelvic inflammatory disease, ectopic pregnancy, breast tenderness, spotting (for copper + first three months in Mirena), nausea, or headache.
   (g) Contraindications: pelvic inflammatory disease, multiple sexual partners, ectopic pregnancy copper allergy, or Wilson's disease (for copper IUD only).
   (h) Correct any myths: "Does not interfere with sex or daily activities." "Uterine perforation is uncommon (0.1—0.3% risk)."

8. **Barrier methods**
   (a) **Male condoms:** Thin sheath of rubber, latex, that should be worn over an erected penis. Effectiveness: 79–97%. Advantages: cheap, readily available, and provides the best protection against STDs, especially the latex and polyurethane type. Side effects: risk of condoms breaking down with oil-based lubricant.
   (b) **Female condoms:** A thin plastic pouch that lines the vagina. It is held in place by a close inner ring at the cervix and an outer ring at the vagina. Effectiveness: 79–97%. It should be placed prior to and kept in for 6–8 hours after the intercourse. Side effects: expensive and no protection against STDs.
   (c) **Diaphragm:** A small dome-shaped device of latex or silicone that fits inside the vagina and covers the cervix. Should be kept in for 6–8 hours postcoital. Effectiveness: 84–94%. Advantages: can be fitted 2–4 hours before intercourse with the ability to increase the period by reapplying spermicide. Side effects: allergy, urinary tract infection (UTI), and toxic shock syndrome if left for more than 24 hrs.
   (d) **Cervical cap:** small plastic dome placed over the cervix and used with spermicide. Effectiveness: in nulliparous 80–90%; in multiparous 60–70%. Advantages: can be fitted 6 hours before intercourse. Side effects: risk of UTI and toxic shock syndrome, should be kept in for 6–8 hours postcoital.
   (e) **Sponge:** Doughnut-shaped device made of soft-coated foam with spermicide. Effectiveness: 84%. Advantages: each sponge allows repeated acts for a 24-hour period. Side effects: risk of toxic shock syndrome, allergy, and vaginal irritation.

9. **Spermicides:**
   (a) Types: Foam, crème, jelly, or suppository.
   (b) Method of use: inserted into the vagina near the cervix no more than 30 mins before having sex.
   (c) Effectiveness: 71–85%.
   (d) Advantages: cheap and readily available.
   (e) Side effects: allergy and vaginitis.
10. **Natural methods:** absenteeism during peri-ovulation period or withdrawal method (effectiveness: 80–99%).
11. **Permanent sterilization:**
    - **Vasectomy for males:** Done through a small incision at the base of the scrotum. There are different techniques to do it, the one with the lowest failure rate is cauterization of the vasa with or without fascial interposition. Effectiveness: 99.85%. Advantages: safer and quicker than tubal ligation. Disadvantage: expensive, surgical risks, and takes time to be effective (confirmed by post-vasectomy semen sample at 12 weeks showing rare, nonmotile sperms if any). Reversal: expensive and success rate is highly variable. Correct any myths: does not increase the risk of prostate and testicular cancer.
    - **Tubal ligation for females:** Advantages: decrease the risk of PID and ovarian cancer. Disadvantages: expensive, surgical risks, and risk of ectopic pregnancy. Effectiveness: 99.5%. Reversal: not evidence based and rarely successful.
5. Assess: compliance of the patient, level of understanding, and any questions or extra clarification needed.
6. Assist:
   (a) Positive reinforcement: "Many others did it before you, you can definitely do it, we are always available to support you."
   (b) Reached to shared understanding and management.
7. Arrange:
   (a) Negotiate appropriate contraception.
   (b) Explain the red flags (unexplained fever, abnormal vaginal discharge with foul smelling, dyspareunia, or pelvic pain).
   (c) Follow up as required.
   (d) Brief assessment of the underlying conditions and age-appropriate screening: vaccination, pap smear, and mammogram.
8. Give away reading material if available.
9. Thank the patient.
10. Communication skills: ensure organized approach, mixed questioning style (open and close-ended questions), active listening, clear language, and reflection on the patient's ICE.

Counseling a Female on Natural Family Planning (Fertility Awareness-Based Method)

Eiman Al Murar, Sumiya Taheri, and Shammah Al Memari

Learning Objectives
- How to take a focused history from females coming for natural family planning?
- How to effectively use the 5 As model to counsel females on natural family planning?
- How to implement good communication skills in counseling females on natural family planning?

Focus areas include a review of the patient's past history to assess the success or failure of prior contraceptive use. Discussion of different types of natural methods (How to use? How long? Failure rate? Side effects? Contraindications?) and helping patients choose the most appropriate method.

1. Introduce yourself and establish a good rapport.
2. Ask:
   (a) Ideas, concerns, and expectations (ICE): Why this method? Any medical contraindications? Currently breastfeeding? Any previous use of contraceptive methods and their success and failure?
   (b) Menstrual history: last menstrual period, regularity, length of cycle, flow, and intermenstrual bleeding.

E. Al Murar · S. Taheri
Ambulatory Healthcare Services, Abu Dhabi, United Arab Emirates

S. Al Memari (✉)
Abu Dhabi, United Arab Emirates

© The Author(s), under exclusive license to Springer Nature Singapore Pte Ltd. 2024
S. Lari et al. (eds.), *Family Medicine OSCE: First Aid to Objective Structured Clinical Examination*, https://doi.org/10.1007/978-981-99-5530-5_124

(c) Obstetric history: number of pregnancies and miscarriages, complications during previous pregnancies and deliveries, and age of the youngest child.
3. Explore the patient's knowledge: "What do you know about the fertile days?"
4. Advise: 'Natural contraceptive methods, as the name implies, use natural ways to prevent pregnancy. They are based on:
    (a) Periodic avoidance of unprotected intercourse during the fertile days. Effectiveness hugely depends on correct use by couples and accurate identification of fertile days. Through the below methods. Refer to Table 124.1 for details.
    (b) Discuss the benefits: no local or systemic adverse effects, no or minimal cost, no delay in return of fertility, and no interactions with other drugs.
    (c) Discuss the barriers to use: no protection against sexually transmitted infections, lack of information sources for patients, not very convenient for patients (to optimally apply the methods) and physicians (to choose the best method for the patient and provide education on application), and duration of abstinence.
5. Assess: couple's ability to follow this advice and any barriers.
6. Assist:
    (a) Set the plan after identifying the fertility days.
    (b) Discuss the emergency contraception in case of having unprotected sex during the fertility period. These are: Plan B: two doses of 0.75 mg levonorgestrel, 12 hrs apart within 3 days or copper intrauterine device (IUD): within 5 days.
7. Arrange: for folic acid supplementation as the failure rate is nonreliable.
8. Communication skills: ensure organized approach, mixed questioning style (open and close-ended questions), active listening, clear language, and reflection on the patient's ICE.

Table 124.1 Methods for identifying fertility and ovulation days: details and effectiveness

Method	Details
Cervical mucus monitoring	Once the cervical mucous appears (copious, whitish, stretchy discharge), avoid sex for 3 days afterward. Might not be effective in women with vaginal discharge or infection.
Basal body temperature	Monitor the temperature every morning waiting for a slight rise (about 0.4 Fahrenheit) that occurs after ovulation. Avoid sex once it goes up and 3 days after. Not appropriate for women with chronically elevated temperature due to chronic illness.
Calendar or rhythm method	(Estimates timing of ovulation by documenting longest and shortest cycle durations over a 6–12-month period); avoid sex from day 8 to 19 of the cycle for women with a cycle length of 26–32 days. Can be used without restriction in women with vaginal discharge or chronically elevated temperature. Restrictions in post-menarcheal, perimenopausal or postpartum women due to irregular menstruation.
LH surge detection using home urine-ovulation test kit	This hormone signals ovulation. If your normal cycle is 28 days, you'll need to test on days 11–14 of the cycle. A positive result means you should ovulate in the next 24–36 hours and must start avoiding sex for 3 days.
Lactation	Gives maximum protection in the first 6 months if the cycle has not resumed yet and no bottle feeds or supplements are introduced.
Symptothermal method	Combines calendar calculations, basal body temperature charting, and cervical mucus monitoring.

Counseling a Female on Early Pregnancy Care

125

Dana Al Marzooqi, Buthaina Al Maskari, and Shammah Al Memari

> **Learning Objectives**
> - How to take a focused history from females coming for early pregnancy care?
> - How to effectively use the 5 As model to counsel females on early pregnancy care?
> - How to implement good communication skills in counseling females on early pregnancy care?

Focus areas include Past medical history for previous high-risk pregnancy, perinatal complications, and chronic illness. Discuss unhealthy habits and risky behaviors and impact on pregnancy (high-risk meds use, illicit drug, alcohol, smoking). Discuss the red flags and address all concerns.

1. Introduce yourself and establish a good rapport: "Congratulations on becoming an expectant parent, this is a very exciting time in your life, even though you may be inclined to feel flat and sick at first" (Rotte & Lopez, 2011).

D. Al Marzooqi
Sheikh Khalifa Medical City, Abu Dhabi, United Arab Emirates

B. Al Maskari
Ambulatory Healthcare Services, Abu Dhabi, United Arab Emirates

S. Al Memari (✉)
Abu Dhabi, United Arab Emirates

2. Ask:
   (a) Explore patient's ideas, concerns and expectations (ICE).
   (b) Past medical history: Any medications? Blood group?
   (c) Gynecological and obstetric history: Last menstrual period (LMP)?
       Regular? Early scans? Aim for correct dating.
   (d) Family (genetic diseases) and social (support, help) histories.
3. Advise: "Your baby is very special and deserves a flying start in life by growing healthy in your womb. As your doctor, I think it's very important for you to understand that the first 12 weeks of pregnancy are the time of organ formations, therefore, some points have to be taken into consideration":
   (a) Nutrition: "Aim for a well-balanced and nutritionally sound diet":
   (b) Folic acid supplements 0.4 mg (as early as possible, preferably 3 months' preconception). If there is a personal or family history of neural tube defects, epileptic, or diabetic, use 5 mg daily. Explain to the patient: "It reduces the risk of having a baby with neural tube defects such as spina bifida."
   (c) Maternal multivitamins, vitamin D, calcium supplements, and iron supplements.
   (d) Limit caffeine consumption to 150–300 mg per day.
   (e) Avoid unpasteurized dietary products and raw eggs, meat, and fish.
   (f) Have moderate amount of liver, avoid shark, swordfish, king mackerel, tilefish, tuna steaks, and saccharin-containing drinks.
   (g) Avoid smoking, alcohol, and illicit drugs (no known safe amount of alcohol consumption during pregnancy).
   (h) Air travel: Safe until 4 weeks before the expected date of delivery (EDD) (hydration, stockings, and mobilization if long trip). Preferably avoided in first and third trimesters.
   (i) Moderate noncontact exercise: greater than or equal to 30 min on most days of the week (avoid activities with risk for falls or abdominal injuries and avoid scuba diving).
   (j) Sexual intercourse: not associated with adverse outcomes.
   (k) Hair treatment and dyes: avoid in early pregnancy (no clear association with fetal malformation).
   (l) Hot tubs and saunas: avoid in first trimester (associated with neural tube defects and miscarriage).
   (m) Medications: avoid nonprescribed medications and herbal remedies.
   (n) Workplace: Favorable demographic and behavioral characteristics. Avoid prolonged standing and exposure to certain chemicals.
   (o) Car seat belts: proper use (the lap strap goes below not on the belly) and risks related to not using them.
   (p) Encourage planning ahead: Labor (what to do when their membranes rupture? What to expect when labor begins? Strategies to manage pain, and the value of labor support and breastfeeding (the best feeding method)?

4. Assess: "What do you think about that?"
   (a) Exclude the red flags (ectopic: abdominal pain or bleeding).
   (b) Depression is related to unwanted pregnancy, low socioeconomic state, neglect, and domestic violence.
5. Assist: "Let's share a plan that is suitable for helping you to keep this pregnancy a nice experience."
   (a) Vaccination for influenza (intramuscular vaccine, killed, and safe in pregnancy).
   (b) Screen for: asymptomatic bacteriuria and sexually transmitted infections, diabetes, ABO and Rh blood typing, and anemia screen (risk of preterm labor, intrauterine growth retardation, and perinatal depression).
   (c) If at risk of preeclampsia: low-dose aspirin prophylaxis and calcium supplementation if dietary intake is low.
   (d) Testing for aneuploidy and neural tube defects (discuss the risks and benefits).
   (e) Change medications to safe alternatives if any and manage smoking or drug abuse.
6. Arrange:
   (a) Positive reinforcement: "Pregnancy is a very normal event in the life cycle and usually goes very smoothly, especially if you have regular medical care."
   (b) Antenatal classes: "Trained therapists will advise you on antenatal exercises, back care, postural advice, relaxation skills, pain relief in labor, general exercises, post-delivery care, and breastfeeding" (Rotte & Lopez, 2011).
   (c) Follow up: every 4–6 weeks until 28 weeks of pregnancy, then every 2 weeks until 36 weeks of pregnancy, then weekly until delivery.
   (d) Safety netting and red flags: "If you develop lower back/abdominal pain, vaginal bleeding, vaginal water gush, or notice a decrease in your baby movements, please come back immediately."
   (e) Age-appropriate screening (pap smear if not done) and give away reading materials.
7. Communication skills: ensure organized approach, mixed questioning style (open and close-ended questions), active listening, clear language, and reflection on the patient's ICE.

Counseling a Female with a High-Risk Pregnancy

126

Eman Al Hayayi, Sumiya Taheri,
and Shammah Al Memari

> **Learning Objectives**
> - How to take a focused history from females with a high-risk pregnancy?
> - How to effectively use the 5 As model to counsel females on a high-risk pregnancy?
> - How to implement good communication skills in counseling females on a high-risk pregnancy?

> **Focus areas** includes medical history highlighting previous high-risk pregnancy, perinatal complications, and chronic illness. Discuss the red flags and address all concerns.

1. Introduce yourself and establish a good rapport (ensure privacy, show empathy, ask if she has a relative with her).
2. Ask:
   (a) Current obstetric history: any vaginal bleeding, fluid leakage, vaginal discharge (meconium stained), premature contractions (three or more in 20 min), preeclampsia symptoms [legs edema, headache, visual changes,

E. Al Hayayi
Etihad Airways Medical Center, Abu Dhabi, United Arab Emirates

S. Taheri
Ambulatory Healthcare Services, Abu Dhabi, United Arab Emirates

S. Al Memari (✉)
Abu Dhabi, United Arab Emirates

© The Author(s), under exclusive license to Springer Nature Singapore Pte Ltd. 2024
S. Lari et al. (eds.), *Family Medicine OSCE: First Aid to Objective Structured Clinical Examination*, https://doi.org/10.1007/978-981-99-5530-5_126

right upper quadrant (RUQ) pain], fetal movement (minimum 12 per day), placenta previa, fetal abnormality, multiple gestation, intrauterine growth restriction (IUGR), or macrosomia and cervical incompetence.

(b) Past obstetric history: preterm delivery, group B strep infection (GBS), gestational diabetes mellitus (GDM), abortions, intrauterine fetal death, fetal abnormality, pre-eclampsia, Rh-isoimmune, previous cesarean section, low birth weight or macrosomia, uterine malformation (fibroid), or uterine scar.

(c) Medical history: GDM, diabetes mellitus (DM), hypertension (HTN), tuberculosis (TB), heart disease, epilepsy, renal disease, current viral infection (chicken pox or active herpes), sexually transmitted disease (STD), human immunodeficiency virus (HIV), syphilis, urinary tract infection (UTI) symptoms, and severe anemia (less than 9 hemoglobin).

(d) Surgical history: previous pelvic surgery, myomectomy, and cerclage.

(e) Drug history and allergies.

3. Advise: according to the history.
4. Assess: understanding and exclude red flags.
5. Assist: "Let's share a plan that is suitable for helping you ..."
6. Arrange:

(a) Check expected date of delivery (EDD): consider induction if post-date.

(b) Examination: refer to Table 126.1 for details

(c) Investigations: hemoglobin level, urine test for albumin and glucose. Vaginal and urine culture for GBS (if positive give antibiotic at labor or after 12 hrs of rapture of membrane (ROM)). Ultrasound to check for fetal well-being: movement, tone, heart sound. Check amniotic fluid index.

(d) Follow up visit and give her time to decide, give away reading material if available, and safety netting: ask the mother to monitor fetal movements.

7. Communication skills: ensure organized approach, mixed questioning style (open and close- ended questions), active listening, clear language, and reflection on the patient's ideas, concerns and expectations (ICE).

Table 126.1 Focus physical examination of females with a high-risk pregnancy

Examination	Details
General	Weight, blood pressure BP, and leg edema.
Abdomen	Fundal level, fetal lie and presentation, head engagement, and fetal heart sound.
Cervical	Dilation, effacement, fetal station, and cervical consistency. Speculum exam to rule out: rupture of membrane (ROM).

Counseling a Pregnant Female on Risk of Having a Baby with Down Syndrome

127

Sumiya Taheri and Shammah Al Memari

> **Learning Objectives**
> - How to take a focused history from females concerned about Down syndrome during pregnancy?
> - How to effectively use the 5 As model to counsel females concerned about Down syndrome during pregnancy?
> - How to implement good communication skills in counseling females concerned about Down syndrome during pregnancy?

Focus areas include medical history highlighting previous high-risk pregnancy, child with Down syndrome, perinatal complications, and chronic illness. Discuss the red flags and address all concerns.

1. Introduce yourself and establish a good rapport.
2. Ask:
   (a) History: patient's age, gestational age, prenatal follow-up, any Down syndrome's screening test performed during this pregnancy, and past obstetric history (any previous child with Down syndrome).
   (b) Ideas, concerns, and expectations (ICE), example: pregnant lady who found out one of her cousins had a baby with Down syndrome and she is worried that she might have a similar baby.

S. Taheri
Ambulatory Healthcare Services, Abu Dhabi, United Arab Emirates

S. Al Memari (✉)
Abu Dhabi, United Arab Emirates

    (c) Patient's knowledge: "What do you know about Down syndrome?" "Has she heard about screening or diagnostic test for Down syndrome?" "Does she expect specific test?"

3. Advise:

    (a) "Being your doctor, I think you should understand that if your cousin had a child with Down syndrome that does not mean that you will have a Down syndrome baby too."

    (b) To ensure we are on the same page, can you tell me what you know about Down syndrome?"

    (c) Explain: Down syndrome is a genetically determined (caused by an extra copy of chromosome 21 resulting from a new mutation or acquired from a carrier), lifelong condition that presents from birth in the form of learning or behavioral problems (varying from mild to severe, the child can take longer to learn how to sit, walk, and talk), as well as other medical problems [obstructive sleep apnea (OSA), stomach, blood, and heart problems].

    (d) Features of Down syndrome: flat face, depressed nasal bridge, extra skin at the back of the neck, eyes that slant up, floppy muscles, and single palmar crease.

    (e) Causes are unknown, and there are no known risk factors that increase a pregnancy risk. Even healthy young women can have a baby with Down syndrome. It occurs in 1: 500 births, and its chances get higher as women get older.

    (f) Early detection and the latest advancement in medicine increased their life expectancy from 25 years in the 1980s to 49 years in 1997. By allowing early treatment of any complications (like heart conditions), many people with Down syndrome live happy and full lives. But they usually need help with some day-to-day tasks.

4. Assess: understand and exclude the red flags: thoughts of aborting herself.

5. Assist: "Let's share a plan that is suitable for helping you …."

    (a) Explore: "Some mothers like to know everything about her expected child before he or she is born to be relieved from any anxiety/prepared for a special child, others choose to wait until the child is born. Which type describes you best?"

    (b) It is important that you understand that there are multiple ways to know if your current fetus has Down syndrome and always discuss the following before performing prenatal screening.

    (c) Discuss and explain the difference between screening and diagnostic tests.

    (d) Discuss the technique, limitations, complications, and ability of screening tests to detect Down syndrome and other abnormalities.

    (e) Discuss the option of no testing.

    (f) Discuss the implications of having a child with Down syndrome.

    (g) Screening options for Down syndrome as follows:

    (h) Cell-free DNA: can be performed at any gestational age after 9–10 weeks' gestation; results may reflect underlying maternal aneuploidy or maternal disease.

(i) First-trimester screening: Performed between 10- and 13 weeks' gestation: "Fetal ultrasound (also called genetic ultrasound) to assess nuchal translucency in combination with measurement of serum analytes (beta-human chorionic gonadotropin and pregnancy-associated plasma protein A [PAPP-A] with or without alpha-fetoprotein). Advantages include one-time testing that allows for early screening, allows for screening of other structural, genetic, or placental disorders. Disadvantages include lower detection rate than tests with first- and second-trimester component."

(j) Second-trimester screening: Performed between 15 and 22 gestations: "Quadruple screening; involves measurement of four maternal serum analytes (human chorionic gonadotropin (hCG), alpha-fetoprotein (AFP), dimeric inhibin A, unconjugated estriol) in combination with maternal factors such as age, weight, race, and presence of pre-gestational diabetes to calculate risk."

(k) Combined first-trimester (10–13 weeks' gestation) and second-trimester (15–22 weeks' gestation) screenings using a combination of serum biomarkers and ultrasound testing: involves obtaining NT on ultrasound plus PAPP-A in the first trimester, then quad screen.

(l) If the above tests are positive, confirmatory test is needed: Chorionic villus sampling (CVS) if 10–13 weeks: During which a needle is put into the mother's uterus and removes a tiny piece from the placenta (the organ that delivers oxygen, nutrients, and carries waste away from the fetus). Risk of miscarriage with the procedure is about 1/200. Amniocentesis if 15–20 weeks: A needle is put into the mother's uterus and removes some of the fluid that is around the baby. Risk of miscarriage with the procedure is about 1/300–1/600. Cordocentesis (percutaneous umbilical blood sampling).

(m) If you choose to have no testing in pregnancy and the baby turns out to have features of Down syndrome, a genetic testing after birth will be done to confirm the diagnosis.

(n) If the child turns out to have Down syndrome, then regular follow-up with screening for common problems: refer to Table 127.1 for details.

Table 127.1 Screening common medical problem in down syndrome patients

Medical problems	Screening method
Growth delay	At first visit, at 2, 4, 6, 12, 18, and 24 months and annually thereafter.
Obstructive sleep apnea	Start screening at first year of age and sleep study by 4 years of age.
Ophthalmology review	At 6 months and annually until the age of 5 years. Every 2 years from 5 to 13 years. Every 3 years from 13 to 21 years.
Hearing abnormalities	At birth, 6 months, then annually.
Thyroid hormone	At birth, 6 months, 12 months, then annually.
Heart defects	Ultrasound before and after baby is born.
Blood disease	Blood test complete blood count (CBC) every year from age 1 to 21 years.
Muscle and nerve problem, joint problem (atlantoaxial instability)	Careful neurological exam annually.

6. Arrange: Positive reinforcement, arrange follow-up, give her the time to decide, give away reading material if available, and safety netting: If she did decide not to have a screening test and then she became anxious and wants to do a screening test to relieve her anxiety, she shall come back.

7. Communication skills: ensure organized approach, mixed questioning style (open and close-ended questions), active listening, clear language, and reflection on the patient's ICE.

Counseling a Female on Epilepsy During Pregnancy

128

Khuloud Al Hammadi, Noora Al Blooshi, and Shammah Al Memari

Learning Objectives
- How to take a focused history from females with epilepsy during pregnancy?
- How to effectively use the 5 As model to counsel females with epilepsy during pregnancy?
- How to implement good communication skills in counseling females with epilepsy during pregnancy?

Focus areas include medical history of previous high-risk pregnancy, perinatal complications, and chronic illness. Discuss the risks of epilepsy vs. the risks of antiepileptic use during pregnancy. Discuss the red flags and address all concerns.

1. Introduce yourself and establish a good rapport.
2. Ask
   (a) Age, work, last menstrual period (LMP), and gestational age.

K. Al Hammadi
Sheikh Khalifa Medical City, Abu Dhabi, United Arab Emirates

N. Al Blooshi
Ambulatory Healthcare Services, Abu Dhabi, United Arab Emirates

S. Al Memari (✉)
Abu Dhabi, United Arab Emirates

© The Author(s), under exclusive license to Springer Nature Singapore Pte Ltd. 2024
S. Lari et al. (eds.), *Family Medicine OSCE: First Aid to Objective Structured Clinical Examination*, https://doi.org/10.1007/978-981-99-5530-5_128

(b) History of epilepsy: medications used, level of control before pregnancy, any previous pregnancies with epilepsy and their outcomes, previous investigations, and their results (MRI, CT, EEG), and previous follow-up with neurology.

(c) Enquire about current, new-onset seizures (the first attack after 20 weeks of gestation, think of eclampsia): How many attacks? Any seizure medications (name, doses, and frequency)? Any other medication (may have interaction)?

(d) Other medical conditions.

(e) Ideas, concerns, and expectations (ICE): the patient is worried about teratogenicity.

3. Advise: "To make sure that we are on the same page, tell me what you know about epilepsy."

(a) What is epilepsy? The most common neurological disorder in pregnancy is characterized by recurring seizures.

(b) What is the risk of having a child with epilepsy? If the mother is epileptic, the risk is less than 5%. If both parents are epileptic, the risk is a bit higher.

(c) What to do when a seizure occurs during pregnancy? Tell your family and friends: In case of a seizure, simply remove potentially harmful objects away. Do not restrain, cover with a blanket, alert the patient (if absence type of seizure), place anything in his/her mouth, or attempt to move to another place. If the attack continues or the patient does not regain consciousness after 20 minutes: Call the ambulance and administer rectal valium (keep at home).

(d) How to decrease the harm to the fetus? Wear a bracelet, necklace, or card that specifies your condition and the details of your medications, your GP, and your hospital phone number.

(e) Advise about the medications: Box 128.1.

(f) Take folic acid 4 mg daily (to prevent neural tube defects).

(g) Avoid precipitating factors: sleep deprivation, extreme hunger, fatigue, constipation, or flickering lights (view smart screens from at least 2 m distance in an illuminated room, if nearer cover one eye with the palm of your hand and use polaroid sunglasses).

(h) Avoid being alone in potentially dangerous places (kitchen, bathroom, near fire/drains) and avoid door locking.

(i) Activities and sport: "You better get engaged in supervised activities only" and avoid activities that may trigger or cause injury.

(j) Driving (according to local driving regulations in different countries and the type of vehicle used, ranges from 1 to 10 years from being seizure free).

(k) Some anticonvulsants increase the risk of hemorrhagic disease; patient's newborns need to be given prophylaxis vitamin K.

4. Assess: level of understanding, ability to adhere to medications, and attendance to follow-up visits.

5. Assist:

(a) Suggest meetings with a close relative for continuous support.

(b) Invite to attend help group associations and foundations.

(c) Postnatally: Counsel regarding breastfeeding and medications (caution if the mother is using phenobarbital, primidone, ethosuximide, or lamotrigine), the safety of the baby (e.g., changing the diaper on the floor), and family planning (progesterone injectable and IUD does not interact with antiepileptic drugs). Antiepileptics reduce the effect of oral contraceptives pills (OCPs), so you might need dual contraceptive methods.

(d) Contraception choices (use LARC or high-dose oral combined pills, avoid a vaginal ring, estrogen implant, or regular oral OCP): antiepileptic drugs are enzyme inducers, thus they decrease the efficacy of contraception.

(e) Lamotrigine or levetiracetam is the drug of choice in childbearing-age women. Valproate should be avoided, but if used must be given in the lowest dose possible.

(f) Lamotrigine, carbamazepine, valproate acid, and phenytoin can be used during breastfeeding.

6. Arrange: "Many mothers did it before you, you can definitely do it, and we are always available to support you".

(a) Follow up a shared plan with the obstetrics medicine clinic (blood levels in each trimester, scans, neurologist meeting, and discussion).

(b) Anticipate complications (safety netting): Contact your doctor if: Seizures change in number, any time you change your medication or take another medication, if you sustain trauma to the tummy or have abdominal pain (think of abruption).

(c) Brief assessment of the underlying conditions and age-appropriate screening.

(d) Give away reading material if available.

7. Communication skills: ensure organized approach, mixed questioning style (open and closed-ended questions), active listening, clear language, and reflection on the patient's ICE.

Box 128.1: Antiepileptic Drug Use in Pregnancy

1. The harm from seizures and resultant hypoxia on the fetus is higher than the side effects of the medications, so it is better to attain the best control with the least medications.

2. All antiepileptic drugs are probably teratogenic.

3. Monotherapy is preferred as polytherapy is associated with a greater risk of teratogenicity. If the patient was well-controlled (seizure-free) in the pre-pregnancy period, the same medication should be continued. If not, then it is best to shift from highly teratogenic (highest risk with valproic acid, phenobarbital) to fewer teratogenic medications (lowest with levetiracetam).

4. Children of mothers with epilepsy have a 4–8% risk of congenital anomalies.

5. "Don't stop your medications suddenly or change the dose by yourself. Continue monitoring blood levels in each trimester when the body's interaction with the drug changes."

Breastfeeding Counseling

129

Reem Al Mansoori, Buthaina Al Maskari,
and Shammah Al Memari

Learning Objectives
- How to take a focused history from mothers regarding breastfeeding?
- How to effectively use the 5 As model to counsel mothers on breastfeeding?
- How to implement good communication skills in counseling mothers on breastfeeding?

Focus areas include breastfeeding benefits, techniques, and any struggles or issues that could lead to failure.

---

1. Introduce yourself and establish a good rapport.
2. Ask:
   (a) Mother's inquiries: Ideas, concerns and expectations (ICE).
   (b) Current situation: Breastfeeding attempts or difficulties, working mother, anyone who helps her in taking care of the child, social support, husband's attitude toward breastfeeding and thoughts from others regarding breastfeeding. Ask about contraception measurements.

R. Al Mansoori
Emirates Medical Association of Family Medicine, Abu Dhabi, United Arab Emirates

B. Al Maskari
Ambulatory Healthcare Services, Abu Dhabi, United Arab Emirates

S. Al Memari (✉)
Abu Dhabi, United Arab Emirates

© The Author(s), under exclusive license to Springer Nature Singapore Pte Ltd. 2024
S. Lari et al. (eds.), *Family Medicine OSCE: First Aid to Objective Structured Clinical Examination*, https://doi.org/10.1007/978-981-99-5530-5_129

    (c) Feeding history: type of feeding, onset, frequency, duration, method (shifting breasts), ask if the child sleeps after feeds, and passes stool and urine.

    (d) Mother's diet, calcium and vitamin D supplements, fluids intake, and maternal medications.

3. Advise: "As your doctor, I encourage you to breastfeed your baby as breastfeeding has multiple benefits for you and your baby."

    (a) Benefits of breastfeeding for the mother and the baby: psychological bonding, increases your baby's immunity, decreases the risk of developing dermatitis, asthma, acute otitis media and gastroenteritis, maternal weight loss and faster uterine recovery, thus reducing postpartum blood loss, lowers the risk of developing diabetes mellitus, hypertension, cardiovascular disease, and breast, ovarian, and endometrial cancers, cost-effective, and easier (no need to prepare).

    (b) Techniques of breastfeeding: (starting breastfeeding best after delivery). Refer to Box 129.1 for details.

4. Address common concerns:

    (a) Pain (ensure good technique and latch), milk supply, and maternal exhaustion

5. Assess:

    (a) Breast examination: inspecting for anatomic abnormalities (scar tissue, previous surgeries, or flat and inverted nipples).

    (b) Understanding of the importance of breastfeeding and excluding red flags (fever, sore breast, bleeding, or discharge from nipples indicating mastitis).

6. Assist (mother in ensuring adequate feeding):

    (a) Recognizing satiety signs like baby's facial and hand muscles are relaxed, and content, not showing feeding cues while awake

    (b) The baby has 6–8 wet diapers per day

    (c) The baby has 3–4 bowel movements per day

    (d) The baby is back up to birth weight by 2 weeks of age and tracking along the growth curve throughout the next few months

    (e) Hearing the baby swallow while breastfeeding with clearly full cheeks

    (f) Milk leaks from one breast when you are feeding the baby from the other

7. Arrange:

    (a) Positive reinforcement ("Many mothers did it and so you can, we are always available to support you"), for example, working mothers: "Still you have enough and excellent time to feed your baby during your maternity leave, even if you plan to stop after, but the best is to continue." "You can use working break hours to feed the baby or pump milk."

    (b) Schedule a follow-up.

    (c) Offer appropriate contraceptive method and consider other options when breastfeeding is stopped.

    (d) Vitamin D drops for the baby and vitamin D with calcium tablets for the mother.

    (e) Safety netting: come back if any fever or sore breast, or redness or greenish discharge.

8. Brief assessment of the underlying conditions and screening for age.

9. Give away reading material if available.

10. Communication skills: ensure organized approach, mixed questioning style (open and close-ended questions), active listening, clear language, and reflection on the patient's ICE.

Box 129.1 Guidelines on Breastfeeding Techniques
- Maintain right position: sit comfortably with back support.
- Baby position: directly facing the nipple without turning his neck, ensuring he is comfortable.
- Ensure good latching by having infant's chin buried in the breast with no areola showing at the bottom, while the areola is visible outside the upper lip and the nose is free.
- Start feeding by compressing the nipple and areola between your thumb and index finger.
- Allow your baby to feed for 10 minutes on each breast.
- Nursing frequency based on baby's demand and look for feeding cues (rooting or turning head, smacking lips, and sucking on fingers and hands).
- It is normal to feel period-like cramps while you feed your baby, it is a normal reflex following breastfeeds, and it indicates that your uterus is going back to its normal pre-pregnancy size.
- If an infant is sleepy at the breast, try arousal techniques such as burping, changing diapers, or rubbing the head, back, arms, or feet, and try to express more milk by breast compression.
- Other advice:
- Milk supply improves with adequate sleep, fluids, relaxed environment, and less stress.
- Clean your breasts with water and keep the nipple dry with loose clothing. Avoid using antiseptics or soaps on the nipple.
- You may need to pump your breast to relieve pain or store milk.
- Engorgement may be helped with a hot shower, massage, milk expression, and supportive bra.
- Counsel about appropriate contraception methods such as progesterone pills. Breastfeeding alone is not an effective contraceptive method.

Counseling a Female on Hormone Replacement Therapy (HRT) Initiation

130

Shaima Lari, Kawthar Al Ameri,
and Shammah Al Memari

Learning Objectives
- How to take a focused history from females interested in hormonal replacement therapy (HRT)?
- How to effectively use the 5 As model to counsel females on HRT?
- How to implement good communication skills in counseling females on HRT?

Hints
- **Bold sentences indicate absolute HRT contraindications.**
- Underlined sentences indicate relative HRT contraindications.

---

1. Introduce yourself and establish a good rapport.
2. Ask:
   (a) Current complaint: hot flushes, sleep disturbances, sexual impairment, reduced activity, and mood swings: "I understand that you are visiting me today because you are disturbed by 'hot flushes.' Can you tell me more about it?"

S. Lari
Sheikh Shakhbout Medical City, Abu Dhabi, United Arab Emirates

K. Al Ameri
Ambulatory Healthcare Services, Abu Dhabi, United Arab Emirates

Faculty of Family Medicine Residency Program, Sheikh Khalifa Medical City, Abu Dhabi, United Arab Emirates

S. Al Memari (✉)
Abu Dhabi, United Arab Emirates

© The Author(s), under exclusive license to Springer Nature Singapore Pte Ltd. 2024
S. Lari et al. (eds.), *Family Medicine OSCE: First Aid to Objective Structured Clinical Examination*, https://doi.org/10.1007/978-981-99-5530-5_130

(b) Identify patient's ideas, concerns, and expectations (ICE).

(c) Explore more: "To be able to help you, I need to ask you further questions": See Box 130.1.

Advise: "I understand how frustrated you are, all the feelings that you are describing point toward menopause. These symptoms can be improved with HRT. HRT is safe when indicated appropriately. In your case, HRT is considered safe because you have no health risks to prevent us from starting HRT and you will benefit from." (Indicate the appropriate type) and clearly explain the advantages and disadvantages of HRTs. See further details in Table 130.1.

3. Assess: Determine your patient's willingness and level of understanding HRT initiation advantages and disadvantages. "So, what do you think about starting you in HRTs?" "Do you think you can cope with those side effects?"

4. Assist:

(a) Choice of the appropriate medication.

(b) Assurance: "To decrease the side effects, we will start you with the smallest dose and use them for the shortest period possible and at that time we will stop it gradually."

(c) Answer questions and clarify concerns: "Do you have any questions for me?"

5. Arrange:

(a) Positive reinforcement and reassurance: "Many others did it before, you can definitely do it and we are always available to support you."

(b) Follow up soon and ensure safety netting.

(c) Screening for age, including booking for mammogram and pap smear.

(d) Give away reading material if available.

6. Communication skills: ensure organized approach, mixed questioning style (open and close-ended questions), active listening, clear language, and reflection on the patient's ICE.

Box 130.1: Key Aspects of History Taking in Counseling Patients on Hormone Replacement Therapy (HRT)

- Ask about decreased concentration and activity, disturbed sleep, night sweats, mood swings, sexual impairment, dyspareunia, dysuria, or incontinence.
- Menstrual history.
- Gynecological problems (**vaginal bleeding**, fibroids, hysterectomy).
- Obstetric history (**current pregnancy or feeding**).
- Past medical history: diabetes mellitus, **cardiovascular diseases** (hypertension, **stroke, deep vein thrombosis**), liver disease, **cancers** (**malignant melanoma, endometrial,** breast, ovarian, colorectal), gall bladder disease, and migraine.
- Family history: osteoporosis, breast, or endometrial cancer.
- Social history: smoking.
- Screening: last mammogram, pap smear (any undifferentiated results), and lipids profile.
- Reflection on life (patient's own feelings and quality of life activity).

Table 130.1 Hormone replacement therapy (HRT)

Advantage	Disadvantage
Decrease hot flushes	GI upset decreased appetite and nervousness
Improve sleep, muscle aches, mood, sexual activity, and vaginal dryness	Breast enlargement, spotting, or vaginal bleeding and acne.
Increase bone mineral density and decrease fracture risk in the forearm, vertebrae, and hip.	Increase risk of uterine cancer. Increase risk of breast cancer especially if obese lady or when used for more than or equal to 3–5 years.
Decrease the risk of colorectal cancer	Increase risk of cardiovascular diseases, stroke, and deep vein thrombosis if used in women 60 years or older.

Part XI

Counseling: Men's Health and Geriatrics

Counseling a Patient on the Use of Performance Enhancers

131

Abeer Al Naqbi, Dana Al Marzooqi, and Shammah Al Memari

Learning Objectives
- How to take a focused history from patients planning to use a performance enhancer?
- How to effectively use the 5 As model to counsel patients on the use of a performance enhancer?
- How to implement good communication skills in counseling patients on the use of a performance enhancer?

Focus areas when evaluating performance-enhancing products include discussing four key factors: the mechanism of action, available research evidence, potential adverse effects, and legality.

1. Introduce yourself and establish a good rapport (show empathy and avoid arguing).
2. Ask:
   (a) Ideas, concerns and expectations (ICE).
   (b) Use of performance enhancers: age at onset/duration, types, route (oral, intranasal, inhalational, trans-buccal, creams/gels, implants, injections), amount, and any previous attempts to quit.

A. Al Naqbi
Ambulatory Healthcare Services, Abu Dhabi, United Arab Emirates

D. Al Marzooqi
Sheikh Khalifa Medical City, Abu Dhabi, United Arab Emirates

S. Al Memari (✉)
Abu Dhabi, United Arab Emirates

(c) Explore motives for use: competition season (use peaks: early preseason, during the season), previous sports injury (use increase after an injury), or desired body image, performance, "What do you want to be?" Do you want to be bigger? Leaner? Have more overall endurance?"

(d) Unusual symptoms (sudden-onset unexplained): sleeping problems, mood/energy/weight changes, or physical symptoms (acne, palpitations).

(e) Past medical history: diabetes mellitus (DM), hypertension (HTN), coronary artery disease (CAD), renal or liver disease (some supplements cause water retention, increase insulin resistance, or exacerbate renal or hepatic failure).

(f) Alcohol or drug use.

(g) Background knowledge about the benefits, harms, and benefits of quitting.

3. Advise: Develop discrepancies between what the athlete wants to have after sports (e.g., want to have kids) and the impact of continued use of the substance:

(a) "As your doctor, I think it is very important for you to be fully informed. It is common for athletes to take substances, including prescription medication in high doses, specifically for the purpose of improving their sports performance (increase their strength, power, speed, endurance (toleration), pain threshold, or to alter their body weight/composition."

(b) "This practice of sports doping is banned by most professional sports associations not only because it is cheating but because of the risks to the athlete him/herself. Unfortunately, most of these risks are based on theoretical medical knowledge or reports from user's doctors, which is all we have. This is because it is difficult to confirm them as it would be unethical to give such high doses to participants in research. The bottom line is that the short-term benefits of these performance enhancers are tempered by many risks. The good news, however, is that most of these side effects are reversible upon discontinuation."

(c) Briefly discuss the supplement used (be aware that they are often combined). Pull out the official website of the specific trade name used and use it while talking the patient through the following facts: Refer to Table 131.1 for details.

4. Assess:

(a) Motivation and willingness to quit (precontemplation, contemplation, preparation, action, maintenance).

(b) Impeders for successful quitting: as peer pressure, "Is there anyone that you are worried to tell that you are quitting?"

5. Assist: "Let's share a plan that is suitable for you to quit supplements":

(a) Set a quit date.

(b) Address psychosocial fears, and family and friends' support.

(c) Use alternatives: See Box 131.1.

6. Arrange:

(a) Positive reinforcement: "Many others did it before you, you can definitely do it, we are always available to support you." "World-class athletes who have the same body as yours, have won champions without enhancers, you can as well."

(b) Follow up soon.

(c) Referral to sport medicine or sports psychologist clinic as needed.

(d) Referral to drug dependency unit if physical dependence is present.

Table 131.1 Performance enhancers in sports—efficacy and side effects

Performance enhancers	Efficacy and side effects

Nutritional supplements (Legal)	• Few studies prove performance enhancement with the following (in small doses):
	  – Carbohydrate-electrolyte beverages
	  – Sodium bicarbonate
	  – Creatine (most popular): A compound that is naturally produced by the body in small amounts (2 mg) to help muscles release energy. Studies demonstrate increased maximum power output, increased lean body mass, and increased endurance. Side effects: increased weight, acute interstitial nephritis, and rapid progression of chronic kidney disease (CKD)

Amino acids (Legal)	Not effective with minimal side effects Side effects: diarrhea and stomach cramps
Beta-hydroxy-beta-methyl butyrate (Legal)	Postulated on decreased protein breakdown. Side effects not known
Chromium (Legal)	Postulated to increase muscle mass. Side effects: rhabdomyolysis, liver, and renal dysfunction
Iron (Legal)	Not effective unless deficiency is present
Growth hormone (GH) (Illegal)	• The only difference between human-derived or animal-derived GH is that the latter has the potential to cause allergic reactions (due to antigenicity), but they both contain the same compound • Limited studies demonstrate an increase in lean body mass, but it does not improve strength and may worsen exercise capacity • Side effects: diabetes, myopathy, cardiomegaly, hepatitis, increased lactate levels, premature epiphyseal closure, fluid retention (soft tissue edema, hypertension, joint pain, carpal tunnel syndrome)

Androgens and anabolic steroids (Illegal)	• Include exogenous testosterone, synthetic androgens (e.g., danazol, nandrolone, stanozolol), androgen precursors (e.g., androstenedione, dehydroepiandrosterone), selective androgen receptor modulators, and other forms of androgen stimulation
	• All increase the testosterone effects that are
	  – Anabolic (increase muscle protein synthesis, promote muscle building, and provide quicker recovery from hard work)
	  – Androgenic (male characteristics: as facial hair, deeper voice)
	• Studies demonstrate that testosterone causes–dose-response increase in muscle strength and mass (not true for androgen precursors)
	• Side effects: tendon rupture, hepatotoxicity, administration-related infections (abscesses, septic arthritis, and hepatitis/HIV), androgenic effects reduce spermatogenesis/fertility, gynecomastia, acne, hirsutism, temporal hair recession, premature closure of epiphysis, cardiovascular system (CVS) effects (reduce HDL, increase LDL, erythrocytosis), and central nervous system (CNS) dysfunction (depression, mania, psychosis, aggression)

(continued)

Table 131.1 (continued)

Performance enhancers	Efficacy and side effects
Stimulants	Include amphetamine, d-methamphetamine, methylphenidate, ephedrine, pseudoephedrine, caffeine (not banned), dimethylamylamine, cocaine, fenfluramine, pemoline, selegiline, sibutramine, strychnine, and modafinil • Studies demonstrate increased endurance, reaction time, and anaerobic performance, and reduced weight and tiredness • Side effects: rhabdomyolysis, autonomic effect (weight loss, headache, nausea, tremor), CVS dysfunction (hypertension, tachycardia, myocardial infarction, stroke, heatstroke), and CNS dysfunction (increased risk two- to threefold, including insomnia, anxiety, panic attacks, agitation, aggression, and psychosis)
Oxygen Transport improvers (Prohibited)	• Include blood transfusions, erythropoiesis-stimulating agents (such as recombinant human erythropoietin and darbepoetin alfa), and hypoxia mimetics that stimulate endogenous erythropoietin production (such as deferoxamine, cobalt, and artificial oxygen carriers) • Transfusions and erythropoiesis-stimulating agents have been shown to increase aerobic power and physical exercise tolerance. However, the ergogenic effects of the other agents are debatable • Side effects: myocardial infarction (MI), stroke, deep vein thrombosis (DVT)/pulmonary embolism, hypertension, and antibody-mediated anemia • Others: beta-agonist and diuretics

(e) Brief assessment of the underlying conditions and age-appropriate screening.

(f) Give away reading material if available.

7. Communication skills: ensure organized approach, mixed questioning style (open and close-ended questions), active listening, clear language and reflection on the patient's ICE.

Box 131.1 Enhancing performance naturally: tips for optimal fitness through sports, balanced diet, and proper nutrition

- "Get involved in regular sports to increase your fitness."
- "Maintain a balanced diet to maintain a blood chemistry necessary to perform at an elite level."
- "Have a pre-exercise meal to ensure that adequate glycogen stores are available for optimal performance."
- "Have a post-exercise meal to enhance recovery and improve your ability to train consistently:
  - Replace fluid loss with water.
  - Take 4:1-gram carbohydrates (such as fruit or juice) to protein ratio. CHO restores your glycogen stores, and proteins will rebuild muscle tissue that is damaged during intense or prolonged exercise."

Counseling a Patient on Male Sterilization

132

Halima Al Shehhi and Shammah Al Memari

Learning Objectives
- How to take a focused history from patients counseled for male sterilization?
- How to effectively use the 5 As model to counsel patients on a male's sterilization procedure?
- How to implement good communication skills in counseling males on sterilization procedure?

1. Introduce yourself and establish a good rapport.
2. Ask:
   (a) Do you have children? Are you planning in future to have more children?
   (b) Have you and your partner tried different methods of contraception?
   (c) What do you know about vasectomy?
   (d) Why do you choose to have a vasectomy?
   (e) Explore the patient's ideas, concerns, and expectations (ICE) about the procedure.
3. Advise:
   (a) "Male sterilization is a very effective way of contraception in which women can take no role at. Out of 100 women, less than one can get pregnant if their partner has a vasectomy in the first 6 months. It is safe and permanent. The procedure is simple and causes only little discomfort. Recovery is quick and

H. Al Shehhi
Ambulatory Healthcare Services, Abu Dhabi, United Arab Emirates

S. Al Memari (✉)
Abu Dhabi, United Arab Emirates

© The Author(s), under exclusive license to Springer Nature Singapore Pte Ltd. 2024
S. Lari et al. (eds.), *Family Medicine OSCE: First Aid to Objective Structured Clinical Examination*, https://doi.org/10.1007/978-981-99-5530-5_132

you can go home on the same day. You should know that it doesn't protect you from sexually transmitted infections."

(b) Vasectomy is typically performed on an outpatient basis with the administration of local anesthesia. The surgeon creates small incisions in the scrotal sac, where the testes are located, and then alters the two tubes responsible for transporting sperm to the penis by either cutting, tying, or blocking them.

(c) While vasectomy is generally well-tolerated, there is a possibility of experiencing swelling, bruising, and discomfort as potential side effects.

(d) Following the procedure, semen production remains unaffected. However, it takes approximately three months for sperm to be fully cleared from the semen. During this interim period, it is advisable to use an alternative method of contraception, such as condoms, until two consecutive tests confirm the absence of sperm.

(e) If you desire to have children in future, it is possible to undergo a reversal surgery. However, it's important to note that this procedure does not guarantee a successful outcome. Alternatively, freezing your sperm for future use can be considered as an option.

(f) Post vasectomy semen analysis is done around 8–16 weeks to confirm the success of the procedure during which the partner should use another contraception because there is still a chance of pregnancy in that period.

4. Assess: understand and correct any wrong knowledge.
5. Assist: "You can take your time and discuss your decision with your partner. We will be happy to meet you again for any further explanation and discuss practicing safe sex as well."
6. Arrange for referral to a surgeon.
7. Communication skills: ensure organized approach, mixed questioning style (open and close-ended questions), active listening, clear language and reflection, and the patient's ICE.

Counseling an Elderly Patient on Health Maintenance

133

Eiman Al Murar, Abeer Al Naqbi, Kawthar Al Ameri, and Shammah Al Memari

> **Learning Objectives**
> - How to conduct a focused history with elderly patients regarding health screening?
> - How to effectively use the 5 As model to counsel an elderly considering health maintenance aspects?
> - How to implement good communication skills in counseling an elderly during regular maintenance visit?

1. Introduce yourself.
2. Establish a good rapport.
3. Ask: Take a brief history:
   (a) Age, work, and marital status.
   (b) Past medical history, including vision, hearing, balance impairment (risk factors for each), chronic diseases and medications and allergies history.
   (c) Surgical history.
   (d) Family and social histories (caregiver support, changes in living arrangement, smoking, alcohol, exercise).
   (e) Risk of elderly abuse and assess caregiver's depression or burnout.

Elderly patient is defined as those who are greater than or equal to 65 years old.

E. Al Murar · A. Al Naqbi · K. Al Ameri
Ambulatory Healthcare Services, Abu Dhabi, United Arab Emirates

S. Al Memari (✉)
Abu Dhabi, United Arab Emirates

© The Author(s), under exclusive license to Springer Nature Singapore Pte Ltd. 2024
S. Lari et al. (eds.), *Family Medicine OSCE: First Aid to Objective Structured Clinical Examination*, https://doi.org/10.1007/978-981-99-5530-5_133

503

(f) Sexual history.

(g) Ideas, concerns and expectations (ICE) (patient often worried about something he or she heard about or have a friend or family member suffering from).

4. Advise (primary prevention):

(a) Avoidance of smoking and alcohol.

(b) Promoting physical activity.

(c) Immunization: influenza, pneumococcal, and diphtheria, tetanus, and acellular pertussis (TdaP) zoster.

5. Assess (secondary and tertiary prevention):

(a) Cognitive impairment: mini-mental status examination and clock test.

(b) Depression: geriatric depression scale.

(c) Hearing (audiometry) or vision impairment (Snellen chart).

(d) Oral health: tooth brushing routine and dental visit.

(e) Malnutrition: nutritional health checklist.

(f) Hypertension, diabetes mellitus, and hyperlipidemia: screening blood pressure measurement, lipid profile, and blood sugar testing.

(g) Abdominal aortic aneurysm (AAA): screen males 65–75 years of age who have ever smoked by abdominal ultrasound once in their lifetime.

(h) Urinary incontinence: take focused history, review fluid intake, and medications history.

(i) Cancer screening: Table 133.1.

(j) Osteoporosis: screen females more than 65 and males more than 75 years old by dual-energy X-ray absorptiometry (DEXA) scan. You may say: "We perform a special type of x-ray, called DEXA scan, to check for osteoporosis, a condition of bone thinning, due to loss of calcium, making them brittle or easily fracture."

(k) Disorders of gait and balance: balance and gait evaluation by "Get up and go" test.

Table 133.1 Cancer screening guidelines

Cervical cancer	21–65 years old by cytology every 3 years, or by combined cytology and human papillomavirus (HPV testing every 5 years; the latter only for greater than or equal to 30 years old)
Breast cancer	40–74 years old by mammography every 2 years
Colorectal cancer	40–75 years old in the UAE, otherwise 50–75 by high-sensitivity fecal occult blood test (FOBT) or fecal immunological test (FIT) test annually, combined sigmoidoscopy every 5 years along with high-sensitivity fecal occult blood test (FOBT) or fecal immunological test (FIT) every 3 years, or colonoscopy every 10 years
Lung cancer	55–80 years old who is smoking greater than or equal to 30 packs per year or have quit it less than or equal to 15 years by annual low-dose computed tomography scan

6. Functional ability: (eating, dressing, bathing), instrumental activities of daily living (cooking, driving, housework, using phone), and ability to drive (movement dysfunction, vision impairment, impaired neck rotation).
7. Assist: "Falls are the most common accidents in older people and most serious in people more than 65 years because our reflexes deteriorate with age. Falls at this age are serious because 5% of them result in a fracture. To avoid them you should":
   (a) Secure rugs by either removing them or firmly affixing them with double-faced tape or nonslip backing.
   (b) Illuminate hallways and stairways by turning on lights. Opt for light bulbs over fluorescent lights for better visibility.
   (c) Clear walkways of clutter, including cords or wires.
   (d) Ensure that handrails are securely attached on both sides of all stairways.
   (e) Install handrails in the bathtub and near the toilet for added safety.
   (f) Place a nonslip rubber mat in the bathtub to prevent slipping.
   (g) Arrange items that are out of reach on lower shelves and cabinets.
   (h) Take your time when transitioning from sitting or lying down to standing.
   (i) Always wear your prescribed eyeglasses. Exercise caution with multifocal glasses, especially when climbing stairs or walking.
   (j) Select shoes with a low heel, secure closures, and nonslip soles. Avoid slippers, backless shoes, or going barefoot.
   (k) Enhance your bone health by taking vitamin D and calcium supplements.
8. Arrange:
   (a) Positive reinforcement: "Many others did it before you, you can definitely do it, we are always available to support you."
   (b) Follow up soon.
   (c) Anticipate complications, safety netting, and address any red flags.
   (d) Brief assessment of underlying conditions and review of the medications.
   (e) Refer for dental checkup or geriatrician as required.
   (f) Give away reading material if available.
9. Communication skills: ensure organized approach, mixed questioning style (open and close-ended questions), active listening, clear language, and reflection on the patient's ICE.

Part XII

Counseling: Mental Health

Counseling a Patient on Sleep Hygiene

134

Shammah Al Memari

Learning Objectives
- How to take a focused history from patients seeking sleep advice?
- How to effectively use the 5 As model to counsel patients on sleep hygiene?
- How to implement good communication skills in counseling patients on sleep hygiene?

Focus areas Examine potential causes of insomnia, considering that 50% of sleeping disorders are secondary in nature.

1. Introduce yourself and establish a good rapport.
2. Ask:
   (a) Sleep history: habits and pattern.
   (b) Medical and drug history: refer to Table 134.1 for details.
   (c) Social history: marital conflict, recent travel with possible jet lag, work, or home-related stress (shiftwork).
3. Advise:
   (a) "The amount of sleep that a person needs for normal health varies with age and differs from person to person. For some adults, 4 hours a night is ample; for others, 10 hours is not enough. The average sleep for a 50-year-old is 7 hours a day".

S. Al Memari (✉)
Abu Dhabi, United Arab Emirates

Table 134.1 Essential historical information for sleep hygiene counseling based on disease differential diagnosis

Disease differential	Presentation
Cardiovascular or respiratory disease	As orthopnea, paroxysmal nocturnal dyspnea, or respiratory as chronic obstructive lung disease, obstructive sleep apnea: "Do you feel short of breath at all? How about when lying flat?"
Gastrointestinal diseases	As a gastro-esophageal reflex disease: "Do you feel any burning sensation in your chest at all?"
Renal diseases	As urinary tract infection, or incontinence: "Do you have any burning sensation in urine?" "Do you wake up at night to go to the toilet? If yes, how often?"
Endocrine diseases	• As hyper- or hypothyroidism, or diabetes: "Do you have difficulty staying still or noted unexplained weight loss?" • "Do you have cold intolerance or constipation?" • "Do you go to the toilet or need to drink frequently?"
Musculoskeletal diseases	• Osteoarthritis of the knee, or back pain: "Do you have any pain from any source?"
Psychiatric problems	• Anxiety, depression, schizophrenia, and delirium: "How do you describe your mood?"
Drug history	• Sedatives such as alcohol, benzodiazepines, and barbiturate. • Stimulants such as amphetamines, and caffeine. • Antihistamines, decongestants, and aminophylline. • Cigarette smoking.

    (b) "The problem arises when lack of sleep or too much sleep interferes with your activities during the day".

    (c) "Insomnia, defined as 'poor sleep,' refers to an insufficient amount of rest, characterized by challenges in initiating sleep, maintaining sleep, or waking up prematurely. In most cases, it is a transient issue often linked to personal challenges. However, at times, it can occur without any apparent cause."

    (d) Symptoms of insomnia might affect the personal life and present with feeling fatigued, having trouble thinking clearly, getting depressed or irritable, having more accidents or mistakes, and worrying about their lack of sleep.

4. Assess:

    (a) Motivation and willingness to follow the abovementioned steps.

    (b) Previous attempts at changing sleeping patterns or taking any medications.

5. Assist: "Let's share a suitable plan to help you sleep better. How about following this program strictly for several weeks to establish an efficient regular sleep pattern?"

    (a) Exercise: "Fit people have better sleep quality. Do regular exercise late afternoon or early evening; avoid strenuous exercise two hours before sleep."

    (b) Diet: "Avoid heavy meals or hunger at bedtime. If the latter occurs, have light snacks, warm milk, or herbal drinks."

    (c) Caffeine: "Limit your consumption of coffee, tea, cola, and chocolate, especially 5–6 hours before bedtime."

    (d) Alcohol: "Avoid drinking 4–6 h before bed, it causes sleep at the beginning, but it soon awakens you."

(e) Environment: "Ensure quiet, secure, well-heated or cooled, and dim-lit bedroom."

(f) "Have a comfortable bed and mattress." "Avoid reading, or watching electronics (television, laptop, or smartphones) in bed and don't use your bed as an office or workroom." "Maintain a regular bed and wake schedule. Set the alarm to the same rising time every day. Avoid naps and recovery sleep to compensate for a previous bad night."

(g) "Every night, set a threshold time after which you should monitor sleepiness. If you are not sleeping within 20–30 mins, get out of bed, sit and relax in another room until you are sleepy or tired again. Repeat this step as often as required."

6. Arrange:

(a) Positive reinforcement: "Many others did it before you, you can definitely do it, we are always available to support you."

(b) Ask the patient to write a log for 2 weeks about their sleeping pattern and follow up soon in 2–4 weeks. If symptoms persist, refer the patient for cognitive behavioral therapy.

(c) Refer; if required for any underlying condition that is causing insomnia.

(d) Brief assessment of underlying conditions and screening for age (vaccination).

(e) Give away reading material if available.

7. Communication skills: ensure organized approach, mixed questioning style (open and close-ended questions), active listening, clear language, and reflection on the patient's ideas, concerns, and expectations (ICE).

Halima Al Shehhi, Noora Al Blooshi,
and Shammah Al Memari

Learning Objectives
- How to take a focused history from patients regarding alcohol misuse?
- How to effectively use the 5 As model to counsel patients on alcohol misuse?
- How to implement good communication skills in counseling patients on alcohol misuse?

1. Introduce yourself and establish a good rapport.
2. Ask:
   (a) Patient's ideas, concerns and expectations (ICE): Any presenting problem? The role of drinking or drug use in it.
   (b) Use one of the questionnaires detailed in Tables 135.1 and 135.2 for assessment: "Now I am going to ask you some questions about your use of alcoholic drinks in the past year."
   (c) Alcohol and other drug use: refer to Table 135.3 for details.
   (d) Effect on the quality of life: relationship, occupation, and driving under alcohol effect.
   (e) Past medical history: diabetes, hypertension, coronary artery disease, and asthma.

H. Al Shehhi · N. Al Blooshi
Ambulatory Healthcare Services, Abu Dhabi, United Arab Emirates

S. Al Memari (✉)
Abu Dhabi, United Arab Emirates

© The Author(s), under exclusive license to Springer Nature Singapore Pte Ltd. 2024
S. Lari et al. (eds.), *Family Medicine OSCE: First Aid to Objective Structured Clinical Examination*, https://doi.org/10.1007/978-981-99-5530-5_135

Table 135.1 AUDIT-C questionnaire

Question	Response options
1. How often do you have a drink containing alcohol?	• Never (0) • Less than or equal to every month (1) • 2–4 times per month (2) • 2–3 times per week (3) • Greater than or equal to four times per week (4)
2. How many drinks containing alcohol do you have on a typical day when you are drinking?	• 1 or 2 (0) • 3 or 4 (1) • 5 or 6 (2) • 7 or 9 (3) • Greater than or equal to 10 (4)
3. How often do you have six or more drinks on one occasion?	• Never (0) • More than every month (1) • Monthly (2) • Weekly (3) • Daily or almost daily (4)

Calculate the final score and interpret the patient's status accordingly (high-risk drinkers' score more than or equal to 5)

Table 135.2 CAGE questionnaire

1. Have you ever felt you needed to **C**ut down on your drinking?
2. Have people **A**nnoyed you by criticizing your drinking?
3. Have you ever felt **G**uilty about drinking?
4. Have you ever felt you needed a drink first thing in the morning (**E**ye-opener) to steady your nerves or to get rid of a hangover?

Calculate the final score and interpret the patient's status accordingly (If an individual answers "yes" to two or more of these questions consider further assessment)

Table 135.3 Detailed history of alcohol use

History item	Description
Duration	Age of onset and duration of alcohol use
Quantify intake in units of alcohol per day and week	• 1 unit equals 1/2 pint (236 ml) of ordinary strength beer, lager or cider equals a small glass of wine, equals a single shot of spirits (including vodka, whiskey, gin equals a small glass of sherry, equals a single measure of aperitifs) • The recommended safe limits are 21 units/week for males and 14 units/week for non-pregnant females
Drinking triggers	Identify specific situations or conditions that trigger alcohol consumption
Features of tolerance	• *"Do you need to increase the amount of alcohol intake to get the desired effects?"*
Features of dependence	• The compulsion to drink, the primacy of drinking over other activities, inability to control use, tolerance, or withdrawal symptoms (anxiety, sweating, nausea, seizures, delirium tremens). History of withdrawal increases the likelihood of withdrawal on quitting
Other drug use	Tobacco, opioids, or illicit drugs

3. Advise: In a nonjudgmental but persuasive manner: "As your doctor, I think it is very important for you to quit drinking." Discuss the 5Rs:
   (a) Relevance: link alcohol misuse to current medical conditions.
   (b) Risks: "Do you know how alcohol abuse can affect your life?" If no, explain:
      Biological effects on gastrointestinal (mainly the liver), cardiovascular, and neurological systems along with the increased risk of trauma or falls.
      Mental problems: violence, suicide risk, depression, anxiety, and psychosis.
      Social function decline: inability to drive, compromise relationships, employment, financial status, and housing, and may lead to legal obligations.
   (c) Rewards: *"I am sure that you will gain many rewards from quitting. It will have a significant impact on your general well-being."*
   (d) Roadblocks: "Set a date and share it with family and friends. Do you think of anyone who can stand between you and this achievement? Are you worried about the reaction of a friend or family to your decision?"
   (e) Repetition: *"Remember it's all about your health, you can do it."*
4. Assess:
   (a) *"On a scale of 0–10, how confident are you that you can quit?"*
   (b) *"On the same scale, how motivated you are to quit?"*
   (c) Stage on behavioral change cycle according to motivation and willingness to quit (pre-contemplation, contemplation, preparation, action, maintenance)
   (d) Examination and investigations:
      Mental state (general presentation, cognition, memory, mood, speech, thought, perception, insight)
      Consider breath alcohol test, and blood tests (liver function test including GGT, full blood count, urea and electrolytes, vitamin B12 level)
5. Assist: "Let's share a plan that is suitable for helping you to reduce drinking."
   (a) Set a quit date or decide to gradually reduce the intake (by switching to low-alcohol beer, alternating alcohol with nonalcoholic drinks, reducing drink size, and eating during drinking sessions).
   (b) Address psychosocial fears, and family and friend's support.
   (c) Identify high-risk situations and practical ways to deal with these. Ask the patient to avoid drinking cues: stress, late-night gatherings, etc.
   (d) Plan an alternative focus for socializing or relaxing.
   (e) Consider pharmacological therapy:
      Treat any withdrawal symptoms with long-term use of low-dose benzodiazepines, clonidine, or anticonvulsant (barbiturate, carbamazepine).
      Treat alcohol dependence with disulfiram (inhibits the desired effect when the patient consumes alcohol; if used, monitor liver function tests), naltrexone (opioid antagonist), acamprosate, and cognitive behavioral therapy (CBT).

6. Arrange:
    (a) Positive reinforcement: "Many others did it before you, you can definitely do it, we are always available to support you."
    (b) Follow up in 2 weeks or earlier if any withdrawal symptoms.
    (c) Refer to a psychologist (controlling drinking strategies, or relapse prevention strategies) and social worker (to coalesce with the family or work).
    (d) Rule out red flags: risk of harm to self or others, serious physical or mental illness, and medico-legal requirements (driving or actions secondary to abuse).
    (e) Brief assessment of the underlying conditions and age-appropriate screening.
    (f) If symptoms of delirium tremens (severe withdrawal) tremors, confusion, seizure, or visual hallucination, refer urgently to the hospital.
    (g) Wernicke encephalopathy is a thiamin deficiency (a triad of nystagmus, ataxia, and confusion).
    (h) Korsakoff syndrome is a thiamin deficiency (ante-/retrograde amnesia, disorientation, and confabulation).
    (i) Give away reading material if available.
7. Communication skills: ensure organized approach, mixed questioning style (open and close-ended questions), active listening, clear language, and reflection on the patient's ICE.

Assessing and Counseling a Patient on Domestic Violence

136

Dhuha Al Ameri, Sumiya Taheri,
and Shammah Al Memari

> **Learning Objectives**
> - How to take a focused history from patients suspecting domestic violence?
> - How to effectively use the 5 As model to counsel patients on domestic violence?
> - How to implement good communication skills in counseling patients on domestic violence?

1. Introduce yourself and establish a good rapport.
2. Explore the reason for attendance and patient's ideas, concerns and expectations (ICE).
3. Before raising the issue: Be nonjudgmental + assure patient about privacy: "Nobody deserves to be hurt by someone else. Anything you tell me will be confidential, and I will not do anything about what you tell me unless you want me to."
4. Use open-ended questions: "Numerous individuals encounter challenges within their households or relationships that may impact their well-being, prompting me to inquire about such matters with all my patients. Can you share with me any concerns you may have about your home life? What are your thoughts regarding your domestic situation? Do you feel secure or apprehensive in your home environment? I'm concerned that you may have experienced harm from someone."

D. Al Ameri · S. Taheri
Ambulatory Healthcare Services, Abu Dhabi, United Arab Emirates

S. Al Memari (✉)
Abu Dhabi, United Arab Emirates

© The Author(s), under exclusive license to Springer Nature Singapore Pte Ltd. 2024
S. Lari et al. (eds.), *Family Medicine OSCE: First Aid to Objective Structured Clinical Examination*, https://doi.org/10.1007/978-981-99-5530-5_136

5. Identify and assess history of violence:
   (a) Current violence: "Do you have any injuries that appear to be the result of rough treatment from someone? Has anyone acted violently towards you recently? Have you experienced physical harm, such as being hit, kicked, punched, or otherwise injured by a partner in the past year, and if so, who was responsible? Do you feel secure in your current relationship? Are you feeling threatened by someone from a previous relationship? Is anyone coercing you into unwanted sexual activities? Are you experiencing any form of stalking or harassment from individuals in your community? Have you ever been in a relationship where you felt frightened or harmed by your partner? Did you experience physical abuse, sexual coercion, or psychological harm, such as being made to feel worthless or unwanted, during your childhood?"
   (b) Previous history of violence.
   (c) General signs and symptoms of distress (fatigue, headache, gastrointestinal or cardiac symptoms).
   (d) Specific signs and symptoms of violence (fracture, burn, bruises, etc.).
6. Social and family history:
   (a) Family dynamics: relationships with husband and children.
   (b) Living situation: Who does the patient live with?
   (c) Explore the situation "We do have to ask you some very personal and painful questions about what happened. I know it will be hard to answer some of these questions, but we are asking them so that we can take care of you to the best of our abilities."
   (d) Physical abuse: *"Is there anyone at home who is hurting you?"*
   (e) Psychological abuse: *"Does he or she belittle you or try to control you?"*
   (f) Sexual abuse: *"Did someone do something to you that you did not want done?"*
   (g) Economical abuse: "Do you feel lonely." "Do you have a lot of arguments with the people you live with?"
   (h) Frequency of abuse, when does it occur, and are alcohols or drugs involved.
   (i) How has he or she been coping? "Are there any children or vulnerable adults involved?"
7. Screen for anxiety, depression, substance use, and risk of suicide: Has it affected his or her mood? Has she or he ever considered harming self or taking own life?
8. Management: Be nonjudgmental, establish the patient's concerns, allow him or her to control the situation, and make decisions. If the patient denies suspected abuse, do not confront or challenge the patient, but express concern. Acknowledge and assure: "It is a very complex situation that must have been difficult for you to disclose."
9. Offer **SOS-DoC** intervention. Refer to Table 136.1 for details.
10. Provide patients with contact numbers of social support programs if available.
11. Thank the patient.
12. Communication skills: ensure organized approach, mixed questioning style (open and close-ended questions), active listening, clear language, and reflection on the patient's ICE.

Table 136.1 SOS-DoC intervention

Intervention	Details
S: offer **Support** and assess **Safety**	(a) **Support**: "I'm sorry this has happened. You have the right to be safe and respected. The violence is not your fault, and no one deserves to be treated that way." "I cannot even imagine what you have gone through. We are going to do everything that needs to be done to help you." * Establish support if they have any friends or family that know or can support them (b) **Safety**: Identify risk markers such as young age, unemployment, prior history of being abusive, alcohol or drugs abuse, depression, low income, and low academic achievement

O: discuss **options**, including safety planning and follow-up	1. Legal tools: Provide information, give handouts and offer referral to police for restraining orders, mandatory arrest, or local domestic abuse services
	2. Counseling social support services: Explain, give handouts, and offer referral to national domestic violence helpline, or women's aid [note that if the victim is an adult with capacity, you can only refer them if they signed the consent (unless a child or vulnerable adult is involved)]
	3. Promote safety planning: Provide information, give handouts, and arrange for refuge if they cannot go home: "If you decided to leave, where could you go?" "Can you keep clothes, money, and copies of keys and important papers in a safe place?" "Where could you go in an emergency?" "How would you get there?" (Rotte and Lopez 2011). Advise about emergency planning:
	   (a) "Preparing an emergency kit with important documents, keys, money, and other essential items, to be stored outside the home in case they need to escape urgently"
	   (b) "A place to go (friends, family, shelter)"
	   (c) "A signal to alert children or neighbors to call 999"
	   (d) "During times of escalating conflict, avoiding rooms with potential weapons (kitchen) or risk for increased injury (hard bathroom surfaces)"

S: identify and validate patient's **strengths**	"I can see that you care deeply about your children. It took courage for you to talk with me today about the violence" (Rotte and Lopez 2011)
Do: document observations, assessment, and plans	(a) Record what the patient said. Use quotation marks to document exact words (b) Objective observations: Describe the injuries you observed, use drawings and photographs: "We need to perform a physical exam and collect samples from your body. This is important because they can be used as evidence against whoever did this to you" (Rotte and Lopez 2011)
C	(a) Offer continuity through follow-up appointments. Encourage the patient to talk about it and seek help. Remind the patient that he or she can come to see you anytime and assess barriers to access (e.g., transportation?): "It is completely up to you if you want to get some help. But if you change your mind we are always here" (Rotte and Lopez 2011)

Counseling a Female with Postpartum Blues

Dhuha Al Ameri, Kawthar Al Ameri, and Shammah Al Memari

Learning Objectives
- How to take a focused history from females with postpartum blues?
- How to effectively use the 5 As model to counsel females with postpartum blues?
- How to implement good communication skills in counseling females with postpartum blue?

1. Introduce yourself, establish a good rapport, and respond to the patient's cues.
2. Ask:
   (a) Patient's ideas concerns and expectation (ICE).
   (b) Screen for depression: Low mood and/or loss of interest or pleasure in life in the last 2 weeks. If yes, ask specifically by using the mnemonic (SIGE CAPS) and confirm the symptom's duration:

   Sleeping disturbance, Loss of **I**nterest or pleasure in life, feeling worthless, hopeless, or overly **G**uilty, Low **E**nergy or motivation to do things, Having difficulty **C**oncentrating, Loss of or increased **A**ppetite with or without unexplained weight loss, **P**sychomotor agitation or retardation (feeling restless, irritable, anxious or tearful with increased crying), **S**uicidality or Homicidally (having thoughts about hurting your baby).

D. Al Ameri · K. Al Ameri
Ambulatory Healthcare Services, Abu Dhabi, United Arab Emirates

S. Al Memari (✉)
Abu Dhabi, United Arab Emirates

© The Author(s), under exclusive license to Springer Nature Singapore Pte Ltd. 2024
S. Lari et al. (eds.), *Family Medicine OSCE: First Aid to Objective Structured Clinical Examination*, https://doi.org/10.1007/978-981-99-5530-5_137

    (c) Effect of the condition: Ask about her ability to cope with the new changes (taking care of her newborn) and whether she is having current family support. Determine any difficulties in breast feeding.

    (d) Past medical history (severe premenstrual syndrome or psychiatric illness), social history (home environment, social support, emotional or financial stressors, marital conflict, domestic abuse, alcohol use), family history, and any taken medications or known allergies. Differentiate a postpartum blues vs. depression. Box 137.1 for definition.

3. Advise: "It is common that mothers develop mood swings (episodes of happiness and crying) after childbirth. They may feel a little depressed, have a hard time concentrating, lose their appetite or find that they cannot sleep well even when the baby is asleep. This starts 2–3 days after delivery and is known as 'baby blues.' But it goes away within 10 days after delivery. However, in some women, these symptoms might last longer or worsen with time; in that case it is called 'postpartum depression.'"

4. Assess: understanding and exclude red flags (suicidality or homicidally).

5. Assist: "This is not your fault, and you are not supposed to suffer alone. We are all here to help you and we will develop a plan to get you in the best state. There are things that you can do that other mothers with postpartum depression have found helpful." Refer to Table 137.1 for details.

6. Arrange:

    (a) Positive reinforcement: "Many others did it before you, you can definitely do it, we are always available to support you."

    (b) Follow up in 1 week.

    (c) Refer to psychotherapy or direct to stress management classes.

Table 137.1 Assisting a patient with postpartum blues

Intervention	Description

Letting it all out	1. "Regularly share your feelings with someone you trust."
	2. "Maintain a daily diary to record your emotions. As you start feeling better, revisit your entries to appreciate your progress and recognize your improvement."
	3. Fulfill your own needs appropriately:
	  (a) "Request support from family or friends for childcare, household duties, and groceries. Carving out time for yourself is crucial to achieving a sense of refreshment."
	  (b) "Prioritize personal time, even if it's just 15 minutes a day. Consider activities such as reading, exercising (a simple walk is beneficial and easy to incorporate), taking a bath, or practicing meditation."

Avoiding stress	1. "The process of giving birth introduces numerous changes, and embracing the role of parenting can be unfamiliar. When you find yourself not feeling like your usual self, these adjustments may appear overwhelming to handle." 2. "Take on only one task at a time, or even consider doing nothing at all. Recognize that each small step is progress in the right direction, and try to avoid being too hard on yourself." 3. "Honestly assess your capacity and don't hesitate to seek assistance from others. You are not expected to embody the ideal of a 'super mom'—asking for help is a strength, not a weakness!"

    (d) If the mother has criteria of postpartum depression, she might need to be started on SSRI.

    (e) Give away reading material if available. Health maintenance (pap smear, contraception).

7. Communication skills: ensure organized approach, mixed questioning style (open and close-ended questions), active listening, clear language, and reflection on the patient's ICE.

Box 137.1 Definition of Postpartum Blues and Postpartum Depression

- Postpartum blues: Mild dysfunction for less than 10 days with an onset within 2–3 days of delivery with prevalence of 80%. No suicidal thoughts.
- Postpartum depression: Moderate to severe dysfunction for less than 2 weeks. Onset is within the first month to the first year. Prevalence: 5–7% with or without suicidality.

Counseling a Patient with Schizophrenia 138

Halima Al Shehhi, Buthaina Al Maskari,
and Shammah Al Memari

> **Learning Objectives**
> - How to take a focused history from patients with schizophrenia?
> - How to effectively use the 5. As model to counsel patients with schizophrenia?
> - How to implement good communication skills in counseling patients with schizophrenia?

Focus areas include positive and negative symptoms, medications and their side effects, and screening for complications from medications.

1. Introduce yourself and establish a good rapport.
2. Ask:
   (a) Explore the reason of clinic visit, onset, associated symptoms [positive symptoms including hallucinations (visual, auditory, somatic, olfactory, or gustatory) or delusions (reference, grandiose, paranoid)], and disorganized speech as well as negative symptoms such as memory impairment, flattened affect, loss of sense of pleasure, loss of will or drive, social or occupational withdrawal, deterioration in hygiene, and grooming, unusual behavior, or outbursts of anger. Symptoms must be present for at least 6 months with

H. Al Shehhi · B. Al Maskari
Ambulatory Healthcare Services, Abu Dhabi, United Arab Emirates

S. Al Memari (✉)
Abu Dhabi, United Arab Emirates

© The Author(s), under exclusive license to Springer Nature Singapore Pte Ltd. 2024
S. Lari et al. (eds.), *Family Medicine OSCE: First Aid to Objective Structured Clinical Examination*, https://doi.org/10.1007/978-981-99-5530-5_138

social or occupational dysfunction, and no other diagnosis explains these symptoms.

(b) Past medical history and hospital admissions, family history, and medications.

(c) Social history: living situation, job, smoking, alcohol, substance use. Criminal history.

(d) Knowledge about schizophrenia.

3. Advise: "As your doctor, I think it's very important for you to know that schizophrenia is a brain disorder that makes you think unclearly. It can cause you to see or hear things that aren't there, or to believe things that aren't true and this all can disturb your daily life activities." Refer to Table 138.1 for details.

Table 138.1 Advice for schizophrenia patients: medications, driving, sports, traveling, and pregnancy

Domain	Advice
Medications (note that when initiating medications for the first time, patient should be referred to a psychiatrist)	(a) Schizophrenia is treated with medications that help in controlling symptoms. There are mainly two types of medications. First-generation (typical) antipsychotics like chlorpromazine and haloperidol (SE): drowsiness, dry mouth, extrapyramidal symptoms, elevated prolactin), second-generation antipsychotic (atypical) like aripiprazole, clozapine, olanzapine, quetiapine, risperidone (SE): hyperprolactinemia, metabolic changes, weight gain) (b) Everyone reacts differently to medications. "You may experience some neurological side effects such as feeling stiff, tremors, fixed upper gaze, neck twisting, or facial muscle spasms. Other symptoms include weight gain. Do not worry you will be given the one that works best for you with the fewest problems, and you will be helped in managing these side effects" (c) "Remember to take your medications regularly. If you suddenly stop them, this could precipitate a relapse, or your symptoms may get worse"
Driving and occupation	(a) Research shows that visual perceptions do not prevent driving, but doctors may assess patients' cognitive function to determine their driving capacity
Sports	(a) Studies encourage sports participation as it has a positive effect on schizophrenia symptoms
Traveling	(a) When traveling, it is important to wear schizophrenia card or bracelet with details of medications, physician name, and hospital number
Female patients	(a) "You can get pregnant when you decide to, many others did it and you can too. But you should let us know as you may need to switch to medication that is less likely to cause problems for your baby" (b) "You might be interested to go off medications to protect your baby. But that could actually do more harm than good" (c) Women who stop their medications before or during pregnancy often get severe schizophrenia symptoms and end up needing more medications than they would have if they had stayed on their medications in the first place

4. Assess:
   (a) Answer any questions and check level of understanding.
   (b) Medication side effects.
   (c) Screen for depression and substance abuse.
5. Assist: "Let's share a plan that is suitable for helping you. I am sorry to say that there is no cure for schizophrenia, but it can be treated and managed in several ways, and we will work in a team with other specialties as needed":
   (a) Starting the appropriate antipsychotic medication.
   (b) Offer psychotherapy approaches, such as cognitive-behavioral therapy, assertive community treatment, and supportive therapy.
   (c) Self-management strategies and education.
6. Arrange:
   (a) Follow up and monitor drug levels, screen for metabolic changes, and cardiovascular risk factors.
   (b) Refer to psychiatric rehabilitation to improve social life and encourage independent living skills.
   (c) Anticipate complications, safety netting, and red flags (suicidal thoughts).
   (d) Provide age-appropriate screening.
   (e) Give away reading materials if available.
7. Communication skills: ensure organized approach, mixed questioning style (open and close-ended questions), active listening, clear language, and reflection on the patient's ideas, concerns and expectations (ICE).

Part XIII

Counselling: Medical Devise Use

Counseling a Patient on Glucometer Use 139

Halima Al Shehhi, Buthaina Al Maskari, and Shammah Al Memari

Learning Objectives
- How to communicate to the patient the purpose of the glucometer device?
- How to recognize the basic steps in using the glucometer?
- Describe the parts of the glucometer device.
- Learn to demonstrate the use of the device to the patient.
- Understand the reading of blood sugar.

1. Introduce yourself.
2. Establish a good rapport (address the patient by name).
3. Explain what the device is used for and what its parts are:
   (a) Name: "Glucometer is a medical device for determining the approximate concentration of glucose in the blood."
   (b) Purpose: "This helps you determine how well controlled your diabetes is."
   (c) Show the patient the glucometer and explain its parts (meter, test strips, lancet, and lancet's pen). Explain: "Always check the expiry date of the lancets and double-check that the meter is working prior to use."
   (d) Explain the steps of usage: **First:** "It is very important to use your glucometer correctly as it will provide you with instant feedback and let you know immediately what your blood sugar level is (too low, too high or in a good range). Keeping a record of your results gives your doctor an accurate pic-

H. Al Shehhi · B. Al Maskari
Ambulatory Healthcare Services, Abu Dhabi, United Arab Emirates

S. Al Memari (✉)
Abu Dhabi, United Arab Emirates

531

ture of how your treatment is working. It is small and easy to take with you. You can test anywhere, and anytime." **Then:** "Wash your hands for 15 seconds, dry them, and get your equipment." "Open the lancet pen and put a lancet in. Adjust the lancet to the shallowest depth that allows the blood drop to flow out freely (avoid squeezing the finger as this will denature the blood and give false readings). Take the cap off the lancet without touching it, and cover the pen." "Pull out a test strip and put it in the meter to turn it on. Double check that the code that appears on the meter's screen matches that on the test strips' bottle." "Wait until a test strip symbol flashes on the screen before you draw the drop of blood."

   (e) Checking blood sugar: "Prick yourself using the lancet pen against the outer or inner borders of one of your fingers (avoid fingertips that are rich with nerves, thus painful). Do not use the same finger or side every time." "Allow the blood drop to form freely, and then approximate the test strip to absorb it. Be sure that the test area on the strip fills completely with blood." "Place the test strip in the meter and wait for the reading to appear on the screen. Record it in your logbook or diary."

   (f) Demonstrate to the patient all the steps.

   (g) Let him or her do it and observe to correct.

   (h) Advise the patient about cleaning up the supplies: "With every use: throw the test strip in the trash, and the needle in a puncture-proof container with a lid (such as an old bleach or detergent bottle)." "Store your equipment or medications away from children and pets."

4. Encourage any questions.
5. Ensure:

   (a) Positive reinforcement: "Many others use it, you can definitely use it correctly." "We are always available to support you."

   (b) Patient understands side effects: risk of infection (decreased by handwashing) and pin-prick pain on needle use.

6. Arrange a follow-up (in 2 weeks) to check the results and adjust medications.
7. Give away reading material if available.
8. Communication skills: ensure organized approach, mixed questioning style (open and close-ended questions), active listening, clear language, and reflection on patient's ideas, concerns and expectations (ICE).

Counseling a Patient on Insulin Use 140

Halima Al Shehhi, Sumiya Taheri,
and Shammah Al Memari

Learning Objectives
- How to communicate to the patient the purpose of insulin use?
- Recognize the basic steps in using insulin.
- Describe the parts of the device.
- Learn to demonstrate the use of the device to the patient.

---

1. Introduce yourself and establish a good rapport (address the patient by name).
2. Explain what the medication is:
   (a) Name: insulin injection or pen.
   (b) Purpose: "Provides the body with the insulin that it lacks in order to regulate its utilization of sugar."
   (c) Show the patient the insulin injection or pen and explain its parts.
3. Explain the steps of use: "The proper technique is very important to ensure that your body benefits from the medication used":
   (a) "Wash your hands for 15 seconds, dry them, and get your insulin ready (cleaning the skin with an alcohol swab is not necessary)."
   (b) *For insulin in syringe:* Box 140.1
   (c) *For insulin pen:* Box 140.2
4. Demonstrate to the patient all the steps.
5. Let him or her do it and observe to correct.

H. Al Shehhi · S. Taheri
Ambulatory Healthcare Services, Abu Dhabi, United Arab Emirates

S. Al Memari (✉)
Abu Dhabi, United Arab Emirates

© The Author(s), under exclusive license to Springer Nature Singapore Pte Ltd. 2024
S. Lari et al. (eds.), *Family Medicine OSCE: First Aid to Objective Structured Clinical Examination*, https://doi.org/10.1007/978-981-99-5530-5_140

6. Advise the patient:
    (a) To decrease the pain: "Keep your insulin out of the refrigerator for 30 minutes prior to use, allow alcohol to dry before pricking yourself, relax the muscle at the injection site, and avoid changing the direction of the needle during insertion and removal."
    (b) Rotating the injection site is very important to avoid complications (lipohypotrophy or lipohypertrophy). "Always keep a distance of 3 centimeters (1.5 inches) from the last injection site."
    (c) "Use a new needle every time you inject insulin and dispose it in your sharp trash after use. Do not store the insulin with the needle attached."
    (d) "Store all your unused medications in the refrigerator (not the fridge). Keep the currently used pen (not insulin vial) at room temperature. At all times keep away from the reach of children."
    (e) "When traveling, your insulin should be kept in your handbag not your luggage (you will need a prescription for the airlines to allow that)."
    (f) "If you are traveling in the car for a long time, use icebags to avoid damaging the insulin."
    (g) "If you forget your insulin in a hot place or where direct sunlight is present, discard it."
    (h) Encourage any questions.
7. Ensure:
    (a) Positive reinforcement: "Many others use it; you can definitely use it correctly." "We are always available to support you."
    (b) Patient understands the doses.
    (c) Patient understands the side effects including hypoglycemia and ways to manage it.
    (d) Arrange follow-up.
    (e) Give away reading materials if available.
8. Communication skills: ensure organized approach, mixed questioning style (open and close-ended questions), active listening, clear language, and reflection on the patient's ideas, concerns and expectations (ICE).

Box 140.1 A Step-By-Step Guide to Insulin Injection/Syringe Administration

- "Get your supplies": insulin vial (double-check that it is the right kind of insulin and that the fluid is clear with no clumps), proper sized syringe (for 50–100 units use 1 mL syringe, for 30–50 units use 0.5 mL syringe, for less than 30 units use 0.3 mL syringe), needles, and alcohol pads.
- "Prepare the insulin injection":
  - Only for intermediate or long-acting insulin: "Gently mix by turning the bottle on its side and rolling or rubbing it between the palms of your hands. Do not shake the bottle because shaking can make the insulin clump together."
  - "Prepare the insulin bottle: If the insulin bottle is new, remove the cap. Clean the top of the insulin bottle with an alcohol pad before you put a needle into it."
  - "Pull air into the syringe and inject it into the vial (to increase its pressure)."
  - "Pull the plunger to fill the syringe with just a little more than the insulin dose you need."
  - "Release any air bubbles from the syringe: Tap the syringe with your finger to make them rise to the top. Slowly push in the plunger just enough to push out the air and the extra insulin."
- "Prepare for injecting the insulin":
  - "Change the needle before injecting yourself (as it gets blunter when it is pushed into the vial)."
  - "Use areas with a good layer of fat under the skin (2.5 centimeters can be pinched between two fingers), as this is the place that you want the insulin to stay and slowly go to the blood. Use the abdomen below the navel, outer part of the thighs, arms, or buttocks."
  - "Lift up or pinch the skin and insert the needle perpendicularly using your dominant hand (hold the syringe between your thumb and middle finger). Push the plunger using your index finger all the way down. Keep the needle in for 10 seconds (to avoid insulin leakage after withdrawal of the needle). Quickly withdraw the needle."
  - "Press down firmly (do not rub or massage) over the injection site for up to 60 seconds."

Box 140.2 A Step-By-Step Guide to Insulin Pen Administration

- "Get your supplies": insulin pen (double-check that it is the right kind of insulin and that the fluid is clear, colorless, with no clumps, and not expired), insulin cartridge (follow the pen manufacturer's instructions for inserting an insulin cartridge into a reusable pen), disposable needles, their cap, and alcohol pads.
- "Attach the disposable needle to the pen":
  - "Remove the pen cap. Clean the rubber seal on the insulin cartridge with a sterile alcohol swab."
  - "Attach the disposable needle to the pen. Remove the outer needle cap and save it to use after your injection. Remove the inner needle cap and throw it away."
- "Prepare the insulin":
  - "Gently mix it by turning the pen upside down 10 times."
  - Prime the pen before each injection. "This releases a small amount of insulin into the needle in order to get rid of any air bubbles and ensure the use of correct dose. Point the needle up. Tap the insulin cartridge to force any air bubbles to the top. Dial 2 units of insulin on the dose selector (for most insulin pens, you will hear a click for each unit of insulin that you have dialed)".
  - Firmly press the plunger until a drop of insulin appears at the needle tip. "Repeat this step if a droplet does not appear or change the needle if you had to repeat it several times."
- "Return your dose selector to 'zero' and dial the correct dose (make sure there is enough insulin in the pen for your full dose)."
- "Lightly pinch a fold of skin and insert the injection perpendicularly. Push the plunger all the way in and keep pressing it for a count of 5–10 before you remove the needle from the skin. Gently apply pressure on the injection site, but do not rub it."

Counseling a Patient on Peak Flow Meter's Use

141

Dana Al Marzooqi, Abeer Al Naqbi,
and Shammah Al Memari

Learning Objectives
- Identify the purpose of the peak flow meter.
- Recognize the basic steps in using the peak flow meter.
- Describe the parts of the device to the patient.
- Learn to demonstrate to the patient how to use the device.
- Understand the reading of the peak flow meter.

1. Introduce yourself.
2. Establish a good rapport (address the patient by name).
3. Explain what the device is used for and what its parts are:
   (a) Name: peak flow meter (PFM).
   (b) Purpose: "Tells you how well your lungs are working with the current medications and serves as an early warning sign of deterioration."
   (c) Show the patient the instrument and explain its parts (clear plastic body, logarithmic scale, internal flow indicator with color zones, mouthpiece).

D. Al Marzooqi · A. Al Naqbi
Ambulatory Healthcare Services, Abu Dhabi, United Arab Emirates

S. Al Memari (✉)
Abu Dhabi, United Arab Emirates

4. Explain and demonstrate to the patient how to use the device:
   (a) Ensure the pointer is at zero.
   (b) Proper posture: standing (sitting will restrain the diaphragm movement by stomach contents giving a false reading), avoid bending your neck down, and no food or gum in the mouth.
   (c) Hold the peak flow meter so that your fingers are clear of the scale.
   (d) Breath in as deeply as possible and hold your breath.
   (e) Place the mouthpiece well into your mouth (bite mouthpiece lightly and seal your lips firmly around it). Ensure that you are not blocking the mouthpiece with your tongue or teeth. Blow as hard and as fast as you can.
   (f) Write down the level (aside) and put the marker back to zero. Repeat the measurement three times and record the highest reading on the chart as your peak expiratory flow (PEF) L\min.
5. Allow the patient to use the PFM on his or her own and tell you what the actual reading is, determine if he or she does that correctly.
   (a) Determining the personal best peak flow number: When the patient gets out of the acute attack, ask the patient to measure his/her PFM daily, between 12–2 pm, between 7–9 am, and 6–8 pm for 2–3 weeks so that they know their best peak expiratory flow rate (PEFR) number. Record any event that has happened and might have exacerbated your cough (e.g., common cold). You will notice that your readings will not form a flat line but more of a zigzag pattern, which is normal.
6. Ensure:
   (a) Positive reinforcement: "Many others use it; you can definitely use it correctly." "We are always available to support you."
   (b) Patient understands how it should be used.
   (c) Arrange follow-up.
   (d) Give away reading materials if available.
7. Communication skills: ensure organized approach, mixed questioning style (open and close-ended questions), active listening, clear language, and reflection on the patient's ideas, concerns and expectations (ICE).

Counseling a Patient in Regard of Metered Dose Inhaler's Use

142

Khuloud Al Hammadi, Sumiya Taheri, and Shammah Al Memari

> **Learning Objectives**
> - Identify the purpose of metered dose inhaler.
> - Recognize the basic steps in using the metered dose inhaler.
> - Describe the parts of the device to the patient.
> - Learn to demonstrate to the patient how to use the device.
> - Understand how to use spacer for kids.

1. Introduce yourself and establish a good rapport (address the patient by name).
2. Explain the device:
   (a) Name: Metered Dose Inhaler (MDI).
   (b) Purpose: either used as a symptom reliever "quick acting medication that opens the airways and resolves your symptoms during an attack" or as a preventer "slow acting medication that prevents the symptoms from occurring in the first place." If both types of inhalers are prescribed, advise the patient to use the symptom reliever first.
   (c) Show the patient the inhaler and explain its parts (cap, mouthpiece, plastic holder, canister, with or without spacer). Emphasize the need to revise the expiry date and double-check that the inhaler is not empty prior to use.

K. Al Hammadi
Sheikh Khalifa Medical City, Abu Dhabi, United Arab Emirates

S. Taheri
Ambulatory Healthcare Services, Abu Dhabi, United Arab Emirates

S. Al Memari (✉)
Abu Dhabi, United Arab Emirates

© The Author(s), under exclusive license to Springer Nature Singapore Pte Ltd. 2024
S. Lari et al. (eds.), *Family Medicine OSCE: First Aid to Objective Structured Clinical Examination*, https://doi.org/10.1007/978-981-99-5530-5_142

3. Explain the steps of use—"It is very important to use your inhaler correctly so that the medication in the spray reaches deep into your lungs to treat your asthma":
   (a) If this is the first time to use the inhaler, then it needs priming (getting it ready for use) by:
   (b) First take the cap off the mouthpiece, then shake the inhaler for 5 s and press down on the canister to spray the medicine into the air (away from your face), repeat these steps three more times
   (c) Sit upright or stand up for better medication delivery.
   (d) Remove the cap and check correct positioning (canister up/L-shape).
   (e) Shake the inhaler for 5 s.
   (f) Breath out slowly and gently through your mouth.
   (g) Put the mouthpiece into your mouth and seal tightly with your lips.
   (h) Tilt your head back slightly with your chin up.
   (i) Start to breathe in slowly through your mouth while pressing the puffer firmly as you do so. Continue breathing in from your mouth as far as you can for 3–5 s.
   (j) When you cannot breathe in any more take the inhaler out of your mouth and hold breath for 10 s, then breathe out gently.
   (k) In case your dose is more than 1 puff; repeat steps c to h as above after 15–30 s.
   (l) Re-cap the inhaler, wash your mouth if steroid inhaler used.
   (m) Let the patient do it and observe to correct.
4. Advise the patient about taking care of the MDI:
   (a) Wash the cap twice a week.
   (b) Ensure that you always have the reliever around in case you need it.
5. Introduce the patient to spacers and their benefits—"Many people who have trouble using inhalers do better when using a special device called a spacer. It is very efficient and cause less irritation of the mouth and throat":
   (a) Indications: children less than 5 years, elderly, or patients who have difficulty coordinating.
   (b) Show the patient the instrument and explain its parts: (inhaler entry port, body, valve, mouthpiece mask and cap).
   (c) Method of use: repeat the instructions above (steps a to f as above) then advise the patient to first; press on the canister once to deliver one puff into the spacer, then take (**4**) normal breaths in and out from the mouthpiece and repeat the above for the number of puffs needed.
   (d) Advise the patient about taking care of the spacer: Prime the spacer by pushing one puff in before first use. Clean by rinsing it with water only once a week. Do not use soap and do not attempt rubbing the spacer from inside, allow the device to dry overnight. Replace the spacer every 6 months.
6. Encourage any questions.

7. Ensure:
   (a) Positive reinforcement—"Many others use it; you can definitely use it correctly." "We are always available to support you."
   (b) Patient understands the doses (reliever: 1–2 puffs every 3–4 h).
   (c) Patient understands side effects of short acting beta agonist: palpitations, tremors.
   (d) Arranging a follow-up.
   (e) Give away reading materials if available.
8. Communication skills: ensure organized approach, mixed questioning style (open and close ended questions), active listening, clear language and reflection on patient's ideas, concerns and expectations (ICE).

Counseling a Healthcare Worker with Needlestick Injury

143

Khuloud Al Hammadi and Shammah Al Memari

Learning Objectives
- Describe the detailed history of the incident.
- Recognize the risk factors of the injury.
- Identify the risk and the treatment after the exposure.

1. Introduce yourself and establish a good rapport.
2. Ask to identify the complaint:
   (a) Details of the injury: What happened, when (date and time), where, and how?
   (b) Ask about occupation, job title, employer, and years of experience.
   (c) Details of source case and procedure: medical history, type of care provided or procedure that took place, type of sharps (scalpel, suture needle, borehole needle), use of safety-engineered device, depth of puncture, body part on which procedure was performed (a vein or artery, SC, IM, surgical site tissues), and any visible blood on the needle,
   (d) Details of injured healthcare worker: Body part involved, visible bleeding, hepatitis B vaccination status, and use of single/double gloves. Also inquire about the precautionary measures implemented immediately (encourage bleeding, squeezing puncture site, washing the hands, reporting to the Occupational Health Department), any assessment or post-exposure prophylaxis given, and history of other exposure incidents.
   (e) Identify other possible contributing factors: refer to Table 143.1 for details.

K. Al Hammadi
Sheikh Khalifa Medical City, Abu Dhabi, United Arab Emirates

S. Al Memari (✉)
Abu Dhabi, United Arab Emirates

© The Author(s), under exclusive license to Springer Nature Singapore Pte Ltd. 2024
S. Lari et al. (eds.), *Family Medicine OSCE: First Aid to Objective Structured Clinical Examination*, https://doi.org/10.1007/978-981-99-5530-5_143

Table 143.1 Possible contributing factors for needlestick injury

Domain	Details
Healthcare workers' personal factors	Fatigue, inexperience, lack of attention, noncompliance with infection prevention control measures, and safe handling of sharps
Environmental factors	Improper setup, inadequate lightening, or device failure
Source or patients' factors	Aggressive, sudden unexpected movement, uncooperative patients or having features suggesting higher risk of blood-borne viral infection (tattoos, venipuncture sites, body pierces, multiple sexual partners, living with a partner with blood-borne viruses)

3. Explore ideas, concerns and expectations (ICEs) and the impact of injury on the quality of life (emotions, interaction with spouse, and close family members).
4. Advise: "As your doctor, I think it's very important for you to know that there are several control measures now implemented at the facility to protect both patients as well as healthcare workers from viral infections, especially the blood-borne ones. Kindly allow me to walk you through the full assessment so that I can provide assurance that is based on objective findings."
5. Assess:
   (a) Explore ongoing problems: past medical history (blood-borne viral infections, chronic liver disease, history of blood transfusions) and past surgical history.
   (b) Question use of any regular medication and allergies.
   (c) Family history of blood-borne infections.
   (d) Social history (marital status, smoking, alcohol consumption).
   (e) Last menstrual cycle and pregnancy status for female healthcare workers.
6. Assist: based on the information obtained, determine the significance of exposure and where possible state the risk and treatment recommendation as detailed in Table 143.2.
7. Arrange: provide relevant reading educational materials.
8. Advice that further follow-up shall be arranged as per the employer's occupational health policies and infectious diseases specialist advice.
9. Check understanding and reflect on ICE.
10. Communication skills: ensure organized approach, mixed questioning style (open and close-ended questions), active listening, clear language, and reflection on the patient's ICE.

Table 143.2 Risk of diseases after a needlestick injury

Disease	Risk
Hepatitis B infection	• If the patient (source) has active replication of the virus (indicated by HBeAg- positive blood test), then the risk of developing clinical hepatitis is as high as 30% • Hep B infection risk is averted by adequate hepatitis B's ab titer documented at >10 mIU/mL at any point in time since employed • Post-exposure prophylaxis: If hepatitis B's ab titer inadequate, post-exposure management includes hepatitis B immunoglobulin (HBIG) administration as soon as possible (within 24 h), in addition to hepatitis B vaccine course initiation
Hepatitis C infection	• The risk of HCV seroconversion after a needlestick injury from a patient infected with HCV is approximately 3% • Post-exposure management: There is no recommended post-exposure prophylaxis. Appropriate follow-up is warranted and counseling about current treatment efficacy if seroconversion takes place • All workers exposed to HCV should undergo HCV antibody testing at 6 weeks, 12 weeks, and 6 months. Some sources recommend testing as well at 12 months post exposure if implied epidemiological factors identified or high-risk features identified with source patient
HIV	• The average risk of seroconversion after a needlestick injury from a confirmed HIV source is approximately 0.3% without post-exposure prophylaxis • Post-exposure prophylaxis (PEP): If indicated, this should be arranged following a consultation with infectious disease and where appropriate the engagement of the employer's occupational health physician. The following are special considerations regarding HIV exposure management • Start post-exposure prophylaxis as soon as possible. PEP is most effective if given within 2 h but can be given up to 72 h later – If the source is determined to be HIV-negative and unlikely in the window period, post-exposure prophylaxis can be discontinued – If the source is determined to be HIV-positive, continue treatment for 4 weeks if tolerated – All workers exposed to HIV should undergo HIV antibody testing at 6 weeks, 12 weeks, and 6 months • The most common regimen is Truvada (emtricitabine/tenofovir) and dolutegravir. There is the possibility of toxicity with antiretrovirals, so use should be restricted to exposures in which reasonable risk of transmission is present • Pregnancy status and current medication uses should be clarified as these can influence the selection of a treatment regimen

Assessment and Counseling of a Truck Driver Seeking Pre-employment Occupational Evaluation

144

Shaima Lari and Shammah Al Memari

> **Learning Objectives**
> - Describe the medical fitness of the truck driver.
> - Recognize the ongoing medical problem.

1. Introduce yourself.
2. Establish a good rapport.
3. Identify the complaint:
   (a) Ask about the new occupation, job title, and employer.
   (b) Details of the new job: part time or full time, nature of duties (regular hours/shift work, office/field work, indoor/outdoor), and significant workplace exposures if any (biological, chemical, physical, ergonomic, psychological).
   (c) Details of previous positions/job: chronologically ask about each job (job title, duration of work, employer, work-related disease or accident/injury).
4. Explore ideas, concerns and expectations (ICE) and the impact of employment on the quality of life (emotions, behavioral changes, work attendance, interactions with manager and coworkers and performance).
5. Explore ongoing problems or past medical/surgical history: inquire about any
   (a) Nervous system conditions: migraine, epilepsy, stroke, altered mental status/syncope, vision and visual field-related problems, balance and hearing-related problems, any condition impacting coordination and/or

S. Lari
Sheikh Shakhbout Medical City, Abu Dhabi, United Arab Emirates

S. Al Memari (✉)
Abu Dhabi, United Arab Emirates

© The Author(s), under exclusive license to Springer Nature Singapore Pte Ltd. 2024
S. Lari et al. (eds.), *Family Medicine OSCE: First Aid to Objective Structured Clinical Examination*, https://doi.org/10.1007/978-981-99-5530-5_144

concentration, memory and judgment, insight and understanding, and psychiatric illness.

(b) Cardiovascular system conditions: dysrhythmia, coronary artery disease, peripheral vascular disease, syncope, and bleeding disorder.

(c) Respiratory system conditions: asthma, chronic obstructive pulmonary disease, recurrent idiopathic pneumothorax, and obstructive sleep apnea.

(d) Musculoskeletal system conditions: any condition having an impact on the range of motion at neck, shoulder, as well as knee/ankle, cervical or lumbar disc disease, upper or lower extremity weakness, and limited range of movement or movement disorders.

(e) Other: diabetes mellitus, essential hypertension, renal disease, and liver disease.

6. Question use of any regular medication and allergies.

7. Family history of any condition of concern, epilepsy, migraine, cardiac diseases, or psychiatric illness.

8. Social history (marital status, smoking, alcohol consumption, or any drug/substance misuse). See Box 144.1.

9. Management and education:

(a) Provide relevant reading educational materials.

(b) Advice that further follow-up shall be arranged as per the employer's occupational health assessment and evaluating/treating specialist advice.

10. Check understanding and reflect on ICE.

Box 144.1 Health and Safety Considerations for Heavy Vehicle Drivers: Understanding Medical Clearance Requirements and Potential Risks

Based on the information obtained, determine the significance of the findings and related health effects.

- Clarify any standards or official guidelines required for pre-employment medical clearance specific to heavy vehicle drivers by the employer and regulatory authorities. Where possible, state the risk associated with any condition found by history or physical examination and refer for further evaluation.
- Generally, anyone with a medical condition likely to cause sudden disabling event associated with incapacitation at the wheel or who is unable to control their vehicle safely for any reason must not drive.
- Individuals with any neurological, cardiovascular, and pulmonary conditions that may have an impact on the level of consciousness or cause sudden disabling event must be first referred to the concerned Medical Specialty for assessment and evaluation of the condition and its impact on the ability to drive.
- Diabetes mellitus is not a disqualifying condition even if treated and controlled by insulin. Heavy vehicle driver's initiating treatment with insulin should not drive on temporary basis until dose adjustment is confirmed and no hypoglycemia is reported. However, episodes of severe hypoglycemia, impaired awareness of hypoglycemia symptoms, seizures provoked by hypoglycemia, and diabetic visual complications affecting visual equity or visual field must not drive unless until evaluated by a specialist.
- Severe anxiety or depression, acute psychotic disorders, mania or hypomania, relapsing/remitting schizophrenia, dementia, and severe learning disabilities or psychiatrist conditions that contraindicate driving.
- Persistent alcohol and/or illicit drugs misuse or dependence on contraindicate driving.
- Color blindness does not contraindicate driving. Monocular vision, diplopia, and defects in the visual field contraindicate driving.
- Obstructive sleep apnea of any severity and any other condition or medication that may cause excessive sleepiness to contraindicate driving.

Assessment and Counseling Attending with a Complaint Related to Office's Ergonomics (in Computer Workstation's Users)

145

Khuloud Al Hammadi and Shammah Al Memari

> **Learning Objectives**
> - Explain the term ergonomics.
> - Describe the tips to adjust the workstations.
> - Identify the risk factors of work-related injuries.

The following ergonomic tips can help you work more comfortably and safely.

1. Introduce yourself and establish a good rapport.
2. Ask:
   (a) Explore the reason for clinic visit and associated symptoms (headache, neck pain, and/or stiffness, shoulder pain, elbow pain, wrist pain, arm or finger numbness, vision changes, fatigue and loss of energy, back pain, lower extremity numbness, and concerns related to memory and concentration).
   (b) Onset of symptoms, and relieving and aggravating factors.
   (c) Past medical and surgical history: ophthalmic conditions, neuro-spinal conditions, head, neck, or back injuries/trauma, or musculoskeletal disorders.
   (d) Social history: smoking, alcohol, and substance use.
   (e) Occupational history: ask about the occupation, job title, employer, part time or full time, and nature of duties (regular hours or shift work, office or field work, Indoor or outdoor).
   (f) Details of previous positions/job: chronologically ask about each job (job title, duration of work, employer, work-related disease, or accident/injury).

K. Al Hammadi
Sheikh Khalifa Medical City, Abu Dhabi, United Arab Emirates

S. Al Memari (✉)
Abu Dhabi, United Arab Emirates

© The Author(s), under exclusive license to Springer Nature Singapore Pte Ltd. 2024
S. Lari et al. (eds.), *Family Medicine OSCE: First Aid to Objective Structured Clinical Examination*, https://doi.org/10.1007/978-981-99-5530-5_145

553

3. Advise: "As your doctor, I think it's very important for you to know that prolong use of computer workstation and number of years spent doing office work have an impact on your physical and mental health, which is what is known as Office Ergonomics."
   (a) "Ergonomics means the study of the physical and cognitive demands of work to ensure a safe and productive workplace by eliminating safety hazards, controlling errors, and preventing awkward postures or movements."
4. Assess:
   (a) Answer any questions and check your level of understanding.
   (b) Screen for any alarming signs or symptoms.
5. Assist: "Let's share some tips that are suitable for helping you to adjust your workstation." Refer to Table 145.1 for further details.
   (a) If you have any concerns and believe modifications or adjustment needed to your workstation, inform your manager, or contact who shall guide you into further steps, e.g., IT support, health and safety team, occupational hygienist, or Occupational Health team.
6. Arrange:
   (a) Follow up and monitor improvement in symptoms.
   (b) Refer to specialty clinic if concerned about major pathology or need for an intervention.
   (c) Give away reading materials if available.
7. Communication skills: ensure organized approach, mixed questioning style (open and close-ended questions), active listening, clear language, and reflection on the patient's ideas, concerns and expectations (ICE).

Table 145.1 Optimizing work ergonomics: advice for office chair, keyboard and mouse, and display screens/work surface

Item	Advice
Office chair	• Your chair should be suitable and stable. • The height, seat, and back of the chair can be adjusted to achieve the posture outlined below. • Your feet are fully supported by the floor when you are seated. • Your chair provides support for your lower back. • When your back is supported, you should be able to sit without feeling pressure from the chair seat on the back of your knees. • Your armrests allow you to get close to your workstation.
Keyboard and mouse	• Ensure your keyboard characters are clear and readable, if not the keyboard may need modification or replacement. • Ensure your keyboard, mouse, and work surface are located at your elbow height. • Ensure your keyboard is close to the front edge, however, allowing space for the wrist to rest on the desk surface. • Ensure your wrists are straight and your upper arms relaxed when using your keyboard and mouse. • Good keyboard techniques also include hands are not bent at the wrist, not hitting the keys too hard and not overstretching the fingers. • Place your mouse at the same level and as close as possible to your keyboard to avoid overreaching and encourage a relaxed arm and straight wrist. • Check if the mouse works smoothly and at a suitable speed.
Display screens/work surfaces	• Ensure the image is stable, free of flickers and jitters, and that the contrast and brightness are appropriate. • The screen should be free from glare and reflections. • Ensure characters are clear and readable and that the screen is clean using appropriate materials. • The text size should be comfortable to read, if not, software/IT setting changes may be needed. • Ensure your monitor is positioned directly in front of you and at least an arm's length away. • Ensure your monitor height is slightly below eye level. • Keep all frequently used items within easy reach.
Breaks	• Take a postural break every 20–30 min, e.g., standing, walking to printer/get water. • Take regular eye breaks by refocusing on distant objects intermittently when working.
Accessories	• Use a headset or speakerphone if you are writing or keying while talking on the phone.

Further Reading

Department of Health standard for Premarital Screening Standard.

Drutz HP. Overview of urinary incontinence in women. Up to date. 2022. https://www.uptodate.com/contents/overview-of-urinary-incontinence-in-women.

Elster N. Adolescent sexual and reproductive health care. Up to date. 2021. https://www.uptodate.com/contents/adolescent-sexual-and-reproductive-health-care.

Jeremiah U, Unwin BK, Greenwald MH. Essential concepts for healthy living. Burlington: Jones & Bartlett Publishers; 2015.

Kaunitz A. Abnormal uterine bleeding: management in premenopausal patients. Uptodate. 2021. https://www.uptodate.com/contents/abnormal-uterine-bleeding-management-in-premenopausal.

Molloy DW, Standish TI. A guide to the standardized mini-mental state examination. Int Psychogeriatr. 1997;9(Suppl 1):87–150. https://doi.org/10.1017/s1041610297004754.

Murtagh JA. Murtagh's patient education, vol. 6. New York: McGraw Hill; 2012.

Randolph TR. Hematology in Rodak's hematology. 6th ed. New York: Elsevier; 2020. p. 394–423. https://doi.org/10.1016/B978-0-323-53045-3.00033-7.

Riley L. Rubella in pregnancy. 2021 [online] up to date. Available at.: <https://www-uptodate-com.eu1.proxy.openathens.net/contents/rubella-in-pregnancy?search=rubella%20pregnancy&topicRef=8301&source=see_link#H11> [Accessed 18 March 2022].

Rotte M, Lopez B. Perfect Phrases for Healthcare Professionals: Hundreds of Ready-to-Use Phrases. McGraw Hill Professional; 2011. http://books.google.ie/books?id=V5m-DGRv9LYC&printsec=frontcover&dq=0071768335+%C2%B7+9780071768337&hl=&cd=1&source=gbs_api.

Vitto C, Del Buono B, Daniel L, Rivet E, Cholyway R, Santen SA. Teaching toolbox: breaking bad news with virtual Technology in the Time of COVID. Journal of cancer education: the official journal of the American Association for Cancer Education. 2022;37(5):1429–32. https://doi.org/10.1007/s13187-021-01975-7.

Workshop notes, Family Medicine Arab Board OSCE Preparatory Course, Dubai Health Authority, Dubai, United Arab Emirates.

Workshop notes, Family Medicine Arab Board Preparatory Course, Ethraa Consultation and Training, Dubai, United Arab Emirates.

GPSR Compliance

*The European Union's (EU) General Product Safety Regulation (GPSR)
is a set of rules that requires consumer products to be safe and our
obligations to ensure this.*

*If you have any concerns about our products, you can contact us on
ProductSafety@springernature.com*

In case Publisher is established outside the EU, the EU authorized
representative is:

Springer Nature Customer Service Center GmbH
Europaplatz 3
69115 Heidelberg, Germany

Batch number: 10091867

Printed by Printforce, the Netherlands